Health
Technology
SOURCEBOOK

First Edition

Health Reference Series

First Edition

Health Technology

SOURCEBOOK

■

Basic Consumer Health Information about Medicine and Technology, Telemedicine, Information Technology and Medicine, Preventive Medicine and Health Technology, Medical Equipment Technology, Diagnostic Technology, Nanotechnology, Neurologics, Health Information Technology, Stem Cell Research, Personal Healthcare Mobile Applications, and Assistive Devices

Along with Information about Digital Innovations in Healthcare, Medical Technology and Law, a Glossary of Related Terms, and a List of Resources for Additional Help and Information.

■

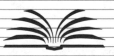

OMNIGRAPHICS

615 Griswold, Ste. 901, Detroit, MI 48226

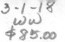

3-1-18
WW
$85.00

Bibliographic Note
Because this page cannot legibly accommodate all the copyright notices, the Bibliographic Note portion of the Preface constitutes an extension of the copyright notice.

* * *

OMNIGRAPHICS
Greg Mullin, *Managing Editor*
***

Copyright © 2018 Omnigraphics

ISBN 978-0-7808-1591-9
E-ISBN 978-0-7808-1592-6

Library of Congress Cataloging-in-Publication Data

Names: Omnigraphics, Inc., issuing body.

Title: Health technology sourcebook: basic consumer health information about medicine and technology, telemedicine, information technology and medicine, health information technology management systems, medical equipment technology, robotics, nanotechnology, smart operating rooms, technological research and healthcare, stem cells research, personal healthcare mobile applications, and assistive devices along with information about digital innovations in healthcare, medical technology and law, a glossary of related terms, and a list of resources for additional help and information.

Description: Detroit, MI: Omnigraphics, [2018] | Series: Health reference series | Includes bibliographical references and index.

Identifiers: LCCN 2017043919 (print) | LCCN 2017048444 (ebook) | ISBN 9780780815926 (eBook) | ISBN 9780780815919 (hardcover: alk. paper)

Subjects: LCSH: Medical technology. | Medical care--Data processing.

Classification: LCC R855.3 (ebook) | LCC R855.3.H437 2018 (print) | DDC 610.285--dc23

LC record available at https://lccn.loc.gov/2017043919

Table of Contents

Preface xiii

Part I: Introduction to Health Technology

Chapter 1 — Understanding Medical Technology 3

Chapter 2 — Telehealth 9

Chapter 3 — Telemedicine and E-Health.................................... 15

Chapter 4 — Types of Telemedicine Technology........................ 21

    Section 4.1 — Real-Time Telehealth 22

    Section 4.2 — Store-and-Forward
        Telehealth 26

    Section 4.3 — Telemedicine and Patient
        Safety... 27

Chapter 5 — Benefits of Telemedicine... 33

Chapter 6 — Health Technology Assessment 35

Chapter 7 — Technology and Healthcare Expenditure.............. 45

Part II: Technology and Preventive Healthcare

Chapter 8 — Digital Health 53

Chapter 9 — Digital Innovations in Preventive
    Medicine 61

    Section 9.1 — Sensors 62

Section 9.2 — Body Area Networks and Pervasive Health Monitoring.................................. 67

Section 9.3 — Wireless Medical Devices 70

Section 9.4 — Wearables and Safety................. 73

Section 9.5 — Remote Patient Monitoring........ 75

Section 9.6 — Continuous Glucose Monitoring................................... 81

Section 9.7 — Mobile Medical Applications...... 85

Chapter 10 — Medical Device Data Systems............................... 91

Chapter 11 — Medical Device Interoperability............................ 97

Chapter 12 — Clinical Decision Support..................................... 101

Chapter 13 — Big Data in the Age of Genomics 107

Chapter 14 — Big Data for Infectious Disease Surveillance 111

Chapter 15 — Screening and Detection Technologies 115

Section 15.1 — Advanced Molecular Detection (AMD) 116

Section 15.2 — Cancer Screening in a Briefcase 118

Section 15.3 — DNA Microchip Technology...... 120

Section 15.4 — Early Detection of Colorectal Cancer..................... 122

Section 15.5 — Genetic Testing 123

Section 15.6 — Sensitive Stroke Detection....... 125

Section 15.7 — Tool to Detect Cardiovascular Disease Risk... 126

Part III: Diagnostic Technology

Chapter 16 — Imaging Services... 131

Section 16.1 — Computed Tomography (CT)..................... 132

Section 16.2—Electrocardiogram (ECG)......... 135

Section 16.3—Functional Near-Infrared
Spectroscopy (fNIRS)................ 137

Section 16.4—Magnetic Resonance
Imaging (MRI)........................... 139

Section 16.5—Mammogram.............................. 143

Section 16.6—Medical X-Ray Imaging............ 145

Section 16.7—Nuclear Medicine...................... 148

Section 16.8—Optical Imaging 151

Section 16.9—Ultrasound 154

Chapter 17—Advances in Imaging 159

Section 17.1—Magnetic Resonance
Electrography........................... 160

Section 17.2—Neuroimaging Technique
to Predict Autism among
High-Risk Infants 161

Section 17.3—Metal-Free MRI Contrast
Agent 162

Section 17.4—Virtual Colonoscopy................. 165

Section 17.5—Advanced Magnetic
Imaging Methods...................... 167

Chapter 18—Advanced Imaging in Laboratory
Technology 169

Section 18.1—Live Cell Imaging 170

Section 18.2—Non-Linear Optical
Imaging 172

Section 18.3—Surface Plasmon
Resonance Imaging................... 174

Chapter 19—Point-of-Care Diagnostic Testing........................ 177

Chapter 20—Precision Medicine for Cancer
Diagnostics... 181

Chapter 21—Food Allergy Lab Fits on Your
Keychain.. 183

Chapter 22—Wireless Patient Monitoring................................ 187

Part IV: Role of Technology in Treatment

Chapter 23—Medical Treatment Technology (MTT)............... 193

Section 23.1—Genomic Medicine..................... 194

Section 23.2—Personalized Medicine.............. 198

Section 23.3—Nanomedicine 200

Section 23.4—Drug Delivery Systems............. 202

Section 23.5—Artificial Pancreas Device
System 205

Chapter 24—Surgical Treatment Technology (STT) 211

Section 24.1—Surgical Robots for Tumor
Treatment 212

Section 24.2—Robotic-Assisted
Surgery (RAS)........................... 214

Section 24.3—Computer-Assisted
Surgical Systems 220

Section 24.4—Technologies Enhance
Tumor Surgery......................... 222

Section 24.5—Smart Operating Rooms of
the Future 225

Chapter 25—Technology and the Future of Mental
Health Treatment................................. 229

Chapter 26—New Technology to Optimize Cancer
Therapy 237

Chapter 27—Nutrigenomics..................................... 241

Chapter 28—Nanotechnology.................................... 245

Section 28.1—Nanotechnology Research
at NIH 246

Section 28.2—Benefits of Nanotechnology...... 249

Section 28.3—Nanotechnology in Cancer 254

Chapter 29—Robotics 259

Section 29.1—Robots for Better Health
and Quality of Life.................... 260

Section 29.2—Robotic Cleaners 261

Section 29.3—Image-Guided Robotic
Interventions.............................. 263

Chapter 30—Advanced Therapies 267

Section 30.1—Tissue Engineering and
Regenerative Medicine 268

Section 30.2—Cartilage Engineering.............. 272

Section 30.3—Regenerative Medicine
Biomanufacturing...................... 274

Section 30.4—New Method Builds Bone......... 275

Section 30.5—Light Therapy and Brain
Function 277

Part V: Rehabilitation and Assistive Technologies

Chapter 31—Rehabilitation Engineering.................................. 283

Chapter 32—Rehabilitation Medicine: Research
Activities and Scientific Advances...................... 287

Chapter 33—Vision and Hearing Loss 295

Section 33.1—Low Vision and Blindness
Rehabilitation 296

Section 33.2—Artificial Retina 299

Section 33.3—Cochlear Implants:
Different Kind of Hearing 302

Chapter 34—Robotics in Rehabilitation 305

Section 34.1—Cybernetics............................... 306

Section 34.2—Prosthetic Engineering............. 310

Section 34.3—New Robotic Wheelchair 314

Chapter 35—Electrical Signals and Stimulations 317

Section 35.1—Electrical Signals to
Restore Functioning 318

Section 35.2—BrainGate................................. 322

Section 35.3—Noninvasive Spinal Cord
Stimulation for Paralysis 326

Chapter 36—Physical Therapists of the Future 333

Chapter 37—Assistive Devices... 337

    Section 37.1—Rehabilitative and Assistive
             Technology: Overview............... 338

    Section 37.2—Assistive Devices for
             Communication....................... 343

    Section 37.3—Hearing Aids 346

    Section 37.4—Mobility Aids............................ 348

Chapter 38—Space Technologies in the
Rehabilitation of Movement Disorders................ 355

Part VI: Health Information Technology

Chapter 39—Understanding Health Information
Technology 361

    Section 39.1—Basics of Health
             Information Technology 362

    Section 39.2—Benefits of Health IT 364

    Section 39.3—Consumer Health IT
             Applications 366

    Section 39.4—Trends in Use........................... 368

Chapter 40—Integrating Technology and
Healthcare... 373

    Section 40.1—Health Information
             Technology Integration............. 374

    Section 40.2—Information and
             Communication Technology 375

    Section 40.3—E-Health.................................. 377

Chapter 41—Digital Health Records 381

    Section 41.1—Blue Button............................. 382

    Section 41.2—Personal Health
             Record (PHR) 389

    Section 41.3—Benefits of Electronic
             Health Records (EHRs) 391

    Section 41.4—E-Prescription........................... 397

Part VII: Medical Technology—Legal and Ethical Concerns

Chapter 42—Health Information Privacy Law and
Policy 403

Chapter 43—Health Information Technology
Legislation and Regulations.............................. 407

Chapter 44—HIPAA Privacy Rule's Right of
Access and Health Information
Technology 411

Chapter 45—Personal Health Records (PHRs) and
the HIPAA Privacy Rule 419

Chapter 46—Privacy, Security, and Electronic
Health Records (EHRs) 427

Chapter 47—Cloning and Law... 431

Part VIII: Future of Health Technology

Chapter 48—Artificial Brains 437

Chapter 49—Computational Modeling..................................... 441

Chapter 50—Stem Cell Research... 447

Chapter 51—Medical Applications of 3D Printing................... 467

Chapter 52—Microneedle Patch for Flu Vaccination 471

Chapter 53—Photonic Dosimetry 475

Part IX: Additional Help and Information

Chapter 54—Glossary of Terms Related to Health
Technology 479

Chapter 55—Directory of Agencies That Provide
Information about Health Technology................. 489

Index... 499

Preface

About This Book

Technology has revolutionized the way healthcare is being delivered today, from preventive medicine to rehabilitation. Future technological innovations will transform healthcare, helping healthcare professionals provide better services with enhanced precision. More than anything, technology drives healthcare, enabling good health and wellness to people all over the world. The emergence of health information technology has made things easier, faster, and simpler to healthcare professionals. It provides information they need with the click of a button. Healthcare technology will surely achieve many more remarkable achievements in the future, changing the face of the healthcare industry completely in the future.

Health Technology Sourcebook, *First Edition* provides facts about health technology, telehealth, telemedicine technology, digital health, innovations in preventive medicine, screening and detection, imaging, and patient monitoring services. It further discusses medical and surgical treatment technologies, nutrigenomics, nanotechnology, rehabilitation and assistive devices, and health information technology. In addition, it details ethical and legal concerns of medical technology, cloning and cloning laws, and the future of health technology. The book concludes with a directory of resources for additional information and a list of suggestions for further reading about health technology.

How to Use This Book

This book is divided into parts and chapters. Parts focus on broad areas of interest. Chapters are devoted to single topics within a part.

Part I: Introduction to Health Technology gives an overview about medical technology, telehealth, telemedicine, and e-health concepts. It also provides information about the benefits of telemedicine, health technology assessment, and technology and healthcare-related expenditures.

Part II: Technology and Preventive Healthcare discusses the use of technology in preventive healthcare. It offers detailed information about digital health concepts and innovations, medical device data systems, medical device interoperability, and clinical decision support systems. Additionally, it discusses about the use of Big Data in healthcare and screening and detection technologies.

Part III: Diagnostic Technology deals with various technologies used in the field of diagnosis such as imaging, diagnostic testing, precision medicine, and wireless patient monitoring systems. It also discusses various advanced imaging concepts and other innovations in diagnostic technology.

Part IV: Role of Technology in Treatment provides information about medical and surgical treatment technologies, nutrigenomics, nanotechnology, and robotics. In addition, it discusses various advanced therapies such as tissue and cartilage engineering, regenerative medicine, and light therapy and brain function.

Part V: Rehabilitation and Assistive Technologies discusses various rehabilitative and assistive technologies such as prosthetic engineering, cybernetics, robotic wheelchairs, and vision, hearing, and mobility aids. It further discusses the role of electrical signals and stimulations in rehabilitation and research and scientific advances in the field.

Part VI: Health Information Technology deals with the basics of health information technology, benefits of health information technology, and trends in use. It also provides details about and communication technologies, e-health, digital health records, and other aspects.

Part VII: Medical Technology—Legal and Ethical Concerns discusses medical records privacy, confidentiality, and health information privacy law and policy. It also discusses cloning and law.

Part VIII: Future of Health Technology gives information about the various health technologies of the future such as artificial brain, computational modeling, stem cell research, and photonic dosimetry. In addition, it discusses medical applications of 3D printing.

Part IX: Additional Help and Information provides a glossary of important terms related to health technologies and a directory of organizations that offer information-related health technologies.

Bibliographic Note

This volume contains documents and excerpts from publications issued by the following government agencies: Agency for Healthcare Research and Quality (AHRQ); Centers for Disease Control and Prevention (CDC); *Eunice Kennedy Shriver* National Institute of Child Health and Human Development (NICHD); Federal Communications Commission (FCC); National Aeronautics and Space Administration (NASA); National Cancer Institute (NCI); National Eye Institute (NEI); National Heart, Lung, and Blood Institute (NHLBI); National Human Genome Research Institute (NHGRI); National Institute of Biomedical Imaging and Bioengineering (NIBIB); National Institute of Diabetes and Digestive and Kidney Diseases (NIDDK); National Institute of Standards and Technology (NIST); National Institute on Deafness and Other Communication Disorders (NIDCD); National Institute on Mental Health (NIMH); National Institutes of Health (NIH); *NIH News in Health*; Office of the National Coordinator for Health Information Technology (ONC); Substance Abuse and Mental Health Services Administration (SAMHSA); U.S. Congressional Budget Office (CBO); U.S. Department of Energy (DOE); U.S. Department of Health and Human Services (HHS); U.S. Department of Homeland Security (DHS); U.S. Department of Justice (DOJ); U.S. Department of Veterans Affairs (VA); U.S. Food and Drug Administration (FDA); and U.S. Library of Congress (LOC).

About the Health Reference Series

The *Health Reference Series* is designed to provide basic medical information for patients, families, caregivers, and the general public. Each volume takes a particular topic and provides comprehensive coverage. This is especially important for people who may be dealing with a newly diagnosed disease or a chronic disorder in themselves or in a family member. People looking for preventive guidance, information about disease warning signs, medical statistics, and risk factors for health problems will also find answers to their questions in the *Health Reference Series*. The *Series*, however, is not intended to serve as a tool for diagnosing illness, in prescribing treatments, or as a substitute for the physician/patient relationship. All people concerned about medical symptoms or the possibility of disease are encouraged to seek professional care from an appropriate healthcare provider.

A Note about Spelling and Style

Health Reference Series editors use *Stedman's Medical Dictionary* as an authority for questions related to the spelling of medical terms and the *Chicago Manual of Style* for questions related to grammatical structures, punctuation, and other editorial concerns. Consistent adherence is not always possible, however, because the individual volumes within the *Series* include many documents from a wide variety of different producers, and the editor's primary goal is to present material from each source as accurately as is possible. This sometimes means that information in different chapters or sections may follow other guidelines and alternate spelling authorities. For example, occasionally a copyright holder may require that eponymous terms be shown in possessive forms (Crohn's disease vs. Crohn disease) or that British spelling norms be retained (leukaemia vs. leukemia).

Medical Review

Omnigraphics contracts with a team of qualified, senior medical professionals who serve as medical consultants for the *Health Reference Series*. As necessary, medical consultants review reprinted and originally written material for currency and accuracy. Citations including the phrase, "Reviewed (month, year)" indicate material reviewed by this team. Medical consultation services are provided to the *Health Reference Series* editors by:

Dr. Vijayalakshmi, MBBS, DGO, MD
Dr. Senthil Selvan, MBBS, DCH, MD
Dr. K. Sivanandham, MBBS, DCH, MS (Research), PhD

Our Advisory Board

We would like to thank the following board members for providing initial guidance on the development of this series:

Health Reference Series *Update Policy*

The inaugural book in the *Health Reference Series* was the first edition of *Cancer Sourcebook* published in 1989. Since then, the *Series* has been enthusiastically received by librarians and in the medical community. In order to maintain the standard of providing high-quality health information for the layperson the editorial staff at Omnigraphics felt it was necessary to implement a policy of updating volumes when warranted.

Medical researchers have been making tremendous strides, and it is the purpose of the *Health Reference Series* to stay current with the most recent advances. Each decision to update a volume is made on an individual basis. Some of the considerations include how much new information is available and the feedback we receive from people who use the books. If there is a topic you would like to see added to the update list, or an area of medical concern you feel has not been adequately addressed, please write to:

Managing Editor
Health Reference Series
Omnigraphics
615 Griswold, Ste. 901
Detroit, MI 48226

Part One

Introduction to Health Technology

Chapter 1

Understanding Medical Technology

It is almost inconceivable to think about providing healthcare in today's world without medical devices, machinery, tests, computers, prosthetics, or drugs. Medical technology can be defined as the application of science to develop solutions to health problems or issues such as the prevention or delay of onset of diseases or the promotion and monitoring of good health. Examples of medical technology include medical and surgical procedures (angioplasty, joint replacements, organ transplants), diagnostic tests (laboratory tests, biopsies, imaging), drugs (biologic agents, pharmaceuticals, vaccines), medical devices (implantable defibrillators, stents), prosthetics (artificial body parts), and new support systems (electronic medical records, e-prescribing, and (telemedicine).

New vaccines may eliminate or greatly reduce the incidence and prevalence of many diseases, and antibiotics and other drugs can treat previously untreatable pathogens. Genetic typing offers the opportunity for early diagnosis and individualized therapies. New technologies can also improve on existing ones, such as new drugs that have fewer

This chapter contains text excerpted from the following sources: Text in this chapter begins with excerpts from "Health, United States, 2009," Centers for Disease Control and Prevention (CDC), 2009. Reviewed December 2017; Text under the heading "Medical Technology Industry in the United States" is excerpted from "Medical Technology Spotlight," U.S. Department of Commerce (DOC), August 9, 2017.

side effects and surgical advances such as laparoscopic techniques, which are less invasive and have a quicker recovery time than traditional surgery. New indications for existing therapies are common, such as fluoxetine, originally used for depression and now also used for premenstrual dysphoria, and atomoxetine, originally used for Parkinson disease and now also used for attention deficit hyperactivity disorder (ADHD). Combinations of technologies can be more effective than individual ones, such as the combination "cocktail" now used to treat HIV/AIDS (human immunodeficiency virus/acquired immunodeficiency syndrome), combination chemotherapy for many types of cancers, and the recent creation of scanning machines that combine positron emission tomography and computed tomography (PET/CT) or PET and magnetic resonance imaging (PET/MRI).

As some technologies become easier to use and less expensive, as equipment becomes more transportable, and as recovery times for procedures are reduced, even complex technologies can diffuse out of hospitals and institutional settings and into ambulatory surgery centers, provider offices, outpatient facilities, imaging centers, and patients' homes, making the technologies more accessible. Technologies have shifted out of institutional settings and into ambulatory surgery centers and from hospitals into the home. Telemedicine, or the use of technology to remotely diagnose and treat conditions through electronic envisioning and data transfer, can provide services to remote or underserved areas.

New types of medical equipment, procedures, and devices have created the need for personnel with specialized training in their use, in some cases creating entirely new professions. Medical specialists such as radiation oncologists, medical geneticists, and surgical subspecialists, as well as allied and support professions such as medical sonographers, radiation technologists, and laboratory technicians, have all been created to use specific types of technology.

The infrastructure necessary to support more complex technologies is also considered to be a part of medical technology. Use of electronic medical records and electronic prescribing are methods for coordinating the increasingly complex array of services provided, as well as allowing for electronic checks of quality to reduce medical errors (for example, drug interactions). The percentage of private office-based physicians who work in offices with fully functional electronic medical records remains low.

Because technologies have diffused into standard medical practice, there are concerns about whether they are consistently being used properly and about the quality of the information provided by tests, imaging, and other technological outputs. To address these concerns, several laws and regulations have been enacted. These include the Clinical Laboratory Improvement Amendments of 1988 (CLIA) and the Mammography Quality Standards Act (MQSA, 1992). In July 2008, Congress passed the Medicare Improvements for Patients and Providers Act (MIPPA). MIPPA requires that "advanced diagnostic imaging services" (diagnostic MRI, CT, and nuclear medicine, including PET) be reimbursed by Medicare only if performed by accredited facilities.

Technologies applied to new populations and conditions generally come at a cost to individuals and to society as a whole. Technologies can be very expensive (e.g., heart transplants, chemotherapy) or very inexpensive (e.g., the Band-Aid). Total expenditures for a given technology, however, are determined by both use and cost; consequently, widely used inexpensive technologies can often have higher aggregate expenditures than rarely used expensive ones. Some new technologies can be cost-saving—for example annual influenza vaccinations in high-risk children. Many technologies, however, contribute to increases in overall healthcare expenditures because they increase utilization (e.g., more doctor visits may be needed to monitor new drug therapies); they may be used on a larger number of patients; they may be more expensive than technologies they replace; or they may increase life expectancy in populations and thus their lifetime healthcare costs. Therefore, although there is general agreement that new technologies and new uses for existing technologies are a major component of increases in healthcare expenditures, the cumulative contribution of all new technologies to rising medical expenditures, and how technology can be used in the most cost-effective manner, is a subject of much debate.

Medical technology expenditures are determined in large part by how technologies are used by practitioners and patients, and, for new technologies, how they diffuse into medical practice. In addition to the potential benefit of using technologies, use is also influenced by provider preferences, patient preferences, legal and regulatory constraints, and costs to both insurers and consumers. Use may be increased relative to what may be considered most cost effective because of overuse, errors in data interpretation, overestimation of the benefits of technology or underestimation of its risks, and defensive medicine. Patient demand may be influenced by advertising or information obtained from friends, the Internet, or other sources, and low tolerance of ambiguity by provider or patient (more information is always better). Negative effects of technologies can include unnecessary expenditures, false positives that can spur additional testing or anxiety, and the inefficient use of resources. Some providers may be inclined to use the more profitable technologies, particularly when these technologies are less invasive or better accepted by patients than alternatives, such as counseling about lifestyle changes, that patients may not accept or implement and over which the provider has less control.

Once diffused into practice, it is often difficult to reduce the use of technologies, even in situations where they have been shown to be ineffective or not superior to less complex or less expensive alternatives. Widespread use of electronic fetal monitoring in low-risk deliveries continues, although there has been evidence for many years that it is unnecessary, perhaps even harmful. Diuretics have been shown to be more successful than newer, more expensive drugs in controlling hypertension for some patients.

In general, Americans—both providers and consumers—appear to be more willing and eager to adopt and use new technologies than people in other countries. More rapid acceptance of new technologies can be beneficial when they are effective, but in some cases harmful effects can be discovered only after widespread use. For example, use of nonsteroidal anti-inflammatory drugs (NSAIDs) increased substantially during the early 2000s, and it was not until reports of complications were reported to the U.S. Food and Drug Administration (FDA) that studies showing adverse effects were publicized and use of these drugs decreased.

Technology diffusion can differ by population group (e.g., by income, race/ethnicity, gender, urbanization, or age), producing inequalities in treatment (overuse or underuse). Women and black persons are significantly underrepresented among Medicare patients with ischemic cardiomyopathy who received implantable cardioverter-defibrillators. Higher spending is not necessarily associated with higher quality, so it is often difficult to determine whether some populations are overusing or underusing specific technologies relative to others.

Technology provides an increasing ability to monitor, prevent, diagnose, control, and cure a growing number of health conditions and to improve quality and length of life. Questions remain, however, about how much innovation and improvement in new and existing technologies is possible when resources are constrained and healthcare expenditures are rising to unacceptable levels, about the opportunity costs of using one technology versus another (or neither), and whether target populations are appropriately and equitably served.

Medical Technology Industry in the United States

The United States remains the largest medical device market in the world with a market size of around $140 billion, and the U.S. market represented about 40 percent of the global medical device market in 2015. U.S. exports of medical devices in key product categories identified by the Department of Commerce exceeded $44 billion in 2015.

According to the most recent Economic Census, conducted in 2012, the sector employed about 356,000 people at approximately 5,800 establishments, and paid median salaries 15 percent higher than the average manufacturing job. More than 80 percent of medical device companies in the United States consist of fewer than 50 employees, and many (notably innovative start-up companies) have little or no sales revenue. Medical device companies are located throughout the country, but are mainly concentrated in regions known for other high-technology industries, such as microelectronics and biotechnology.

U.S. medical device companies are highly regarded globally for their innovations and high technology products. R&D spending continues to represent a high percentage of medical device industry expenditures, averaging 6.7 percent of revenue from 2011–2016. Compared to several other industries including automotive, defense, and telecom, the medical device industry invests a higher percentage of yearly revenues into product innovation. This reflects the competitive nature of the industry, and constant innovation and improvement of existing technologies.

The medical device industry relies upon several industries where the United States holds a competitive advantage, including microelectronics, telecommunications, instrumentation, biotechnology, and software development. Collaborations have led to recent advances including neuro-stimulators, stent technologies, biomarkers, robotic assistance, and implantable electronic devices. Innovation fuels the medical device sector's ongoing quest to improve and maintain the health of the world. Coupled with life expectancy increases and the growing population of the elderly, the medical device market is expected to see positive growth for the foreseeable future.

Chapter 2

Telehealth

What Is Telehealth?

Telehealth is broadly defined as the use of communications technologies to provide and support healthcare at a distance. Telehealth has become a valuable tool for improved health thanks to combined advances in a number of areas including communications, computer science, informatics, and medical technologies.

Telehealth can be as simple as two doctors talking on the phone about a patient's care or as complex as the use of robotic technology to perform surgery from a remote site. Nowadays, telehealth is often associated with remote monitoring of a patient's condition; for instance, blood pressure, heart rate, and other measurements of health status can be obtained by a device worn by the patient and electronically sent to medical personnel.

This chapter contains text excerpted from the following sources: Text beginning with the heading "What Is Telehealth?" is excerpted from "Science Education—Telehealth," National Institute of Biomedical Imaging and Bioengineering (NIBIB), November 2016; Text under the heading "Importance of Telehealth Services" is excerpted from "E-Health and Telemedicine," U.S. Department of Health and Human Services (HHS), August 12, 2016.

Telehealth Technologies: Types and Their Contribution in Improving Medical Care

Teleconsultations

Teleconsultations allow a physician in a rural area to receive advice from a specialist who may be in a distant location, about patients with special or complex conditions. Such consultations can be as simple as a phone call. Increasingly, they involve more sophisticated sharing of medical information such as computed tomography (CT), magnetic resonance imaging (MRI), or ultrasound scans. These images can be taken by the local physician, incorporated into an electronic medical record, and sent to the specialist for diagnosis and treatment recommendations.

Remote Patient Monitoring (RPM)

This is a technology enabling patients to be monitored outside of conventional clinical settings, such as in the home. RPM requires sensors on a device that wirelessly transmits or stores physiological data for review by a health professional. Incorporating RPM into chronic disease measurement can significantly improve an individual's quality of life, particularly when patients are managing complex processes, such as home hemodialysis. For example, in diabetes management, the real-time transmission of blood glucose and blood pressure readings enables immediate alerts for patients and healthcare providers to intervene when needed.

Intraoperative Monitoring (IOM)

This technique that allows a surgeon to perform continuous checking, recording, and testing during a difficult surgical procedure. In neurological surgeries, IOM is used to detect potentially damaging changes in brain, spinal cord, and peripheral nerve function prior to irreversible damage. Staff in rural hospitals rarely have the expertise to perform this type of monitoring. Remote IOM uses systems to transmit data, voice, and images over the Internet to a site for monitoring by an expert. The expert can then let the on-site surgeons know if any problems arise as the surgery progresses.

Telehomecare (THC)

Telehomecare (THC) provides the remote care and reassurance needed to allow people with chronic conditions, dementia, or a high risk of falling to remain living in their own homes. The approach focuses on reacting to emergency events and raising a help response quickly. Deterioration can be spotted at an early stage before an accident occurs.

Advanced systems use sensors to monitor serious changes in chronic conditions as well as other health risks including floods, fires, and gas leaks. Such sensors can also alert caregivers if a person with dementia leaves the house. When a sensor is activated, a radio signal is sent to a central unit in the user's home. This signal automatically calls a monitoring center where appropriate action can be taken such as contacting a caregiver, family member, or doctor, or sending emergency services.

Medical Diagnosis and Treatment at the "Point-of-Care"

This refers to the ability to test and treat patients rapidly at sites close to where they live, rather than coming to the doctor or hospital for tests, waiting days or weeks for results, and then returning to the doctor for treatment. Point-of-care medicine is particularly useful for communities with limited access to large healthcare facilities, such as rural or low-resource areas.

Point-of-care medicine relies on portable diagnostic and monitoring devices that can be delivered to remote areas, combined with telehealth technologies. Such systems allow healthcare workers in remote areas to test patients and instantly send the results to experts to make a diagnosis and send back instructions for proper care. Portable devices have been developed that can measure blood gases, electrolytes, blood chemistries, glucose levels, and even detect cancer. This capability greatly enhances healthcare for patients in remote and underserved areas.

Developments in Telehealth

Smartphone-Based Device Provides Rapid Cancer Diagnosis at Low Cost

National Institute of Biomedical Imaging and Bioengineering (NIBIB)-funded researchers have developed a smartphone-based device that can diagnose cancer in less than an hour at a cost of under $2 per patient. Certain types of cancer can be detected using biological fluids such as blood, saliva, or other aspirates. The device could enable point-of-care cancer diagnostics in remote areas where a local clinic collects patient samples and must send them out to a central service that reports the results in several days—a system that often results in patients never returning to the clinic for follow-up care because they have to travel a long distance or cannot take off work. With the new device, biological fluid from patients is mixed with microbeads coated with antibodies that capture cancer cells. The smartphone, with a snap-on imaging module, then takes pictures of the cell-bead mixture. The pictures are transmitted to Massachusetts General Hospital (MGH) where, within seconds, computer analysis classifies the sample as high-risk, low-risk, or benign. This enables the patient to receive a diagnosis and initiation of treatment in a single trip to the clinic. The research team is bringing the system to small village clinics in Botswana to train local healthcare workers to screen for lymphoma.

Wearable Sensors Gather Mobile Health Data to Enable Treatment

A multi-center effort known as Mobile Sensor Data-to-Knowledge (MD2K) is under development to use wearable sensors to conduct large-scale clinical trials by collecting data remotely. One project in its initial phase is the remote monitoring of individuals who are trying to quit smoking. Participants wear a chest strap that measures heart rhythm and can detect inhalation and even stress. A motion sensor on the arm tracks movements as the person smokes and eats. They also wear smart eyeglasses to record their surroundings, which might reveal visual exposure to smoking triggers, such as cigarette advertising. All of this remotely collected data will be used to identify when a person is about to smoke. Smartphones apps are being developed that can automatically send "just-in-time" stress interventions to help the person abstain from smoking. The MD2K consortium of 12 universities and centers work together to develop and test software systems that collect and analyze health data, which will be openly available to researchers. The consortium also provides training to expand the number and expertise of researchers interested in developing mobile sensor strategies for managing a wide range of diseases and disorders.

Simple Computer Test for Early Stages of Alzheimer Disease

Alzheimer disease affects an estimated 5.3 million Americans, and is expected to increase in the coming decade. A critical goal of Alzheimer disease research is to improve methods of diagnosis so affected individuals can be identified sooner and begin treatment in the early stages of the disease. NIBIB-funded scientists are developing an automated, web-based, behavioral screening test for early cognitive decline and memory loss. The goal is to adapt the visual paired comparison (VPC) test of memory loss so that it can be performed with the subject viewing images on a computer screen. The VPC currently requires an eye tracking device that is expensive, requires specially trained personnel, and is not widely available. The researchers are developing a version of the VPC that uses simple methods to determine the eye movements of the test subject. The new automatic screening system will then be tested in the field for screening elderly individuals in various healthcare settings. If successful, it has potential to dramatically simplify current methods for diagnosing memory loss and enable millions of patients to take the test as part of a routine checkup.

Importance of Telehealth Services

In general, telehealth holds promise as a means of increasing access to care and improving health outcomes. Some analysts also see the potential for telehealth to reduce costs. Telehealth has existed in some form for decades. For instance, radiologists and dermatologists have relied on store-and-forward techniques, for instance transmission of videos or digital imagery (e.g., X-rays) through a secure electronic communications system, since the 1980s. However, significant advances in telecommunications, including the improvement of high-resolution imaging and greater access to broadband, have accelerated the use and availability of telehealth by a broad array of physicians and clinicians. For instance, it is estimated that 61 percent of healthcare institutions currently use some form of telehealth, and between 40–50 percent of all hospitals in the United States currently employ some form of telehealth. This figure includes rural/critical access hospitals, academic medical centers, and urban institutions. In 2013, the market for telehealth generated annual revenue of $9.6 billion, a 60-percent growth from 2012. Moreover, the ubiquity of Internet linked mobile computers, such as iPads, and video platforms, such as Skype, enable "direct" consultations between providers and patients located hundreds of miles apart.

The availability of telehealth is of particular interest for patients who live in areas that are inadequately served. Access to certain medical specialties, such as oncologists, is limited in rural areas. Currently, 59 million Americans reside in Health Professional Shortage Areas (HPSAs), rural and urban areas with shortages of primary care providers. Of special concern are rural individuals who have higher mortality rates; a greater chance of being unnecessarily hospitalized;

and have one-third as many specialists per capita as do persons living in cities.

Telehealth appears to hold particular promise for chronic disease management. Almost 50 percent of all adults in the United States have at least one chronic illness. Chronic disease accounts for approximately 75 percent of all healthcare expenditures and contributes to about 70 percent of all deaths in this country. Many persons with chronic conditions are elderly, and therefore have mobility limitations. Moreover, people with multiple chronic conditions typically require frequent visits to clinicians. Ensuring ready access to care for such individuals may help avert costly emergency room visits or hospital stays. However, aside from care for mental health, the majority of telehealth provided for chronic conditions to date has been limited to asynchronous monitoring.

Chapter 3

Telemedicine and E-Health

There are many factors, such as a shortage of healthcare professionals and greater incidence of chronic conditions that are driving the need to develop tools and solutions to improve healthcare delivery. One possible tool is the electronic exchange of medical information, which is commonly referred to as Health Information Technology ("Health IT"). Health IT plays a key role in digitizing and transmitting health information electronically that can improve patient outcomes. Health IT processes can also include:

1. Use of electronic health records (for patients, physicians, insurers, hospitals, and clinics);

2. Health information exchange across industries and geographies;

3. Use of electronic health information to detect trends in population and public health; and

4. Transmission of medication refills and a patient's prescription history.

A key part of Health IT is increasing the frequency and use of technology-driven remote monitoring and consultation to treat patients. This area of Health IT is commonly referred to as "telemedicine." There

---

This chapter includes text excerpted from "Telemedicine: An Important Force in the Transformation of Healthcare," International Trade Administration (ITA), U.S. Department of Commerce (DOC), June 25, 2009. Reviewed December 2017.

is no universally accepted definition of telemedicine; however, the American Telemedicine Association (ATA), a leading trade association, defines the term as follows:

Telemedicine is the use of medical information exchanged from one site to another via electronic communications to improve patients' health status. Closely associated with telemedicine is the term 'tele-health,' which is often used to encompass a broader definition of remote healthcare that does not always involve clinical services.

Videoconferencing, transmission of still images, e-health including patient portals, remote monitoring of vital signs, continuing medical education, and nursing call centers are all considered part of telemedicine and telehealth.

Products and Services within the Telemedicine Sector

Telemedicine involves a combination of medical products and services. Accordingly, there are numerous products and services comprising telemedicine, ranging from medical devices to delivery systems.

Products: Many medical devices capable of collecting and electronically transmitting information (either immediately or in the future) can be digitized to be used in telemedicine applications. These include blood glucose meters, pulse oximeters, blood pressure cuffs, CT scanners, and MRI machines. Some of these devices are targeted toward home healthcare and the needs/wants of patients interested in closely monitoring their health status, while others facilitate the exchange of information between hospitals, clinics, and physicians.

Key industry associations and stakeholders involved in these types of products include the Advanced Medical Technology Association (AdvaMed), the Medical Industry Technology Alliance (MITA), and the Medical Device Manufacturers Association (MDMA).

Services: The use of medical products with electronic exchange capabilities allows for the provision of a wide range of telemedicine-related services. These include store-and-forward technology for documents and images; remote monitoring of a patient's vital signs; secure messaging; e-mail exchange of data, alerts and reminders between physicians and patients; and having a specialist remotely available by videoconference to observe and diagnose a patient's condition and recommend treatment. Electronic exchange of prescription information between physicians, pharmacies, and consumers is an additional service. Other telemedicine services include transmitting information to alert communities about pandemics and other widespread health threats.

The key trade associations and stakeholders involved in telemedicine services include the American Telemedicine Association (ATA), the Healthcare Information and Management Systems Society (HIMSS), and the American Health Information Management Association (AHIMA).

The availability of innovative medical products and new applications of existing products and services can enhance the application of telemedicine. For example, more frequent information exchange of basic personal information remotely, including glucose level, pulse rate, and heart rate can lead to improved health for many patients, especially those with chronic conditions.

Potential Benefits of Telemedicine

There are several benefits that can be realized by an increased use of telemedicine, and there are multiple factors driving the need for telemedicine. Benefits can range from increased compliance in taking medications, to improved healthcare delivery in rural and underserved areas, to improved delivery of healthcare services outside hospitals and clinics, and better utilization of healthcare professionals.

Manage chronic diseases effectively: Chronic conditions such as diabetes, congestive heart failure, and obstructive pulmonary disease require long-term treatment and use of multiple specialists, all of which significantly increase costs.

These patients account for roughly 75 percent of total healthcare expenditures. Widespread telemedicine adoption will allow vital sign information and monitoring to be gathered frequently (instead of only during periodic physician visits). Messages can then be simultaneously transmitted to the treatment team, allowing for possible early intervention (a physician or hospital visit) if a patient's condition deteriorates.

Improve care of elderly, home-bound, and physically challenged patients: Use of telemedicine to reduce the frequency of visits to physician offices and hospital emergency rooms can potentially lead to greater convenience and compliance for elderly and home-based patients. By reducing the frequency of visits by remote monitoring and e-mail information exchange, more timely patient intervention can occur before acute care treatment is necessary.

Empower patients regarding their own health: Raising the responsibility level of patients to take their medicines and report basic health metrics to their physician(s) by using telemedicine represents an opportunity for patients and caregivers to play a greater role in their own care. By giving the patient the ability to directly see the correlation between adherence to treatment regimen and improvement in health, patients will more likely comply with treatment protocols, leading to faster recovery.

Improve competitiveness of U.S. industry by controlling healthcare costs: With rising healthcare costs, telemedicine can provide a tool for companies and insurers to better control and manage healthcare spending by enabling greater use of remote monitoring of a patient's condition to minimize the need for acute care intervention, and more efficient deployment of healthcare professionals (discussed further below).

Improve community and population health: Electronic sharing of images and video consults (a component of telemedicine) allows for: an easier exchange of information between public health services about a rare or unusual health condition; better measurement of chronic disease in a population; and the addressing of a public health crisis such as pandemic flu or anthrax. Faster awareness of current threats will help public health providers make better decisions regarding population health in these situations.

Enhancing VC awareness of potential new telemedicine applications for medical devices could further advance the prospects for companies across the medical device and related industries.

Address possible future shortages of healthcare professionals: Telemedicine services, such as videoconferencing and remote consults, better utilize current staff, whether at a hospital, physician's office, or via home-care. The availability of telemedicine technologies and procedures can also alleviate potential shortages of healthcare professionals by enabling remote consultations by physicians and nurses for patients located in other states or countries.

Reduce deaths, injuries, and infections: Increased use of telemedicine across all settings could reduce the incidence of adverse events caused by treatment and medication errors arising from piecemeal or inaccurate patient information, leading to more consistent patient treatment by limiting the number of hospital visits and reducing exposure to illness from other patients. In addition, electronic prescribing can help reduce errors in dispensing medicines by eliminating the need to decipher handwritten prescriptions.

Extend reach to underserved/rural communities in the United States: Many regions of the United States (both urban and rural) do not have a full range of healthcare services available. The presence of telemedicine services in rural areas has been shown to improve care by decreasing transportation costs; more efficiently deploying healthcare professionals and specialists; and offering timely healthcare delivery without the obstacles presented by lakes, forests, and mountains.

Challenges to Telemedicine

The telemedicine sector currently faces a number of challenges and barriers. This partly stems from healthcare providers having greater interest in using Health IT to implement electronic health records (EHRs) and reduce administrative costs rather than use these technologies to make more healthcare-related services widely available. The root cause of this limited application seems to be the financial investment that is needed for full development and, more importantly, the lack of adequate reimbursement opportunities for such investment. In addition, several other barriers have slowed the development of telemedicine, including:

- Reimbursement policies of third-party payers.

- Concerns about security and privacy.

- Lack of common standards and certification decreasing the likelihood of interoperability between medical devices, videoconferencing, and other systems.

- Availability of broadband Internet, medical access, and education, especially in rural and underserved areas.

- Medical liability and malpractice issues.

- Variable and exclusive state licensure requirements.

- Mismatch of telemedicine costs and benefits between physicians and insurers.

- Limited Congressional funding for telemedicine.

Chapter 4

Types of Telemedicine Technology

Chapter Contents

Section 4.1—Real-Time Telehealth... 22

Section 4.2—Store-and-Forward Telehealth 26

Section 4.3—Telemedicine and Patient Safety 27

Section 4.1

Real-Time Telehealth

This section contains text excerpted from the following
sources: Text in this section begins with excerpts from "Clinical Video
Telehealth (CVT)," U.S. Department of Veterans Affairs (VA), July
2015; Text under the heading "What Are the Components of CVT?"
is excerpted from "VHA Clinical Video Telehealth Technology,"
U.S. Department of Veterans Affairs (VA), June 25, 2013.
Reviewed December 2017.

Clinical video telehealth (CVT) uses video conferencing technology to conveniently, securely, and quickly provide Veterans with access to healthcare services from remote facilities. CVT instantly connects a Veteran in one location with a healthcare provider in a different location. This connection allows for real-time interaction between patient and provider. Specialty equipment provides a safe, reliable, and accurate way for providers to assess a patient and manage their treatment without physically being in the same location.

What Is CVT like to Use?

CVT appointments feel a lot like traditional face-to-face appointments.

When you come to your scheduled appointment, a staff member will escort you to the CVT equipped room.

The television monitors and cameras will be set up so that you and your provider can both see and hear each other clearly.

When your visit is over, you will let the staff know your session is complete. If a follow-up appointment is needed, you will go to scheduling to set up your next appointment.

Why Should I Use CVT?

Clinical video telehealth (CVT) helps you access the best healthcare without having to make long trips to see a specialist in person.

Using advanced technology, our doctors can provide you with the care you need by CVT as effectively as they can with a traditional face-to-face appointment.

What Are the Components of CVT?

1. **CODEC**

   CODEC is short for Coder-Decoder. The CODEC compresses (codes) the two-way audio and video streams so that they can be sent over the communications link, then decodes incoming signals from the far side. CODECs can be dedicated hardware "boxes" running proprietary software, or can be based on a personal computer.

2. **Video Camera**

   The CVT system camera and Web cam for computers are specially designed for videoconferencing applications. Some offer pan (side to side) and tilt (up and down) controls so that the user can easily point the camera at the appropriate subject. It also offers control of the zoom for a wider or tighter angle of view. The CVT systems provide multiple camera connections to facilitate additional specialized diagnostic cameras.

   Many systems allow control of the camera on the far end of the connection. This is especially useful because the consultant has direct control over the view so the consultant can frame the subject as needed. Far-end camera control has become standard on newer systems.

3. **Video Monitor**

   Each CVT system has at least one video monitor. Systems with a dedicated CODEC most often use a standard video monitor. Computer-based CODECs generally use a computer monitor, although some newer systems use a combination of one video monitor and one computer monitor for data display.

4. **Microphone**

   Each end has at least one microphone to pick up the sound for transmission to the far end.

5. **Speakers**

   Speakers allow the user to hear the sound from the far end.

6. **Accessories**

CVT system accessories are available for virtually any specialized application. Some key accessories often used in telehealth applications include document cameras to share ECG's, X-rays, graphs, and other static materials. Diagnostic peripherals adapted for use with videoconferencing equipment include dermascope, ENT scope, digital stethoscope, still camera, etc.

Polytrauma

Linking the four Polytrauma Rehabilitation Centers (PRC's) in Minneapolis, Palo Alto, Richmond, and Tampa with each other and the 17 Polytrauma Network Sites (PNS's) with the express intent of improving access to care for combat wounded. Polytrauma Rehabilitation Centers bring together a critical mass of relevant clinical expertise to assess, treat and rehabilitate the physical, mental and psycho social problems that accompany polytrauma.

TeleMental Health

VHA uses information technology and telecommunication modalities to augment care provided by its Mental Health clinicians to Veterans throughout the United States. VHA TeleMental Health is the delivery of services using virtual linkages between VHA patients and Mental Health providers separated by distance or time.

TeleRehabilitation

The delivery of services using virtual linkages like using video teleconferencing to link a speech pathologist located at the urban VA medical center with a poststroke Veteran patient located at the local VA community-based outpatient clinic, or using home telehealth technologies to connect with Veterans at home to monitor their functional status and equipment needs.

TeleSurgery

The main need VHA is meeting via telesurgery is not for operative surgery support but for specialist consultation to remote sites. The diagnosis of surgical conditions, the coordination of care for many surgical conditions and the triage of surgical patients can be favorably influenced by the availability of telesurgical consultation. Additionally, the use of telehealth can provide intra-operative consultation, patient and staff education as well as pre- and postoperative assessment.

Additional Clinical Video Telehealth Specialties

New telehealth specialties are being added up as the technology improves, allowing telehealth technologies to integrate into more areas of Veteran care.

- TeleCardiology
- TeleGenomics
- TeleICU
- TeleNeurology
- TeleNutrition
- TelePrimary Care
- TelePulmonology (Sleep Services)
- TeleRehabilitation
- TeleAmputation Clinics
- TeleKinesiology
- TeleOccupational Therapy
- TeleSpinal Cord Injury/Disorder
- TeleMOVE!

These video technologies make it possible for Veteran patients to come to many of VA's community-based outpatient clinics and connect to a specialist physician or other practitioner who may be in a hospital that is dozens, or hundreds or even thousands of miles away.

Clinical Video Telehealth means that instead of having the cost and inconvenience of traveling by road, rail or air to see a specialist in the hospital the specialist comes to you. If Veteran's need medication prescriptions changed or if the veteran needs to see the specialist in person, have special investigations or come into hospital then this can even be arranged through Clinical Video Telehealth.

Section 4.2

Store-and-Forward Telehealth

This section includes text excerpted from "VA Telehealth
Services—Store-And-Forward Telehealth," U.S. Department of
Veterans Affairs (VA), June 3, 2015.

You have probably heard the expression that a picture is worth
a thousand words? In some areas of healthcare, pictures can be
worth thousands of clinic visits. Three areas of healthcare where
this is becoming commonplace are: radiology, dermatology, and
checking for the effects of diabetes on the retina in the back of the
eye.

Store-and-Forward Telehealth involves the acquisition and storing of clinical information (e.g., data, image, sound, video) that is
then forwarded to (or retrieved by) another site for clinical evaluation. For many years, local and regional Store-and-Forward Telehealth programs have been providing consultation to Veterans Health
Administration (VHA) sites in need of specialty expertise. VHA's first
national Store-and-Forward Telehealth program was a primary care-
based model that screens veterans with diabetes for retinopathy using
teleretinal imaging that expedite referral for treatment and provide
health information.

TeleDermatology

Dermatology (skin) problems are common and often a source of
discomfort and concern to patients. The diagnosis of a skin problem
can often be made from a digital picture if it is sent to a skin specialist
(dermatologist) to see. A report with recommendations for treatment
can then be sent back to a patient's primary care, or other, physician.
The recommendation may be for treatment in the form of a medication
or may be a referral to a dermatology clinic for more detailed assessment. VA is using TeleDermatology to improve access to skin care for
veteran patients who live in remote and other areas to save having to
travel to a dermatology clinic.

TeleRetinal Imaging

Diabetes can cause problems with the blood vessels in the back of the eye (retina), especially if the diabetes is poorly controlled. A special camera is now available that can take pictures of the retina of the eye without needing to put drops in the eye to widen the pupil of the eye. The picture that is taken is then sent to an eye care specialist to review and a report is sent back to the patient's primary care physician who then follows-up if treatment to prevent blindness is required. This investigation does not replace a full eye exam and is not suitable for people who already have complications of diabetes but makes it does mean that those at risk of eye problems from diabetes can be assessed easily and conveniently in a local clinic.

The ability to acquire, store, and then forward digital images for reporting is a crucial area of care coordination development within VHA. VA's computerized patient record called VistA has a component called VistA Imaging. VistA Imaging. VistA Imaging enables the communication of clinical images throughout VA. Using VistA Imaging VA is able to undertake.

Section 4.3

Telemedicine and Patient Safety

This section includes text excerpted from "Telemedicine and Patient Safety," Agency for Healthcare Research and Quality (AHRQ), U.S. Department of Health and Human Services (HHS), September 2016.

A paradigm shift is ongoing in the healthcare sector. The traditional model of episodic and hospital-based care is being replaced by a patient-centric approach, in which patients are constantly connected to their healthcare providers. This shift is driven by the need to optimize the performance of the healthcare system and enabled by advances in technology.

Advanced communications and monitoring technologies facilitate the exchange of a patient's information between two or more sites.

These technologies are now commonly applied in virtually every medical specialty to educate, monitor, offer self-management support for patients, and provide clinicians with clinical decision support for diagnosis and ongoing care. A variety of terms telemedicine, telehealth, connected health, eHealth, mHealth are used to describe this model of care delivery. The more general term, telemedicine, will be used in this section.

The evidence supporting the role of telemedicine is strong. Studies have shown that telemedicine promotes continuity of care, decreases the cost of care, and improves patient self-management and overall clinical outcomes. For example, a synthesis of evidence from 15 systematic reviews published between 2003 and 2013 demonstrated that heart failure telemonitoring reduced all-cause mortality by 15–40 percent and heart failure related hospitalizations by 14–36 percent. Another systematic review found that, compared with usual care, telemonitoring for patients with heart failure was associated with significant cost reductions, ranging from 1.6–68.3 percent. This body of evidence is driving the increased adoption of telemedicine services. For instance, the heart failure telemonitoring program (Connected Cardiac Care Program) at Partners Healthcare, which has consistently achieved significant reductions in 30-day readmissions, started as a small pilot project in 2007. Since then, the program has been deployed as a population health management tool across Partners' network of hospitals.

Telemedicine can also help in identifying and preventing treatment-related errors between clinic visits. As one example, a number of studies have shown that medication errors can be significantly reduced by telemedicine. One study utilized real-time videoconferencing consultations between physicians in rural emergency departments (EDs) and pediatric critical care physicians in a large academic medical center to manage treatment of children with serious illness or injury in eight rural EDs in California. They found that the frequency of physician-related medication errors was at least three times higher in patients who didn't receive telemedicine consultation than in those who did. Similar reductions in medication errors have been reported in telepharmacy programs.

Furthermore, telemedicine surveillance applications can detect preventable treatment-related adverse events that may otherwise go unnoticed by care providers. For instance, a study of ambulatory patients with diabetes found that a weekly interactive, automated telephone application that provided patient education and self-management support with targeted nurse follow-up detected more (59%)

treatment-related adverse events than either nurse elicitation (30%) or patient detection (11%) alone. Another similar application is used for monitoring patients with implantable cardioverter defibrillators to prevent inappropriate defibrillator shock.

These studies create a body of evidence that supports a positive impact of telemedicine on patient outcomes, particularly in the management of discrete disease states like heart failure or for specific situations such as the use of defibrillators. However, the overall impact of telemedicine on safety is less well studied, and some have raised concerns. Like any innovation that affects care delivery, telemedicine must face the same standards and thoughtful evaluation as traditional care. Some argue that telemedicine should be subject to even closer scrutiny because the absence of the traditional face-to-face encounter could increase the risk of medical errors.

Moreover, in an effort to improve clinical efficiency, telemedicine could be employed in situations that are inappropriate. For example, even telemedicine advocates would not argue that patients with chest pain should be managed via email or over the telephone. One key component of the telemedicine research agenda is to determine these boundaries. One concerning study reviewed 32 cases that ended in catastrophic outcomes, including deaths and malpractice settlements amounting to more than $12 million. Telephone communication was implicated as a significant root cause, raising issues regarding the importance of face-to-face visits in some circumstances.

The exponential growth of mobile medical applications raises new safety concerns. Telemedicine has evolved from simple telephone communications to more complex algorithmic-driven smartphone-based applications. Many developers lack medical training, and some fail to involve clinicians in the mobile application development or implementation process. On top of that, many of these applications are marketed directly to consumers without any formal safety or efficacy testing. For example, one study investigated the accuracy of a top-selling mobile application that promised personal assistance with management and diagnosis of skin cancer.

In the study, the authors tested the application's ability to detect melanoma by using it to evaluate 93 photos of biopsy-proven melanoma. Disconcertingly, it correctly classified only 10.8 percent of the lesions. Other examples include applications that, based on inputting the diet of patients with diabetes, calculate that patient's insulin dose. The U.S. Food and Drug Administration (FDA) and the Federal Trade Commission (FTC) are fast at work trying to evaluate medical mobile applications to determine if they are safe and effective. However, with the tally of mobile health applications now exceeding 100,000, the task is a mammoth one.

Given these concerns, should we suspend telemedicine implementations until we can address these issues? In the spirit of "not throwing the baby out with the bathwater," we argue that the answer is "no." New technologies and care models come with attendant risks. Telemedicine has demonstrated many positive effects on care. Rather than stop the forward progress, we argue for a more thoughtful, continuous safety improvement process that could start from the moment of project conception.

Suggestions to increase patient safety in telemedicine include:

1. patient safety awareness should permeate all phases of the telemedicine project life cycle;

2. integrate safety testing as part of usability and efficacy trials, such evaluations should not be limited to academic medical settings;

3. use the latest data security and encryption systems to protect patient privacy;

4. increase regulatory, professional, and healthcare organizations' involvement in creating consensus-driven guidelines, operational protocols, and standards, all of which should be updated regularly;

5. full disclosure of possible risks prior to patient enrollment in telemedicine interventions;

6. create systems for clinicians to document telemedicine services and integrate them as part of regular workflow; and

7. increase efforts to lessen social risks by creating more solutions for patients with low health literacy, along with solutions for non-English speakers.

On the whole, telemedicine is improving the health of patients and has the promise to revolutionize healthcare delivery. The current rise in adoption and integration into clinical workflows will no doubt continue. The constant advances in technological innovations present new opportunities for care delivery innovation as well as new challenges. Although some telemedicine programs can prevent medical errors, known and emerging threats to patient safety are real.

Therefore, there is a need to increase research efforts evaluating the impact of telemedicine on patient safety. Ultimately, we need to balance our commitment to the ethical principle of nonmaleficence (do no harm) with the need to adopt technology-driven innovations in healthcare to enhance quality and efficiency. Doing so should allow us to use these technologies to improve patient safety.

Chapter 5

Benefits of Telemedicine

Telemedicine is a broad term within health information technology (Health IT) that encompasses methods for electronically transmitting medical information to sustain and/or improve a patient's health status. These methods can include: store-and-forward technology for documents and images; remote monitoring of a patient's vital signs; secure messaging; e-mail exchange of data, alerts and reminders between physicians and patients; and the ability to observe, diagnose and recommend treatment via videoconference.

There are multiple products and services and respective industries that are involved in developing the various applications of telemedicine, including information technology vendors, medical device manufacturers, pharmacies, hospitals, nursing homes, and venture capitalists, among others. In the current environment of a shortage of healthcare professionals, greater incidence of chronic conditions, and rising healthcare costs, telemedicine offers a potential tool to improve efficiency in the delivery of healthcare.

The need for telemedicine is further compounded by the following factors:

- Significant increase in the U.S. population—estimated growth of 20 percent (to 363 million) between 2008-2030

This chapter includes text excerpted from "Telemedicine: An Important Force in the Transformation of Healthcare," International Trade Administration (ITA), U.S. Department of Commerce (DOC), June 25, 2009. Reviewed December 2017.

- Shortage of healthcare professionals being educated, trained, and licensed

- Increasing incidence of chronic diseases around the world, including diabetes, congestive heart failure, and obstructive pulmonary disease

- Need for efficient care of the elderly, homebound, and physically challenged patients

- Lack of specialists and health facilities in rural areas

- Adverse events, injuries and illness at hospitals and physician's offices

- Need to improve community and population health

Telemedicine can play an important role in providing solutions to these challenges. For instance, telemedicine maximizes the use of existing healthcare professionals by allowing them to remotely diagnose, monitor and recommend treatment for patients located in rural areas. In addition, telemedicine limits patient exposure to infections by eliminating or limiting the need to visit a hospital or a physician's office for healthcare services.

Despite these potential benefits, there are a number of barriers that have hindered the expansion of telemedicine in the U.S. market, including:

- Reimbursement policies of third-party payers

- Concerns about security and privacy

- Lack of common standards and certification decreasing the likelihood of interoperability between medical devices, videoconferencing, and other systems

- Limited availability of broadband Internet, medical access, and education, especially in rural and underserved areas

- Medical liability and malpractice issues

- Variable and exclusive state licensure requirements

- Mismatch of telemedicine costs and benefits between physicians and insurers

- Limited Congressional funding for telemedicine

These barriers must be sufficiently overcome to accelerate the development and application of telemedicine.

Chapter 6

Health Technology Assessment

Health technology assessment (HTA) is the systematic evaluation of properties, effects, or other impacts of health technology. The main purpose of HTA is to inform policymaking for technology in healthcare, where policymaking is used in the broad sense to include decisions made at, e.g., the individual or patient level, the level of the healthcare provider or institution, or at the regional, national, and international levels. HTA may address the direct and intended consequences of technologies as well as their indirect and unintended consequences. HTA is conducted by interdisciplinary groups using explicit analytical frameworks, drawing from a variety of methods.

Purposes of HTA

HTA can be used in many ways to advise or inform technology-related policies and decisions. Among these are to advise or inform:

- Regulatory agencies about whether to permit the commercial use (e.g., marketing) of a drug, device, or other regulated technology

This chapter includes text excerpted from "Introduction to Health Technology Assessment," U.S. National Library of Medicine (NLM), 2014. Reviewed December 2017.

- Payers (healthcare authorities, health plans, drug formularies, employers, etc.) about technology coverage (whether or not to pay), coding (assigning proper codes to enable reimbursement), and reimbursement (how much to pay)

- Clinicians and patients about the appropriate use of health-care interventions for a particular patient's clinical needs and circumstances

- Health professional associations about the role of a technology in clinical protocols or practice guidelines

- Hospitals, healthcare networks, group purchasing organizations, and other healthcare organizations about decisions regarding technology acquisition and management

- Standards-setting organizations for health technology and healthcare delivery regarding the manufacture, performance, appropriate use, and other aspects of healthcare technologies

- Government health department officials about undertaking public health programs (e.g., immunization, screening, and environmental protection programs)

- Lawmakers and other political leaders about policies concerning technological innovation, research and development, regulation, payment, and delivery of healthcare

- Healthcare technology companies about product development and marketing decisions

- Investors and companies concerning venture capital funding, acquisitions, and divestitures, and other transactions concerning healthcare product and service companies

- Research agencies about evidence gaps and unmet health needs

Many of the types of organizations noted above, including government and commercial payers, hospital networks, health professional organizations, and others, have their own HTA units or functions. Many HTA agencies are affiliated with national or regional governments or consortia of multiple organizations. Further, there are independent not-for-profit and for-profit HTA organizations.

HTA contributes in many ways to the knowledge base for improving the quality of healthcare, especially to support development and updating of a wide spectrum of standards, guidelines, and other healthcare policies. For example, in the United States, the Joint Commission (formerly, JCAHO) and the National Committee for Quality Assurance (NCQA) set standards for measuring quality of care and services of hospitals, managed care organizations, long-term care facilities, hospices, ambulatory care centers, and other healthcare institutions. The National Quality Forum (NQF) endorses national evidence-based consensus standards for measuring and reporting across a broad range of healthcare interventions.

Health professional associations (e.g., American College of Cardiology, American College of Physicians, American College of Radiology) and special panels (e.g., the U.S. Preventive Services Task Force, the joint Department of Veterans Affairs/Department of Defense Clinical Practice Guidelines program) develop clinical practice guidelines, standards, and other statements regarding the appropriate use of technologies. The Guidelines International Network (G-I-N) of organizations and individual members from more than 40 countries supports evidence-based guideline development, adaptation, dissemination, and implementation toward reducing inappropriate practice variation throughout the world. The National Guideline Clearinghouse (NGC, sponsored by the U.S. Agency for Healthcare Research and Quality), is a searchable database of evidence-based clinical practice guidelines. Among the criteria for a new guideline to be included in NGC effective June 2014 is that it be based on a carefully documented systematic review of the evidence, including a detailed search strategy and description of study selection.

Standards-setting organizations such as the American National Standards Institute (ANSI) and the American Society for Testing and Materials coordinate development of voluntary national consensus standards for the manufacture, use, and reuse of health devices and their materials and components. For example, ANSI has developed standards and specifications for electronic information sharing and interoperability in such areas as laboratory results reporting, medication management, personalized healthcare, immunizations, and neonatal screening.

As noted above, HTA can be used to support decision making by clinicians and patients. The term evidence-based medicine refers to the use of current best evidence from scientific and medical research, and the application of clinical experience and observation, in making decisions about the care of individual patients. This prompted the appearance of many useful resources, including:

- Evidence-Based Medicine, a guide to the field, recently updated

- Evidence-Based Medicine (a joint product of the American College of Physicians and the BMJ Publishing Group), a journal digest of articles selected from international medical journals

37

- "Users' guides to the medical literature," a series of more than 30 articles by the Evidence-Based Medicine Working Group, originally published in the Journal of the American Medical Association, starting in the 1990s and more recently assembled and updated

- Centre for Evidence-Based Medicine

Basic HTA Orientations

The impetus for an HTA is not necessarily a particular technology. Three basic orientations to HTA are as follows.

- *Technology-oriented assessments* are intended to determine the characteristics or impacts of particular technologies. For example, a government agency may want to determine the clinical, economic, social, professional, or other impacts of cochlear implants, cervical cancer screening, PET scanners, or widespread adoption of electronic health record systems.

- *Problem-oriented assessments* focus on solutions or strategies for managing a particular disease, condition, or other problem for which alternative or complementary technologies might be used. For example, clinicians and other providers concerned with the problem of diagnosis of dementia may call for HTA to inform the development of clinical practice guidelines involving some combination or sequence of clinical history, neurological examination, and diagnostic imaging using various modalities.

- *Project-oriented assessments* focus on a local placement or use of a technology in a particular institution, program, or other designated project. For example, this may arise when a hospital must decide whether or not to purchase a PET scanner, considering the facilities, personnel, and other resources needed to install and operate a PET scanner; the hospital's financial status; local market potential for PET services; competitive factors; etc.

These basic assessment orientations can overlap and complement one another. Certainly, all three types could draw on a common body of scientific evidence and other information. A technologyoriented assessment may address the range of problems for which the technology might be used and how appropriate the technology might be for different types of local settings (e.g., inpatient versus outpatient). A problem-oriented assessment may compare the effectiveness, safety, and other impacts of alternative technologies for a given problem, e.g., alternative treatments for atrial fibrillation (e.g., drug therapy, surgery, or catheter ablation), and may draw on technology-oriented assessments of one or more of those alternatives as well as any direct ("head-to-head") comparisons of them. A projectoriented assessment would consider the range of impacts of a technology or its alternatives in a given setting, as well as the role or usefulness of that technology for various problems. Although the information used in a project-oriented assessment by a particular hospital may include findings of pertinent technology- and problem-oriented assessments, local data collection and analysis may be required to determine what is appropriate for that hospital. Thus, many HTAs will blend aspects of all three basic orientations.

Properties and Impacts Assessed

What does HTA assess? HTA may involve the investigation of one or more properties, impacts, or other attributes of health technologies or applications. In general, these include the following.

- Technical properties

- Safety

- Efficacy and/or effectiveness

- Economic attributes or impacts

- Social, legal, ethical, and/or political impacts

The properties, impacts, and other attributes assessed in HTA pertain across the range of types of technology. Thus, for example, just as drugs, devices, and surgical procedures can be assessed for safety, effectiveness, and cost effectiveness, so can hospital infection control programs, computer-based drug-utilization review systems, and rural telemedicine networks.

Technical properties include performance characteristics and conformity with specifications for design, composition, manufacturing, tolerances, reliability, ease of use, maintenance, etc.

Safety is a judgment of the acceptability of risk (a measure of the probability of an adverse outcome and its severity) associated with using a technology in a given situation, e.g., for a patient with a particular health problem, by a clinician with certain training, or in a specified treatment setting.

Efficacy and effectiveness both refer to how well a technology works, i.e., accomplishes its intended purpose, usually based on changes in one or more specified health outcomes or "endpoints" as described below. A technology that works under carefully managed conditions does not always work as well under more heterogeneous or less controlled conditions. In HTA, efficacy refers to the benefit of using a technology for a particular problem under ideal conditions, e.g., within the protocol of a carefully managed RCT, involving patients meeting narrowly defined criteria, or conducted at a "center of excellence." Effectiveness refers to the benefit of using a technology for a particular problem under general or routine conditions, e.g., by a physician in a community hospital for a variety of types of patients. Whereas efficacy answers the question, "Can it work?" (in the best conditions), effectiveness answers the question "Does it work?" (in real-world conditions).

Clinicians, patients, managers, and policymakers are increasingly aware of the practical implications of differences in efficacy and effectiveness. Researchers delve into registers, databases (e.g., of thirdparty payment claims and administrative data), and other epidemiological and observational data to discern possible associations between the use of technologies and patient outcomes in general or routine practice settings. As these are observational studies, their validity for establishing causal connections between interventions and patient outcomes is limited compared to experimental studies, particularly RCTs. Even so, observational studies can be used to generate hypotheses for experimental trials, and they can provide evidence about effectiveness that can complement other evidence about efficacy, suggesting whether findings under ideal conditions may be extended to routine practice.

Economic attributes or impacts of health technologies can be microeconomic and macroeconomic. Microeconomic concerns include costs, prices, charges, and payment levels associated with individual technologies. Other concerns include comparisons of resource requirements and outcomes (or benefits) of technologies for particular applications, such as cost effectiveness, cost utility, and cost benefit. Health technology can have or contribute to a broad range of macroeconomic impacts. These include impacts on: a nation's gross domestic product, national healthcare costs, and resource allocation across healthcare and other industrial sectors, and international trade. Health technology can also be a factor in national and global patterns of investment, innovation, competitiveness, technology transfer, and employment (e.g., workforce size and mobility). Other macroeconomic issues that pertain to health technologies include the effects of intellectual property policies (e.g., for patent protection), regulation, third-party payment, and other policy changes that affect technological innovation, adoption, diffusion, and use.

Ethical, legal, and social considerations arise in HTA in the form of normative concepts (e.g., valuation of human life); choices about how and when to use technologies; research and the advancement of knowledge; resource allocation; and the integrity of HTA processes themselves. Indeed, the origins of technology assessment called for the field to support policymakers' broader considerations of technological impacts, such as the "social, economic, and legal implications of any course of action" and the "short- and long-term social consequences (for example, societal, economic, ethical, legal) of the application of technology." More recently, for example, an integral component of the Human Genome Project of the U.S. National Institutes of Health is the Ethical, Legal and Social Implications (ELSI) Research Program. One recently proposed broader framework, "HELPCESS," includes consideration of: humanitarian, ethical, legal, public relationships, cultural, economic, safety/security, and social implications.

Whether in healthcare or other sectors, technological innovation can challenge certain ethical, religious, cultural, and legal norms. Current examples include genetic testing, use of stem cells to grow new tissues, allocation of scarce organs for transplantation, and life-support systems for critically ill patients. For example, the slowly increasing supply of donated kidneys, livers, hearts, lungs, and other solid organs for transplantation continues to fall behind the expanding need for them, raising ethical, social, and political concerns about allocation of scarce, life-saving resources. In dialysis and transplantation for patients with end-stage renal disease, ethical concerns arise from patient selection criteria, termination of treatment, and managing noncompliant and other problem patients. Even so, these concerns continue to prompt innovations to overcome organ shortages, such as techniques for improving transplantation success rates with organs from marginal donors, organs from living donors, paired and longer chain donation, xenotransplantation (e.g., from pigs), stem cells to regenerate damaged tissues, and the longer-range goal of whole-organ tissue engineering.

Technologies that can diminish or strengthen patient dignity or autonomy include, e.g., end-of-life care, cancer chemotherapy, feeding devices, and assistive equipment for moving immobilized patients. Greater involvement of patients, citizens, and other stakeholders in

41

healthcare decisions, technology design and development, and the HTA process itself is helping to address some concerns about the relationships between patients and health technology. Ethical questions also have led to improvements in informed consent procedures for patients involved in clinical trials.

Allocation of scarce resources to technologies that are expensive, misused, not uniformly accessible, or noncurative can raise broad concerns about equity and squandered opportunities to improve population health. The same technologies can pose various challenges in the context of different or evolving societal and cultural norms, economic conditions, and healthcare system delivery and financing configurations. Even old or "mainstream" technologies can raise concerns in changing social contexts, such as immunization, organ procurement for transplantation, or male circumcision. In addition to technologies, certain actual or proposed uses of analytical methods can prompt such concerns; many observers object to using actual or implied cost per quality-adjusted life year (QALY) thresholds in coverage decisions.

Methods for assessing ethical, legal, and social implications of health technology have been underdeveloped relative to other methods in HTA, although there has been increased attention in recent years to developing frameworks and other guidance for these analyses. More work is needed for translating these implications into policy, such as for involving different perspectives in the HTA process in order to better account for identification of the types of effects or impacts that should be assessed, and for values assigned by these different perspectives to life, quality of life, privacy, choice of care, and other matters.

As a form of objective scientific and social inquiry, HTA must be subject to ethical conduct, social responsibility, and cultural differences. Some aspects to be incorporated or otherwise addressed include: identifying and minimizing potential conflicts of interest on the part of assessment staff and expert advisors; accounting for social, demographic, economic, and other dimensions of representativeness and equity in HTA resource allocation and topic selection; and patient and other stakeholder input on topic selection, evidence questions, and relevant outcomes/endpoints.

The terms "appropriate" and "necessary" often are used to describe whether or not a technology should be used in particular circumstances. These are judgments that typically reflect considerations of one or more of the properties and impacts described above. For example, the appropriateness of a diagnostic test may depend on its safety and effectiveness compared to alternative available interventions for particular patient indications, clinical settings, and resource constraints, perhaps as summarized in an evidence-based clinical practice guideline. A technology may be considered necessary if it is likely to be effective and acceptably safe for particular patient indications, and if withholding it would be deleterious to the patient's health.

HTA inquires about the unintended consequences of health technologies as well an intended ones, which may involve some or all of the types of impacts assessed. Some unintended consequences include, or lead to, unanticipated uses of technologies.

Chapter 7

Technology and Healthcare Expenditure

Contribution of Technological Change to the Growth of Healthcare Spending

On the basis of a review of the economic literature, Congressional Budget Office (CBO) concludes that roughly half of the increase in healthcare spending during the past several decades was associated with the expanded capabilities of medicine brought about by technological advances.

Expanded Capabilities of Healthcare from Technological Change

CBO defines technological advances as changes in clinical practice that enhance the ability of providers to diagnose, treat, or prevent health problems. Technological advances take many forms. Examples include new drugs, devices, or services, as well as new clinical applications of existing technologies (providing a particular service to a broader set of patients, for example). Other technological changes are newly developed techniques or additions to knowledge.

This chapter includes text excerpted from "Technological Change and the Growth of Healthcare Spending," Congressional Budget Office (CBO), 2008. Reviewed December 2017.

Medical breakthroughs occasionally create new types of therapies that enable providers to treat conditions they previously could not treat or could not treat effectively or aggressively. In such cases, new financial costs are incurred where little or no costs had been incurred before. Other advances in knowledge or technical capabilities bring the benefits of existing methods or services to much wider patient populations, increasing spending.

Even when technological innovation leads to a decline in the cost of a given service, net spending rises if the use of services increases sufficiently. Innovation can also make older treatments more costly than they would otherwise be.

New curative therapies with one-time costs could reduce spending if they obviated the need for costlier treatments. Many advances in medical science, however, do not fall into that category. In fact, many of the most notable medical advances in recent decades involve ongoing treatments for the management of chronic conditions such as diabetes and coronary artery disease.

Can New Technology Reduce Spending?

Advances in medical care can reduce spending in some instances. Some vaccines, for example, may offer the potential for savings, and certain types of preventive medical care may help some patients avoid costly hospitalizations for acute care. But, overall, examples of new treatments for which long-term savings have been clearly demonstrated are few. Many medical advances to date have increased spending because they made treatments available for conditions that were previously impossible to treat or were not aggressively treated. Furthermore, improvements in medical care that decrease mortality by helping patients avoid or survive acute health problems paradoxically increase overall spending on healthcare because surviving patients live longer and therefore use health services for more years.

Future advances—in molecular biology and genetics, in particular—may one day offer the possibility of savings if they make curative therapies available. Continued advances in understanding the genetic origins of disease offer the credible possibility that future providers will accurately predict the health risks faced by individual patients and design therapies tailored specifically to them. Some therapies may involve the insertion of healthy genes into tissue in order to compensate for damaged or missing genes; others might be aimed at the signaling processes within and between cells that initiate cell growth

46

or metabolic activity. Major illnesses such as cancer, Lou Gehrig's disease, Huntington disease, epilepsy, cystic fibrosis, and glaucoma may be targeted at their genetic origins. Treatment for coronary artery disease may include therapies that target the genes that regulate cholesterol; other therapies may stimulate repairs to damaged heart muscle or new vessel growth for vascular disease. Compared with some existing therapies that manage—often over many years—the effects of chronic disease, new therapies that target the genetic origins of disease may yield savings, but predicting how they would affect spending is very difficult. And most of these therapies are not likely to be a practical reality in the near term.

Advances in Medical Technology That Increase Healthcare Spending

Advances in medical science during the past several decades have greatly increased the set of available medical services, allowing practitioners to treat patients in ways that were not previously possible. Most health policy analysts agree that the long-term increase in healthcare spending is principally the result of the healthcare system's incorporation of these new services into clinical practice. Although compiling an exhaustive list of technological advances that have affected medical costs is not possible, a qualitative discussion of selected major scientific advances and the changes in clinical practice that followed them can help illustrate how technological progress has been accompanied by more spending.

Bone Marrow (Stem Cell) Transplantation. A number of illnesses can prevent the body from producing vital platelets and blood cells. One such condition, aplastic anemia, was treated successfully with bone marrow transplantation for the first time in the late 1960s. A bone marrow transplant, or stem cell therapy, involves transferring healthy cells from donors into patients whose bodies cannot produce blood cells. Initially, this procedure was used in treating the relatively small number of patients with aplastic anemia, as well as some patients with leukemia or certain disorders of the immune system, and few patients over the age of 40 were viewed as candidates for the procedure. Over time, technological advances have broadened the set of patients who can be treated to include those with multiple myeloma, lymphoma, sickle cell disease, and other conditions. One major advance in the 1990s was the development of autologous transplantation, which enables providers to obtain "donor" cells from the patient. This advance has greatly expanded the set of patients who are candidates for this type of therapy.

Neonatal Intensive Care. Many years ago, the healthcare system spent very little on low-birthweight babies because few effective therapies were available. Today, many valuable treatments are available. Ventilators suitable for infant care have been improved. Delivery of nutrition to very sick infants has been aided by advances in intravenous methods. Clinical monitoring of the heart, blood pressure, and other vital indicators is far more advanced today than in decades past. Estimated costs for low birthweight infants today are about 10 times those for infants of normal weight, principally because of the use of advanced treatments.

Joint Replacement. Since the introduction of the first successful hip replacements in the 1960s, newer metals and plastics have allowed the development of stronger, longer-lasting materials that are less subject to corrosion and produce better long-term outcomes. In part because of the availability of better artificial joints and improved outcomes, surgery for total or partial hip replacement and knee replacement is increasingly common in the United States. During the 25 years from 1979 to 2004, the number of hip and knee replacements per year increased substantially.

Diagnostic Imaging. Before today's noninvasive diagnostic imaging methods became available, reliable diagnoses often required exploratory surgery, which posed clinical risks and caused patients considerable discomfort. Recent technological advances, however, have led to powerful new diagnostic imaging capabilities. Newly developed diagnostic scans may be far less costly per procedure than exploratory surgery, but by their nature they invite much greater use and therefore tend to increase total spending compared with previous methods. Computed axial tomography imaging, which produces a digital cross-section image, or "slice," of the body, came into use in the 1970s. The imaging process was slow at first, but subsequent improvements in computing power and imaging speed made it possible to create hundreds of images in just seconds. Magnetic resonance imaging, which can produce images of superior quality in some cases, became available in the 1980s.

The introduction and continual improvement of these imaging techniques effectively reduced the cost of producing a diagnostic image of any given level of quality. Improvements in quality and rapid growth in the use of those techniques, however, led to higher total spending on diagnostic services. To understand how these new imaging techniques affected healthcare spending, it is instructive to draw a comparison with personal computer technology and information technology in general. As technological innovations enabled more powerful computer processing at a fraction of the previous cost, total spending on computers did not decrease. Instead, it increased dramatically as more consumers made greater use of what became available. Similarly, continued innovation in imaging technology tended to increase total spending, even as the effective cost of diagnostic imaging fell. Advances in diagnostic capability, by furnishing more detailed clinical information, may also indirectly increase spending by spurring the provision of a greater quantity of therapeutic services than would have been provided otherwise.

Part Two

Technology and Preventive Healthcare

Chapter 8

Digital Health

The 21st Century Cures Act (12/13/2016) clarified U.S. Food and Drug Administration's (FDA) regulation of medical software. The law amended the definition of "device" in the Food, Drug, and Cosmetic Act (FD&C) to exclude certain software functions.

The FDA is developing draft guidance for public comment to help industry and FDA staff understand how the 21st Century Cures Act affects FDA's oversight of medical device software.

The broad scope of digital health includes categories such as mobile health (mHealth), health information technology (IT), wearable devices, telehealth and telemedicine, and personalized medicine.

Providers and other stakeholders are using digital health in their efforts to:

- reduce inefficiencies,

- improve access,

- reduce costs,

- increase quality, and

- make medicine more personalized for patients.

Patients and consumers can use digital health to better manage and track their health and wellness related activities.

This chapter includes text excerpted from "Medical Devices—Digital Health," U.S. Food and Drug Administration (FDA), September 6, 2017.

The use of technologies such as smartphones, social networks, and Internet applications is not only changing the way we communicate, but is also providing innovative ways for us to monitor our health and well-being and giving us greater access to information. Together these advancements are leading to a convergence of people, information, technology, and connectivity to improve healthcare and health outcomes.

Why Is the FDA Focusing on Digital Health?

Many medical devices now have the ability to connect to and communicate with other devices or systems. Devices that are already FDA-approved or cleared are being updated to add digital features. New types of devices that already have these capabilities are being explored.

Many stakeholders are involved in digital health activities, including patients, healthcare practitioners, researchers, traditional medical device industry firms, and firms new to FDA regulatory requirements, such as mobile application developers.

FDA's Center for Devices and Radiological Health (CDRH) is excited about these advances and the convergence of medical devices with connectivity and consumer technology. The following are topics in the digital health field on which the FDA has been working to provide clarity using practical approaches that balance benefits and risks:

- Wireless medical devices
- Mobile medical apps
- Health IT
- Telemedicine
- Medical Device Data Systems
- Medical device interoperability
- Software as a Medical Device (SaMD)
- General wellness
- Cybersecurity

How Is the FDA Advancing Digital Health?

CDRH has established the Digital Health Program which seeks to better protect and promote public health and provide continued regulatory clarity by:

- Fostering collaborations and enhancing outreach to digital health customers, and

- Developing and implementing regulatory strategies and policies for digital health technologies.

Digital Health Criteria

Software as a Medical Device (SaMD)

Software intended for one or more medical uses that may run on different operating systems or in virtual environments. Software run on a hardware medical device is a SaMD when not part of the intended use of the hardware medical device. Software is not SaMD if it drives or controls the hardware medical device.

This can include standalone software that is intended to run on general purpose computers or mobile platforms (e.g., smartphone, tablet). Other examples include:

- SaMD that uses the microphone of a smart device to detect interrupted breathing during sleep and sounds a tone to rouse the sleeper.

- SaMD that analyzes heart rate data intended for a clinician as an aid in diagnosis of arrhythmia.

Advanced Analytics

A device or product that can identify, analyze, and use big data and large complex data sets from a variety of sources. The product extracts new and relevant information or patterns to use for medical purposes. Required for artificial intelligence devices.

Advanced Analytics may include the use of statistical modeling and analytical techniques that provide insights, predictions, and recommendations based on its analysis. In that respect, devices including Advanced Analytics may have an overlap with those including Artificial Intelligence. However, Advanced Analytics techniques typically analyze large and varied datasets that cannot normally be analyzed by humans without specialized software tools, and often discover new patterns in data.

Examples include:

- An imaging system conducts an analysis of a patient's melanoma by comparing it to a repository of data from past melanoma cases (including images, diagnosis, treatment plans). The system then provides a diagnosis and generates a treatment plan for the patient.

- A software program uses data from a standard CT to create a personalized 3D model of the coronary arteries and analyzes the impact that blockages have on blood flow.

Artificial Intelligence

A device or product that can imitate intelligent behavior or mimics human learning and reasoning. Artificial intelligence includes machine learning, neural networks, and natural language processing. Some terms used to describe artificial intelligence include: computer-aided detection/ diagnosis, statistical learning, deep learning, or smart algorithms.

One rapidly growing area of Artificial Intelligence is machine learning. Machine learning is used to design an algorithm or model without explicit programming but through the use of automated training with data (e.g., a regression function or deep learning network). Devices that include Adaptive Algorithms, i.e., algorithms that continue to learn and evolve in time, are also another area of Artificial Intelligence.

Terms or jargon used to describe artificial intelligence include computer-aided detection/diagnosis, statistical learning machines/ algorithms, classifier, indicator/index/indices, support vector machine, deep learning, and smart algorithm.

Examples include:

- An imaging system that uses algorithms to provide diagnostic information for malignant melanoma or skin cancer in patients.

- A smart electrocardiography (ECG) device that estimates the probability of acute cardiac ischemia (ACI), a common form of heart attack.

Cloud

A device or product with Internet-based computing that provides computer processing resources and data on demand. The cloud is a shared pool of configurable resources (e.g., computer networks, servers, storage, applications, and services). Computing and data storage resources include: servers, operating systems, networks, software, applications, services, and storage equipment.

Examples include:

- SaMD being executed in the cloud.

- A mobile colposcope that stores images taken on the cloud for future retrieval and review in the doctor's office.

- A picture archiving and communications system consists of cloud-based, web-accessible software that analyzes cardiovascular images acquired from magnetic resonance (MR) scanners.

Cybersecurity

A device or product that can prevent unauthorized access, modification, misuse, or denial of use, or the unauthorized use of information which is stored, accessed, or transferred from a medical device to an external recipient.

Examples of security functions for protection include:

- Limited access to devices or products through the authentication of users (e.g., user ID and password, smartcard, biometric).

- Use of automatic timed methods to terminate sessions within the system where appropriate for the use environment.

Interoperability

A device or product that can exchange and use information through an electronic interface with another medical/nonmedical product, system, or device.

Examples include:

- An infusion pump has been designed to receive patient data from any pulse oximeter and uses this data to change infusion pump settings.

- A centralized patient-monitoring system receives patient data from several devices and uses this data to command and control a ventilator to adjust pressure, volume, and flow settings that are appropriate for the patient.

Medical Device Data System (MDDS)

Hardware or software that can transfer, store, convert data formats, or display medical device data without controlling or altering the functions or parameters of any connected medical device.

Examples include:

- The electronic transfer or exchange of medical device data. For example, this would include software that collects output from a ventilator about a patient's CO_2 level and transmits the information to a central patient data repository.

- The electronic storage and retrieval of medical device data. For example, software that stores historical blood pressure information for later review by a healthcare provider.

- The electronic conversion of medical device data from one format to another in accordance with a preset specification. For example, software that converts digital data generated by a pulse oximeter into a digital format that can be printed.

- The electronic display of medical device data. For example, software that displays a previously stored electrocardiogram for a particular patient.

Please note that MDDS does not include devices intended for active patient monitoring (i.e., any device that is intended to be relied upon in deciding to take immediate clinical action or where a timely response is required).

Mobile Medical App (MMA)

A software application that meets the definition of a medical device. The MMA transforms a mobile platform into a regulated medical device or is an accessory to a regulated medical device.

Examples include:

- Mobile apps that transform the mobile platform into a regulated medical device by using attachments, display screens, or sensors or by including functionalities similar to those of currently regulated medical devices

- Mobile apps that are an extension of one or more medical devices by connecting to such device(s) for the purposes of controlling the device(s) or for use in active patient monitoring or analyzing medical device data

- Mobile apps that become a regulated medical device (i.e., SaMD) by performing patient-specific analysis and providing patient-specific diagnosis, or treatment recommendations

Wireless

A device or product that uses wireless communication of any form to perform at least one function.

Examples include Wi-Fi, Bluetooth, and Near Field Communication.

Novel Digital Health

A device or product that includes new, unfamiliar, or unseen digital health technology never submitted, cleared, or approved by the FDA. The technology could potentially be a de Novo, have a new intended use, or have different technological characteristics. This also includes digital health technology or topic areas that have no agreed upon or established definition by industry or FDA.

Examples of novel digital health technologies include but are not limited to:

- Virtual reality

- Gaming

- Medical body area network (MBAN) wearable or implanted wireless devices

Chapter 9

Digital Innovations in Preventive Medicine

Chapter Contents

Section 9.1—Sensors.. 62

Section 9.2—Body Area Networks and Pervasive
Health Monitoring.. 67

Section 9.3—Wireless Medical Devices...................................... 70

Section 9.4—Wearables and Safety 73

Section 9.5—Remote Patient Monitoring 75

Section 9.6—Continuous Glucose Monitoring 81

Section 9.7—Mobile Medical Applications................................. 85

Section 9.1

Sensors

This section includes text excerpted from "Science Education—
Sensors," National Institute of Biomedical Imaging and
Bioengineering (NIBIB), October 2016.

What Are Sensors?

In medicine and biotechnology, sensors are tools that detect specific biological, chemical, or physical processes and then transmit or report this data. Some sensors work outside the body while others are designed to be implanted within the body.

Some monitoring devices consist of multiple sensors that measure a number of physical or biological parameters. Other devices may be multifunctional, incorporating sensors and then delivering a drug or intervention based on the sensor data obtained. Sensors may also be components in systems that process clinical samples, such as increasingly common "lab-on-a-chip" devices.

Sensors help healthcare providers and patients monitor health conditions and ensure that they can make informed decisions about treatment. Sensors are also often used to monitor the safety of medicines, food, environmental conditions, and other substances we may encounter.

How Are Sensors Used in Current Medical Practice?

Many different types of sensors are already used in healthcare, including self-care at home. Thermometers translate the expansion of a fluid or bending of a metal strip in response to heat into a number corresponding to body temperature. Paper-based home pregnancy tests contain a substance that changes color in the presence of hormones indicating pregnancy. In hospitals and other provider-based settings, you can find more complex types of sensors like pulse oximeters (also known as blood-oxygen monitors), which measure changes in the body's absorption of special types of light to provide information on a patient's heart rate and the amount of oxygen in the blood.

How Might Novel Sensors Improve Medical Care or Biomedical Research?

Advances in technology, engineering, and materials science have opened the door for increasingly sophisticated sensors to be used in medical research. A group of National Institute of Biomedical Imaging and Bioengineering (NIBIB)-funded researchers developed a compact, wireless, implantable brain sensor that can record and transmit brain activity data. Building on previously developed brain-computer interfaces that used wired connections, this new sensor may someday lead to unobtrusive, thought-controlled prosthetics and other assistive devices for people with amputated limbs, paralysis, or other movement impairments.

Researchers at NIBIB aim to improve existing sensors through a variety of means, such as making fluorescent probes easier to see and increasing the capabilities and enhancing efficiency of individual sensors.

Some scientists are exploring biological sensors, which rely on substances that occur naturally in the body, or artificial compounds that mimic natural substances, to capture molecules that are important to measure in the body. Biosensors may provide insights into disease processes that are hard to detect directly, such as dysfunctions in brain chemistry that are thought to play a role in many mental disorders.

For example, one method for studying chemical processes in real-time uses engineered cells that can be "programmed" with receptors that latch onto specific brain chemicals. The resulting chain of activity causes a protein within the cell to change color that researchers can detect with a certain type of laser microscope. The biosensors remain active in the brain for several days, allowing scientists to study changes in brain chemistry over time, which may help inform efforts to improve drug treatments for mental disorders.

While many advanced sensors aren't practical for routine medical care, they allow researchers to study the basic foundations of disease in more detail than previously possible, and to develop new technologies that could dramatically improve the quality of life of people with severe disabilities.

What Technologies Are NIBIB-Funded Researchers Developing with Sensors?

Sensors play key roles in all aspects of healthcare—prevention, diagnosis, disease monitoring, treatment monitoring—and the range of research involving sensors is equally broad. In addition to health-related applications, NIBIB funds studies to test new materials and technologies for building sensors, to develop new sensors that can advance medical research, and to promote healthy independent living through home-based and wearable sensors.

New Materials and Technologies

Good health requires not only protecting our bodies but safeguarding things we put into our bodies as well. NIBIB-funded researchers developed a sensor using a thin membrane made from of a special kind of plastic. The researchers loaded the membrane with a compound that creates a voltage difference across the membrane in the presence of oversulfated chondroitin sulfate (OSCS), a potentially deadly contaminant sometimes found in preparations of the commonly used blood thinner heparin. OSCS is inherently highly charged and interacts with the compound-loaded membrane without the need to apply an external electrical current. By measuring the voltage, scientists can quickly identify OSCS-contaminated samples before the heparin is administered to a patient. The reaction between OSCS and the membrane is also reversible, so the sensors can be used repeatedly.

Another NIBIB grant supported research to develop an instrument to detect and monitor levels of vapor phase hydrogen peroxide (VPHP). VPHP is much stronger than the type of hydrogen peroxide commonly used in first aid care but has a similar use: to disinfect and sterilize pharmaceutical manufacturing equipment and facilities. After sterilization procedures, manufacturers have to ensure VPHP levels are reduced back to a minimum to protect workers and product quality. The researchers developed a sensor that uses a new type of highly efficient and extremely sensitive laser to continuously monitor VPHP levels throughout the sterilization process. The sensor can also detect how much VPHP has been absorbed by packaging and other materials within the facility, such as sterile isolators or other protective barriers.

Advancing Medical Research

Many illnesses develop and progress as a result of faulty regulation or dysfunction of a range of hormones, neurotransmitters, or other important body chemicals. Tracking such chemical activity is key to unraveling disease processes, but current sensors are generally limited in the number of chemicals that can be analyzed at one time or require those chemicals to be labeled first, thus greatly increasing the time, cost, and complexity of sensing. NIBIB-funded researchers seek to improve on biosensors in a variety of ways, such as creating novel types of coatings that improve sensor sensitivity, selectivity, and stability; and developing a fluorescence-based strategy for detecting proteins in living organisms and in real time.

Healthy Independent Living

Environmental and mobile sensors are already a part of many people's everyday lives. For example, faucets that automatically start when you place your hands under them and shut off when you're done washing. Lights that turn themselves on when you enter a room. Wearable bands that track your daily activity, perhaps even coordinating with your smartphone to allow you to track data over time or share your information with others. NIBIB supports initiatives to develop improved sensor and related information technologies for home and mobile use that will sustain wellness and facilitate coordinated management of chronic diseases. For example, one research team is working to improve the ability of "smart homes" to make sense of real-time sensor data and to recognize changes in a resident's activity patterns that may signal changes in well-being, such as a fall or disrupted meal schedule.

What Are Important Areas for Future Research on Sensors?

The types of sensors being developed and studied currently may play key roles in expanding and greatly changing the delivery of healthcare. One area in particular that may benefit from sensor research is point-of-care (POC) technologies.

Point-of-care refers to the place where patients receive healthcare, which may be anywhere from primary care offices or community clinics to emergency rooms or even patients' own homes. POC research seeks to address barriers to healthcare that have arisen from the concentration of services in highly specialized medical centers and labs. POC technologies may allow providers to diagnose and treat a particular health condition in a single visit, so patients don't need to make additional appointments or wait for test results.

Besides funding studies seeking to improve the manufacturing process for low-cost POC technologies, NIBIB-funded efforts are already underway to develop cost-effective POC solutions for detecting a range of medical conditions, including H5N1 influenza and allergies and other autoimmune diseases. Miniature, implantable sensors could continuously monitor a person's health status, providing more accurate information than conventional disease screening and a clearer sense of when a doctor's visit is needed. Integrating compact, wireless sensing technologies into medical devices or chronic treatments like long-term oxygen therapy may help lower treatment costs and be easier for patients to use. Such technologies may also be compatible with mobile devices, allowing for remote monitoring and assessments in real-time.

Some of the challenges to sensor research include simplifying and automating the preparation of patient samples to be used at the point-of-care and overcoming the body's natural rejection response to implantable or minimally invasive sensors.

Integrated Sensor Monitoring Systems in Pediatrics

National Institute of Biomedical Imaging and Bioengineering (NIBIB) launched the Pediatric Research Using Integrated Sensor Monitoring Systems program (PRISMS) in 2015 to develop integrated and sensor-based health monitoring systems to study environmental, physiological, and behavioral factors that aid epidemiological studies of asthma in pediatrics and a few other chronic diseases.

(Source: "Pediatric Research Using Integrated Sensor Monitoring Systems," National Institute of Biomedical Imaging and Bioengineering (NIBIB).)

Section 9.2

Body Area Networks and Pervasive Health Monitoring

This section includes text excerpted from "Body Area Networks and Pervasive Health Monitoring," National Institute of Standards and Technology (NIST), April 3, 2017.

Recent advances in microelectronics and wireless networking are moving closer to turning devices once thought of as science fiction into clinical reality. Ultra-small medical sensors/actuators can be either worn or implanted inside the body to collect or deliver a variety of medical information and services. The networking ability between these body devices and also possible integration with existing IT infrastructure could result into a pervasive environment that can convey health-related information between the user's location and the healthcare service provider. This flexibility for greater physical mobility (i.e., mHealth) directly translates into a significantly higher healthcare experience; and therefore, higher quality of life.

Body area network (BAN) is a technology that allows communication between ultra-small and ultra low-power intelligent sensors/devices that are located on the body surface or implanted inside the body. In addition, the wearable/implantable nodes can also communicate to a controller device that is located in the vicinity of the body. These radio-enabled sensors can be used to continuously gather a variety of important health and/or physiological data (i.e., information critical to providing care) wirelessly. Radio-enabled implantable medical devices offer a revolutionary set of applications among which we can point to smart pills for precision drug delivery, intelligent endoscope capsules, glucose monitors and eye pressure sensing systems. Similarly, wearable sensors allow for various medical/physiological monitoring (e.g., electrocardiogram, temperature, respiration, heart rate, and blood pressure), disability assistance, human performance management, etc.

A simple example of BAN application would be a device equipped with a built-in reservoir and pump. This device can administer just the right amount of insulin to a diabetic person based on wirelessly

67

received glucose level measurements from another body sensor. Having such novel uses in pervasive healthcare, BAN is regarded as a promising interdisciplinary technology that could have a huge impact on advancing Health-IT and telemedicine with its widespread commercialization. Although, the technology to create miniature-size devices for these applications is within reach, there are still several technical challenges, including interference issues, reliability, energy efficiency, and security issues that need to be addressed.

RF Propagation from Wearable and Implantable Medical Sensors

Knowledge of propagation media is a key step toward a successful transceiver design. Such information is typically gathered by conducting physical experiments — measuring and processing the corresponding data to obtain channel characteristics. With implantable medical sensors, this process could be extremely difficult, if not impossible. To overcome this challenge, National Institute of Standards and Technology (NIST) has designed and developed an innovative immersive visualization environment that allows for more natural interaction between experts with different backgrounds, such as engineering and medical sciences. This virtual environment can be used as a scientific instrument that offers researchers the ability to observe Radio frequency (RF) propagation from medical implants inside a human body. Additionally, since obtaining large amounts of propagation data for many scenarios and use-cases is difficult for wearable medical sensors, a detailed simulation platform can be extremely beneficial in highlighting the propagation behavior of the body surface and determining the best scenarios for limited physical measurements. Therefore, NIST researchers are using the immersive visualization environment to study RF propagation over the surface of a human body.

Modeling and Characterization of Harvestable Kinetic Energy for Wearable Medical Sensors

RF-enabled wearable and implantable wireless sensors are fast becoming a promising interdisciplinary research area in pervasive health information technology. These sensors offer an attractive set of e-health applications, including medical and physiological monitoring (e.g., temperature, respiration, heart rate, blood pressure). Due to their small size, such sensors might have a very limited battery-enabled power supply. As frequent recharge or even sensor replacement is not a practical solution for all applications, energy harvesting can be used as a technology to prolong the battery lifetime of these sensors. Exploiting such auxiliary sources of energy could directly impact the everyday use of sensors and significantly help their commercial applications in remote monitoring of physiological signals (i.e., telemedicine). In this project, NIST intends to study the statistical characteristics of the harvestable kinetic energy generated from the human motion. This knowledge could help researchers to design efficient energy management protocols for low-power wearable medical sensors.

Interference Analysis and Mitigation for Body Area Networks

A body area network (BAN), which consists of radio-enabled wearable or implantable sensor nodes, is a technology that enables pervasive monitoring and delivery of health-related information and services. While this technology can be integrated with existing IT infrastructure to extend the coverage of healthcare service providers to the user location, it can also facilitate independent living for people that require constant health monitoring. Therefore, it can transform and significantly enhance the patient healthcare experience. Considering the high quality of service required for the operation of such networks, interference among multiple BANs and also from other existing wireless systems (Wi-Fi, Ultra-wideband (UWB), Bluetooth, etc.) could cause a serious problem on the reliability of their operation. NIST researchers are developing tools that can help to study the interference on wearable and implantable wireless medical sensors.

Smart Autonomous Sensors and Environments

Sensor networks are used for gathering, processing, and delivering information about the desired targets or the physical environments surrounding them. A mobile sensor network is typically comprised of devices equipped with battery-powered wireless sensors capable of motion through the environment. Each device in a mobile sensor network usually has limited mobility and data processing capability. Limitations on the physical resources of each individual node (i.e., energy consumption, bandwidth and mobility) make optimization of the network performance a critical condition in the ability of the network to complete its function. In addition to these limits, the lack of centralized control and dynamic and unpredictable nature of the environment contribute to challenges in the performance optimization and evaluation of such networks. NIST is conducting research to examine the optimal deployment of sensor devices (with controlled mobility) and the relevant possible trade-offs between coverage (i.e., connectivity) and information sensing. Mobile patient positioning and tracking in hospitals is an example of a practical application of this research.

Section 9.3

Wireless Medical Devices

This section includes text excerpted from "Medical Devices—
Wireless Medical Devices," U.S. Food and Drug
Administration (FDA), August 29, 2017.

Radio frequency (RF) wireless medical devices perform at least one function that utilizes wireless RF communication to support health-care delivery. Examples of functions that can utilize wireless include transferring patient data from the device to another source, device control and programming, and monitoring patients remotely. As this technology continues to evolve, it is increasingly incorporated in the design of medical devices.

Examples of the technologies that utilize RF wireless technology include:

- Radio frequency identification (RFID)

- Wireless medical telemetry

Coordination with Federal Communications Commission (FCC)

The Federal Communications Commission (FCC) oversees the use of the public radio (RF) spectrum within which RF wireless technologies operate. The U.S. Food and Drug Administration (FDA) coordinates our policies on wireless medical device with the FCC to improve government efficiency in the oversight of broadband and wireless enabled medical devices. Our continued work with the FCC will provide medical devices manufacturers with more predictability and a better understanding of regulatory requirements for medical devices that utilize this technology.

Benefits and Risks

Incorporation of wireless technology in medical devices can have many benefits including increasing patient mobility by eliminating wires that tether a patient to a medical bed, providing healthcare professionals the ability to remotely program devices, and providing the ability of physicians to remotely access and monitor patient data regardless of the location of the patient or physician (hospital, home, office, etc.). These benefits can greatly impact patient outcomes by allowing physicians access to real-time data on patients without the physician physically being in the hospital and allowing real-time adjustment of patient treatment. Remote monitoring can also help special populations such as seniors, through home monitoring of chronic diseases so that changes can be detect earlier before more serious consequences occur.

As wireless developers and device manufacturers increasingly utilize RF wireless technology, they should consider the following:

- Selection of wireless technology

- Quality of service

- Coexistence

- Security

- Electromagnetic compatibility (EMC)

Information for Patients

The use of RF wireless technology can translate to advances in healthcare, but patients should be informed about the safe and effective use of these devices in the course of daily life.

If you are sent home with a RF wireless medical device, talk with your physician or healthcare provider about any restrictions when it comes to the use of personal computers, cellular phones, or any other personal electronic devices that are commonly used in home environments, as they can interfere with signals coming from medical devices that also use wireless technology. In addition, the home electronic devices can add additional burdens on available wireless capabilities (e.g., bandwidth).

Information for Healthcare Facilities: Risk Management

Most well-designed and maintained RF wireless medical devices perform adequately. But, an increasingly crowded RF environment could impact the performance of RF wireless medical devices, which makes risk management an important part of integrating RF wireless technology into medical systems.

Information for Industry: RF Wireless Developers and Manufacturers

Medical devices that incorporate wireless technology introduce some unique risks that should be addressed. The Radio Frequency Wireless Technology in Medical Devices focuses on considerations that should be taken into account to support safe and effective wireless medical devices. Medical device manufacturers are encouraged to read this document to help in the development, testing, regulatory submission and use of wirelessly enabled medical devices.

RF Wireless Coexistence Challenges

All types of wireless technology face challenges coexisting in the same space. For example, devices operating under FCC Part 15 rules must accept any interference from primary users of the frequency band. (Note: FCC Part 15 is applicable to certain types of low-power, nonlicensed radio transmitters, and certain types of electronic equipment that emit RF energy unintentionally.)

The FDA recommends that you periodically consult the FCC website for new specifications and updated information. Mobile wireless equipment can also transmit on an unlicensed basis in frequency bands such as the Industrial, Scientific, Medical (ISM) bands. ISM bands include 900 MHz, 2.4 GHz, 5.2 GHz, and 5.8 GHz and are commonly used for cordless phones and wireless data network equipment.

Section 9.4

Wearables and Safety

This section includes text excerpted from "Wearable Computers and Wearable Technology," Centers for Disease Control and Prevention (CDC), December 7, 2015.

What Are Wearable Computers and Wearable Technology?

Wearable computers and wearable technology are small devices using computers and other advanced technology that are designed to be worn in clothing or directly against the body. These devices are usually used for entertainment and other tasks like monitoring physical activity.

Wearable technology typically uses low-powered radiofrequency (RF) transmitters to send and receive data from smartphones or the Internet. RF transmitters emit radiowaves, a type of nonionizing radiation.

Most devices use low-powered Bluetooth technology similar to that used in "hands free" headsets for cell phones and many other wireless consumer devices. Some devices may use Wi-Fi or other communication technologies as well.

What Are Some Examples of Wearable Computers and Wearable Technology?

Familiar examples of wearable computers or wearable technology include "smartwatches" and fitness trackers. Future devices could include head-mounted displays and a wide variety of personal health monitors.

Wearable Technology and Safety

RF transmitters in wearable technology expose the user to some level of RF radiation. RF radiation is a form of nonionizing radiation made up of radiowaves.

RF transmitters in wearable devices operate at extremely low power levels and normally send signals in streams or brief bursts (pulses) for a short period of time. As a result, wearable devices expose the user to very small levels of RF radiation over time.

How Much RF Radiation Am I Exposed To?

To be sold in the United States, equipment that transmits RF radiation must meet exposure limits set by the Federal Communications Commission (FCC). These limits are designed to reduce exposure to RF radiation.

While the FCC guidelines were adopted in 1996, they are similar to international guidelines that are presently in effect in many other countries. Wearable devices expose the user to small amounts of RF radiation compared to these international exposure limits.

Wearable Technology Can Distract You

If you use wearable devices, it could be a source of distraction and raise a number of safety and other issues unrelated to RF radiation exposure. This is a major concern if you are driving a car or participating in other activities that require close attention.

What You Need to Know

- Most wearable devices include low-powered RF transmitters to enable them to communicate with other devices.

- To be sold in the United States, all such devices must meet FCC limits for human exposure to RF radiation.

- Wearable devices expose the user to lower amounts of RF radiation compared to international exposure limits.

- Wearable electronics may distract the user and increase the chances of injury while driving or using dangerous equipment.

Wearables of the Future

The next generation "wearables" may allow people to access and monitor more than 250,000 bodily measurements a day. When combined with standard laboratory tests, this data can play an important role in early detection of serious medical conditions or infections.

(Source: "Built for the Future. Study Shows Wearable Devices Can Help Detect Illness Early," National Institutes of Health (NIH).)

Section 9.5

Remote Patient Monitoring

This section contains text excerpted from the following sources: Text
in this section begins with excerpts from "Healthcare Telehealth and
Remote Patient Monitoring Use in Medicare and Selected Federal
Programs," U.S. Government Accountability Office (GAO), April
2017; Text under the heading "Effects of Remote Patient Monitoring
on Heart Failure Management" is excerpted from "Effects of Remote
Patient Monitoring on Heart Failure Management," ClinicalTrials.
gov, National Institutes of Health (NIH), September 30, 2010.
Reviewed December 2017; Text under the heading "Effects of Remote
Patient Monitoring on Chronic Disease Management" is excerpted
from "Effects of Remote Patient Monitoring on Chronic Disease
Management," ClinicalTrials.gov, National Institutes of Health
(NIH), April 25, 2017; Text under the heading "Remote Monitoring of
Patient Health and Safety" is excerpted from "Medical Device
Privacy Consortium (MDPC)," Federal Trade Commission (FTC),
June 1, 2013. Reviewed December 2017.

Remote patient monitoring (RPM) refers to a coordinated system
that uses one or more home-based or mobile monitoring devices that
transmit vital sign data or information on activities of daily living that
are subsequently reviewed by a healthcare professional. This process
can enable providers to closely track a patient's condition and provide
earlier intervention to potential problems. According to a report by
the Agency for Healthcare Research and Quality (AHRQ), remote
patient monitoring has been shown to produce positive outcomes,
such as reduced hospitalization, when used as a part of care management for chronic conditions such as diabetes and congestive heart
failure. Remote patient monitoring is helpful for treating patients
with chronic diseases. Medicare models, demonstrations, and a new
payment program have the potential to expand the use of remote
patient monitoring.

For certain individuals, such as those who live in remote areas or
cannot easily travel long distances, access to healthcare services can
be challenging. Telehealth and remote patient monitoring can provide
an alternative to healthcare provided in person at a physician's office.

Telehealth can be used to provide clinical care remotely by two-way video for services such as psychotherapy or the evaluation and management of conditions. Remote patient monitoring can be used to monitor patients with chronic conditions, such as those with congestive heart failure, hypertension, diabetes, and chronic obstructive pulmonary disease, and it can also be used as a diagnostic tool, such as for some heart conditions. Although the literature is mixed on the effectiveness of telehealth and remote patient monitoring, a 2016 review of studies by the AHRQ—an agency within the U.S. Department of Health and Human Services (HHS)—found that the most consistent benefit of telehealth and remote patient monitoring occurs when the technology is used for communication and counseling or to remotely monitor chronic conditions such as cardiovascular and respiratory disease, with improvements in outcomes such as mortality, quality of life, and reductions in hospital admissions.

Federal Government and Remote Patient Monitoring

The federal government uses remote patient monitoring in various healthcare programs, including the following:

- Medicare, which provides healthcare coverage for people age 65 or older, certain individuals with disabilities, and individuals with end-stage renal disease;

- Medicaid, a joint federal-state healthcare financing program for certain low-income and medically needy individuals;

- Department of Defense ((DoD)), which provides services through its regionally structured healthcare program to active duty personnel and their dependents, medically eligible Reserve and National Guard personnel and their dependents, and retirees and their dependents and survivors; and

- U.S. Department of Veterans Affairs (VA), which delivers medical services to veterans primarily through an integrated healthcare delivery system.

- Other federal agencies—within and outside of U.S. Department of Health and Human Services (HHS).

Medicare and Remote Patient Monitoring

According to Centers for Medicare and Medicaid Services (CMS) officials, Medicare fee-for-service does not have an explicit definition of remote patient monitoring. Rather, Medicare pays separately for some services that are used to remotely monitor patients, as well as for other remote monitoring (RM) bundled with other services. For example, separate payment may be made for services used to remotely monitor patients' conditions, such as services that use devices to monitor, record, and relay data on a patient's heart activity to a provider for analysis. Additionally, Medicare pays for remote services as bundled parts of other services, such as elements of monthly care management services.

CMS does not have a separate category for remote patient monitoring services, as it does with telehealth, and these services may be bundled with other services, CMS has not conducted a separate analysis of remote patient monitoring services. Therefore, the number of Medicare beneficiaries who use this service is unknown. While the number of beneficiaries who use remote patient monitoring is not identified, Medicare Payment Advisory Commission (MedPAC) reported information on Medicare spending on remote patient monitoring for selected services. Specifically, MedPAC reported that Medicare spent $119 million on remote cardiac monitoring services for 265,000 beneficiaries in calendar year 2014. MedPAC also reported that in calendar year 2014, Medicare spent $70 million on remote patient monitoring for 639,000 beneficiaries to remotely monitor heart rhythms through implantable cardiac devices, such as pacemakers, and to evaluate the function of these devices.

Medicaid—Telehealth and Remote Patient Monitoring Requirements

CMS does not limit the use of telehealth and remote patient monitoring in Medicaid, which has around 70 million enrollees. Therefore, individual states determine any restrictions and limitations. For example, states have the option to determine:

- whether to cover telehealth;

- what types of telehealth to cover;

- how it is provided or covered;

- which types of telehealth providers may be covered or reimbursed, as long as such providers are recognized and qualified according to Medicaid statute and regulation; and

- how much to reimburse for telehealth services, as long as such payments do not exceed other requirements.

77

Department of Defense (DoD) and Remote Patient Monitoring

DOD also utilizes remote patient monitoring devices to provide care for eligible beneficiaries for a range of services. These services include the diagnosis and treatment of cardiac conditions, including ambulatory blood pressure monitoring and pacemakers, and continuous glucose monitoring for patients with diabetes. According to DOD officials, the department does not have policies that specifically govern the use of remote patient monitoring devices, but instead DOD leaves the determination of use to clinical practice guidelines or to professional society guidance or recommendations.

U.S. Department of Veteran Affairs (VA)—Telehealth and Remote Patient Monitoring

VA, which serves about 6.7 million patients, allows remote patient monitoring using mobile and in-home technologies assigned to veterans based on individual needs. According to officials, VA does not restrict the use of telehealth or remote patient monitoring by type of service, provider, or location. Telehealth in VA can take place in various originating and distant site locations throughout the country, such as between two VA medical centers; a VA medical center and a community based outpatient clinic; two community-based outpatient clinics; from the provider's site and the veteran's home, a community living center, or a contract nursing home; and a provider's home and sites such as a VA medical center or community-based outpatient clinic. In recent years, VA has taken steps to increase the use of telehealth. As part of VA's fiscal year 2009 to fiscal year 2013 telehealth transformational initiative, VA recruited over 970 telehealth clinical technicians and purchased equipment for over 900 sites of care.

Effects of Remote Patient Monitoring on Heart Failure Management

Poor management of heart failure (HF) has added to the high costs and negative health outcomes from this chronic illness, including frequent hospitalization. HF patients require close monitoring to detect worsening health and to optimize their treatment. However, many patients visit their HF clinicians only once every few months, and perform minimal or no self-monitoring.

Remote patient monitoring is a potential tool to help clinicians and the patients better manage HF. A remote patient monitoring system (home monitoring of vital signs and symptoms) that has been developed with extensive clinician and patient input and testing, will be studied to determine its effects on HF management. Half of one hundred patients from the University Health Network Heart Failure Clinic will be randomly placed into the RM group and the other half will be in the control group. Patients in the RM group will monitor their weight, blood pressure, electrocardiography (ECG), and symptoms at home for six months. This information will be automatically sent from the medical devices wirelessly through Bluetooth to a mobile phone, which will send the information to the data servers. Both clinicians and patients will have access to the data. Patients will get automated reminder telephone calls if they do not take the number of measurements prescribed by their doctors.

Effects of Remote Patient Monitoring on Chronic Disease Management

Remote patient monitoring is a potential component for the management of chronic conditions that may provide reliable and real-time physiological measurements for clinical decision support, alerting, and patient self-management. Certain studies provide patients with complex chronic conditions a mobile phone and commercial home medical devices, such as a blood pressure monitor and weight scale. The measurements from the medical devices will be automatically sent to the mobile phone, and from there to a data server at the hospital for analysis and storage. Both clinicians and patients will be able to access these data and will be sent alerts by the system if the measurements are outside of the normal range. The system will be evaluated through interviews and comparing outcomes between the intervention and control groups.

Remote Monitoring of Patient Health and Safety

Remote patient monitoring technologies can be effective in managing chronic disease and postacute care. They can also be used to alert caregivers to situations requiring immediate attention. Many medical devices on the market today come with remote communication abilities embedded or available as optional attachments. For example, many implanted cardiac devices (pacemakers, cardioverter defibrillators, etc.) allow for data to be transmitted to the manufacturer and then made accessible to the patient's healthcare provider through a web interface. Some devices passively collect this data before transmitting it to the manufacturer (e.g., a wireless peripheral in the patient's home automatically receives information from the device) while others require some action by the patient (e.g., holding a wand near the body to upload information from the implanted device to a peripheral). The data may then be transmitted over an analog phone line, global system for mobile communication (GSM) network, or via an Internet service provider (ISP). Some remote patient monitoring technologies can be connected to multiple peripheral devices (e.g., blood pressure cuff, scale, glucose monitor, pulse oximeter, pedometer, etc.). The connections between the communicator and the peripheral devices may be wired or wireless. Any number of wireless transmission protocols or technologies may be used (e.g., Bluetooth™, Zigbee™, WiFi™, WiMax™, RFID, etc.).

As indicated, typically a web interface enables the patient's healthcare provider to view, print, and/or download information transmitted to the manufacturer from the remote patient monitoring technology. The healthcare provider may be able to configure periodic reports to be automatically transmitted. In addition, acute events may trigger an alert to the healthcare provider via email, fax, text message, or phone. Patients may be able to access some or all of the data related to them via patient-directed websites. Security of data generated or transmitted by remote patient monitoring technologies is a priority. Manufacturers' websites typically employ firewalls and encryption to protect patient data.

Users must register and are provided, or prompted to create, access credentials (username, password, etc.). With respect to the medical devices themselves, security requirements based on the risks must be incorporated into device design. For devices that employ wireless communication, the wireless signal could be subject to interception of data, and there is the potential for external interference (intentional or otherwise) which could impact device performance. For manufacturers, these security risks must be managed while keeping in mind design limitations. For example, implanted medical devices may require emergency access modes that bypass a subset of security features.

The Medical Device Privacy Consortium (MDPC), a group of leading companies addressing health privacy issues affecting the medical device industry, launched a new working group on medical device product security. The MDPC's product security working group aims to advance industry dialogue and information sharing on how to protect medical devices from security threats and address related privacy concerns. The working group intends to monitor, analyze, and influence global standards and guidelines on medical device product security, and develop practical tools that can be used to enhance product security. Further, the working group intends to liaise with other medical device industry stakeholders to gather and share intelligence regarding industry-wide efforts related to product security.

At the regulatory level, both U.S. Food and Drug Administration (FDA) medical device regulations and regulations promulgated by the HHS Office for Civil Rights (OCR) under the Health Insurance Portability and Accountability Act (HIPAA) can be relevant to remote patient monitoring privacy and security. As part of the FDA's premarket approval (PMA) process for Class III medical devices, the FDA considers various risks, which can include information security risks. Recommendations concerning the FDA's consideration of information security risks were recently the subject of a report by the U.S. Government Accountability Office (GAO). When patches are necessary to update the software on a medical device in response to a security vulnerability, the patch must undergo thorough assessment and testing before it can be released.

Section 9.6

Continuous Glucose Monitoring

This section includes text excerpted from "Managing Diabetes—
Continuous Glucose Monitoring," National Institute of Diabetes and
Digestive and Kidney Diseases (NIDDK), June 2017.

What Is Continuous Glucose Monitoring?

Continuous glucose monitoring automatically tracks blood glucose levels, also called blood sugar, throughout the day and night. You can see your glucose level anytime at a glance. You can also review how your glucose changes over a few hours or days to see trends. Seeing glucose levels in real time can help you make more informed decisions throughout the day about how to balance your food, physical activity, and medicines.

How Does a Continuous Glucose Monitor (CGM) Work?

A CGM works through a tiny sensor inserted under your skin, usually on your belly or arm. The sensor measures your interstitial glucose level, which is the glucose found in the fluid between the cells. The sensor tests glucose every few minutes. A transmitter wirelessly sends the information to a monitor.

The monitor may be part of an insulin pump or a separate device, which you might carry in a pocket or purse. Some CGMs send information directly to a smartphone or tablet. Several models are available and are listed in the American Diabetes Association's (ADA) product guide.

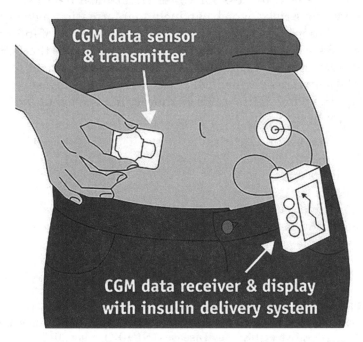

Figure 9.1. *Continuous Glucose Monitor*

A tiny CGM sensor under the skin checks glucose. A transmitter sends data to a receiver. The CGM receiver may be part of an insulin pump, as shown here, or a separate device.

Special Features of a CGM

CGMs are always on and recording glucose levels—whether you're showering, working, exercising, or sleeping. Many CGMs have special features that work with information from your glucose readings:

- An alarm can sound when your glucose level goes too low or too high.

- You can note your meals, physical activity, and medicines in a CGM device, too, alongside your glucose levels.

- You can download data to a computer or smart device to more easily see your glucose trends.

Some models can send information right away to a second person's smartphone—perhaps a parent, partner, or caregiver. For example, if a child's glucose drops dangerously low overnight, the CGM could be set to wake a parent in the next room.

Currently, one CGM model is approved for treatment decisions, the Dexcom G5 Mobile. That means you can make changes to your diabetes care plan based on CGM results alone. With other models, you must first confirm a CGM reading with a finger-stick blood glucose test before you take insulin or treat hypoglycemia.

Special Requirements Needed to Use a CGM

Twice a day, you may need to check the CGM itself. You'll test a drop of blood on a standard glucose meter. The glucose reading should be similar on both devices.

You'll also need to replace the CGM sensor every 3–7 days, depending on the model.

For safety it's important to take action when a CGM alarm sounds about high or low blood glucose. You should follow your treatment plan to bring your glucose into the target range, or get help.

Who Can Use a CGM?

Most people who use CGMs have type 1 diabetes. Research is underway to learn how CGMs might help people with type 2 diabetes.

CGMs are approved for use by adults and children with a doctor's prescription. Some models may be used for children as young as age 2. Your doctor may recommend a CGM if you or your child:

- are on intensive insulin therapy, also called tight blood sugar control

- have hypoglycemia unawareness

- often have high or low blood glucose

Your doctor may suggest using a CGM system all the time or only for a few days to help adjust your diabetes care plan.

What Are the Benefits of a CGM?

Compared with a standard blood glucose meter, using a CGM system can help you:

- better manage your glucose levels every day
- have fewer low blood glucose emergencies
- need fewer finger sticks

A graphic on the CGM screen shows whether your glucose is rising or dropping—and how quickly—so you can choose the best way to reach your target glucose level.

Over time, good management of glucose greatly helps people with diabetes stay healthy and prevent complications of the disease. People who gain the largest benefit from a CGM are those who use it every day or nearly every day.

What Are the Limits of a CGM?

Researchers are working to make CGMs more accurate and easier to use. But you still need a finger-stick glucose test twice a day to check the accuracy of your CGM against a standard blood glucose meter.

With most CGM models, you can't yet rely on the CGM alone to make treatment decisions. For example, before changing your insulin dose, you must first confirm a CGM reading by doing a finger-stick glucose test.

A CGM system is more expensive than using a standard glucose meter. Check with your health insurance plan or Medicare to see whether the costs will be covered.

Section 9.7

Mobile Medical Applications

This section includes text excerpted from "Medical Devices—
Mobile Medical Applications," U.S. Food and Drug
Administration (FDA), September 22, 2015.

The widespread adoption and use of mobile technologies is opening new and innovative ways to improve health and healthcare delivery.

Mobile applications (apps) can help people manage their own health and wellness, promote healthy living, and gain access to useful information when and where they need it. These tools are being adopted almost as quickly as they can be developed. According to industry estimates by 2018, 50 percent of the more than 3.4 billion smartphone and tablet users will have downloaded mobile health applications. These users include healthcare professionals, consumers, and patients.

The U.S. Food and Drug Administration (FDA) encourages the development of mobile medical apps that improve healthcare and provide consumers and healthcare professionals with valuable health information. The FDA also has a public health responsibility to oversee the safety and effectiveness of medical devices—including mobile medical apps.

What Are Mobile Medical Apps (MMAs)?

Mobile apps are software programs that run on smartphones and other mobile communication devices. They can also be accessories that attach to a smartphone or other mobile communication devices, or a combination of accessories and software.

Mobile medical apps are medical devices that are mobile apps, meet the definition of a medical device and are an accessory to a regulated medical device or transform a mobile platform into a regulated medical device.

Consumers can use both mobile medical apps and mobile apps to manage their own health and wellness, such as to monitor their caloric intake for healthy weight maintenance. For example, the National Institutes of Health's (NIH) LactMed app provides nursing mothers

85

with information about the effects of medicines on breast milk and nursing infants.

Other apps aim to help healthcare professionals improve and facilitate patient care. The Radiation Emergency Medical Management (REMM) app gives healthcare providers guidance on diagnosing and treating radiation injuries. Some mobile medical apps can diagnose cancer or heart rhythm abnormalities, or function as the "central command" for a glucose meter used by an insulin-dependent diabetic patient.

How Will the FDA Regulate MMAs?

The FDA will apply the same risk-based approach the agency uses to assure safety and effectiveness for other medical devices. A guidance document provides examples of how the FDA might regulate certain moderate-risk (Class II) and high-risk (Class III) mobile medical apps. The guidance also provides examples of mobile apps that are not medical devices, mobile apps that the FDA intends to exercise enforcement discretion, and mobile medical apps that the FDA will regulate.

FDA encourages app developers to contact the FDA—as early as possible—if they have any questions about their mobile app, its level of risk, and whether a premarket application is required.

What Are the MMAs That the FDA Will Regulate

The FDA is taking a tailored, risk-based approach that focuses on the small subset of mobile apps that meet the regulatory definition of "device" and that:

* are intended to be used as an accessory to a regulated medical device, or

* transform a mobile platform into a regulated medical device.

Mobile apps span a wide range of health functions. While many mobile apps carry minimal risk, those that can pose a greater risk to patients will require FDA review.

For a list of what is considered a mobile medical application, manufacturers and developers of mobile applications can search FDA's database of existing classification by type of mobile medical application (for example diagnostic). Approved/cleared mobile medical applications will also be listed in FDA's 510(k) and PMA databases and on the FDA's Registration and Listing Database.

FDA's mobile medical apps policy does not require mobile medical app developers to seek Agency re-evaluation for minor, iterative product changes.

Mobile Apps for Which the FDA Intends to Exercise Enforcement Discretion

For many mobile apps that meet the regulatory definition of a "device" but pose minimal risk to patients and consumers, the FDA will exercise enforcement discretions and will not expect manufacturers to submit premarket review applications or to register and list their apps with the FDA. This includes mobile medical apps that:

- Help patients/users self-manage their disease or condition without providing specific treatment suggestions;

- Provide patients with simple tools to organize and track their health information;

- Provide easy access to information related to health conditions or treatments;

- Help patients document, show or communicate potential medical conditions to healthcare providers;

- Automate simple tasks for healthcare providers; or

- Enable patients or providers to interact with Personal Health Records (PHR) or Electronic Health Record (EHR) systems.

Does the FDA Regulate Mobile Devices and Mobile App Stores?

FDA's mobile medical apps policy does not regulate the sale or general consumer use of smartphones or tablets. FDA's mobile medical apps policy does not consider entities that exclusively distribute mobile apps, such as the owners and operators of the "iTunes App store" or the "Google Play store," to be medical device manufacturers. FDA's mobile medical apps policy does not consider mobile platform manufacturers to be medical device manufacturers just because their mobile platform could be used to run a mobile medical app regulated by FDA.

Does the Guidance Apply to Electronic Health Records?

FDA's mobile medical app policy does not apply to mobile apps that function as an electronic health record (EHR) system or personal health record system.

Examples of Mobile Medical Apps (MMAs) the FDA Regulates

This list provides examples of mobile apps that are considered medical devices (i.e., mobile medical apps), on which FDA will focus its regulatory oversight. These mobile apps meet the definition of medical device in the Federal Food, Drug, and Cosmetic Act (FD&C Act) and their functionality poses a risk to a patient's safety if the mobile app were to not function as intended. Each example below provides a list of possible relevant product code(s) and/or regulation number.

Mobile apps that transform a mobile platform into a regulated medical device and therefore are mobile medical apps:

These mobile apps use a mobile platform's built-in features such as light, vibrations, camera, or other similar sources to perform medical device functions (e.g., mobile medical apps that are used by a licensed practitioner to diagnose or treat a disease). Possible product codes: Varies depending on the intended use and function of the mobile medical app; see additional examples below.

- Mobile apps that use a sensor or lead that is connected to a mobile platform to measure and display the electrical signal produced by the heart (electrocardiograph or ECG).

- Mobile apps that use a sensor or electrode attached to the mobile platform or tools within the mobile platform itself (e.g., microphone and speaker) to electronically amplify and "project sounds associated with the heart, arteries and veins and other internal organs" (i.e., an electronic stethoscope).

- Mobile apps that use a sensor or electrode attached to the mobile platform or tools within the mobile platform itself (e.g., accelerometer) to measure physiological parameters during cardiopulmonary resuscitation (CPR) and give feedback about the quality of CPR being delivered. Mobile apps that use a sensor attached to the mobile platform or tools within the mobile platform itself to record, view, or analyze eye movements for use in the diagnosis of balance disorders (i.e., nystagmograph).

- Mobile apps that use tools within the mobile platform (e.g., speaker) to produce controlled levels of test tones and signals intended for use in conducting diagnostic hearing evaluations and assisting in the diagnosis of possible otologic disorders (i.e., an audiometer).

- Mobile apps that use a sensor attached to the mobile platform or tools within the mobile platform itself (e.g., accelerometer) to measure the degree of tremor caused by certain diseases (i.e., a tremor transducer).

- Mobile apps that use a sensor attached to the mobile platform or tools within the mobile platform itself (e.g., accelerometer, microphone) to measure physiological parameters (e.g., limb movement, electrical activity of the brain (EEG)) during sleep and are intended for use in diagnosis of specific diseases or conditions such as sleep apnea.

- Mobile apps that use an attachment to the mobile platform to measure blood oxygen saturation for diagnosis of specific disease or condition.

- Mobile apps that present donor history questions to a potential blood donor and record and/or transmit the responses to those questions for a blood collection facility to use in determining blood donor eligibility prior to collection of blood or blood components.

- Mobile apps that use an attachment to the mobile platform to measure blood glucose levels. Mobile apps that use that use an attachment to the mobile platform (e.g., light source, laser) to treat acne, reduce wrinkles, or remove hair.

- Mobile apps that use a microphone or speaker within a mobile platform to serve as a audiometer to allow healthcare providers to determine hearing loss at different frequencies.

- Mobile apps that analyze an image of a skin lesion using mathematical algorithms, such as fractal analysis, and provide the user with an assessment of the risk of the lesion.

Mobile apps that connect to an existing device type for purposes of controlling its operation, function, or energy source and therefore are mobile medical apps:

These mobile apps are those that control the operation or function (e.g., changes settings) of an implantable or body worn medical device. Possible product codes: Varies depending on the intended use and function of the parent medical device; see additional examples below.

- Mobile apps that alter the function or settings of an infusion pump.

- Mobile apps that act as wireless remote controls or synchronization devices for computed tomography (CT) or X-ray machines.

- Mobile apps that control or change settings of an implantable neuromuscular stimulator.

- Mobile apps that calibrate, control, or change settings of a cochlear implant.

- Mobile apps that control the inflation or deflation of a blood-pressure cuff.

- Mobile apps that are used to calibrate hearing aids and assess the electroacoustic frequency and sound intensity characteristics emanating from a hearing aid, master hearing aid, group hearing aid or group auditory trainer.

Mobile apps that display, transfer, store, or convert patient-specific medical device data from a connected device and therefore are mobile medical apps:

- Mobile apps that connect to a nursing central station and display medical device data to a physician's mobile platform for review. (i.e., a medical device data system or MDDS).

- Mobile apps that connect to bedside (or cardiac) monitors and transfer the data to a central viewing station for display and active patient monitoring.

- Mobile apps that connect to a perinatal monitoring system and transfer uterine contraction and fetal heart rate data to another display to allow for remote monitoring of labor progress.

- Mobile apps that are intended to display images for diagnostic review may be regulated as a picture archiving and communications system.

Chapter 10

Medical Device Data Systems

Medical device data systems (MDDS) are hardware or software products that transfer, store, convert formats, and display medical device data. An MDDS does not modify the data or modify the display of the data, and it does not by itself control the functions or parameters of any other medical device. MDDS are not intended to be used for active patient monitoring.

Examples of MDDS include:

- software that stores patient data such as blood pressure readings for review at a later time;

- software that converts digital data generated by a pulse oximeter into a format that can be printed; and

- software that displays a previously stored electrocardiogram for a particular patient.

The quality and continued reliable performance of MDDS are essential for the safety and effectiveness of healthcare delivery. Inadequate quality and design, unreliable performance, or incorrect functioning of MDDS can have a critical impact on public health.

This chapter includes text excerpted from "Medical Device Data Systems," U.S. Food and Drug Administration (FDA), June 9, 2017.

MDDS Rule

In the Federal Register of February 15, 2011 (76 FR 8637), the FDA issued a final rule to reclassify MDDS from Class III (subject to premarket approval) to Class I (subject to general controls).

Devices that were not in commercial distribution prior to May 28, 1976, are generally referred to as postamendment devices, and are classified by operation of law under section 513(f) of the Food Drug and Cosmetic Act (21 U.S.C. 360c(f)) as Class III devices. Center for Devices and Radiological Health (CDRH) evaluates such postamendment devices to establish the appropriate degree of regulatory controls needed to provide reasonable assurance of their safety and effectiveness. CDRH may decide to classify such a device as Class I (requiring general controls), Class II (requiring special controls), or Class III (requiring premarket approval).

Risks associated with MDDS include the potential for inaccurate, incomplete, or untimely data transfer, storage, conversion, or display of medical device data. In some cases, this can lead to incorrect patient diagnosis or treatment. Based on evaluation of these risks, the FDA has determined that general controls such as the Quality System Regulation (21 CFR part 820), will provide a reasonable assurance of safety and effectiveness. Therefore, special controls and premarket approval are not necessary.

What Is an MDDS?

The Federal Register notice provides the following definition of a medical device data system:

§ 880.6310 Medical device data system.—(a) Identification.

1. A medical device data system (MDDS) is a device that is intended to provide one or more of the following uses, without controlling or altering the functions or parameters of any connected medical devices:

- The electronic transfer of medical device data;

- The electronic storage of medical device data;

- The electronic conversion of medical device data from one format to another format in accordance with a preset specification; or

- The electronic display of medical device data.

2. An MDDS may include software, electronic or electrical hardware such as a physical communications medium (including wireless hardware), modems, interfaces, and a communications protocol. This

identification does not include devices intended to be used in connection with active patient monitoring.

In practice, a medical device data system (MDDS) is a medical device intended to provide one or more of the following functions:

- The electronic transfer or exchange of medical device data from a medical device, without altering the function or parameters of any connected devices. For example, this would include software that collects output from a ventilator about a patient's CO_2 level and transmits the information to a central patient data repository.

- The electronic storage and retrieval of medical device data, without altering the function or parameters of connected devices. For example, software that stores historical blood pressure information for later review by a healthcare provider.

- The electronic conversion of medical device data from one format to another in accordance with a preset specification. For example, software that converts digital data generated by a pulse oximeter into a digital format that can be printed.

- The electronic display of medical device data, without altering the function or parameters of connected devices. For example, software that displays the previously stored electrocardiogram for a particular patient.

MDDS include the following, provided the intended use is consistent with the MDDS regulation:

- Any assemblage or arrangement of network components that includes specialized software or hardware expressly created for a purpose consistent with the intended use in the MDDS regulation.

- Products specifically labeled (per 21CFR 801) by the manufacturer as an MDDS, provided such products do not provide additional functionality.

- Custom software that is written by entities other than the original medical device manufacturer (for example, hospitals, third-party vendors) that directly connects to a medical device, to obtain medical device information.

- Modified portions of software or hardware that are part of an IT infrastructure created and/or modified for specific MDDS functionality. For example, when modifying software (writing and compiling software source code), the modified portion is considered MDDS.

What Is Not an MDDS?

General-purpose IT infrastructure used in healthcare facilities that is not altered or reconfigured outside of its manufactured specifications. Modifications within the off-the-shelf parameters of operation are still considered general IT infrastructure and not MDDS. For example, components with the following functions by themselves are NOT considered MDDS if they are used as part of general IT infrastructure even though they may transfer, store, display, or convert medical device data, in addition to other information:

- The electronic transfer of medical device data;
  - network router
  - network hub
  - wireless access point
- The electronic storage of medical device data;
  - network attached storage (NAS)
  - storage area network (SAN)
- The electronic conversion of medical device data from one format to another in accordance with a preset specification;
  - virtualization system (ex: VM Ware)
  - PDF software
- The electronic display of medical device data.
  - computer monitor
  - big screen display

Networks used to maintain medical devices to see which systems are running or malfunctioning, or other similar uses that do not meet the definition of medical device under 201(h) of the FD&C Act.

Standard IT software that is not specifically sold by the manufacturer as a MDDS, which may have MDDS functionality such as reading serial numbers, barcodes, Unique Device Identification (UDI), or other data from a medical device, but is not used in providing patient care.

Off-the-shelf passive network sniffing software that is generally used to monitor any network performance by reading TCP/IP (Transmission Control Protocol/Internet Protocol) packets on a network if this software is not intended to connect directly to a medical device.

Chapter 11

Medical Device Interoperability

From acute care clinical settings, to vital-sign monitoring, and devices that make telemedicine an accurate diagnostic and treatment discipline, medical devices are playing an ever-increasing role in transforming healthcare delivery. These devices have the ability to capture critical medical data, available (perhaps) multiple times per second, on a per-patient basis. However, for the most part, they are unable to communicate with one another and offer almost no plug-and-play interoperability. Lack of reference implementations for existing device interface standards and unanswered questions regarding the safety and performance of networked systems-of-systems are among the challenges to achieve such interoperability. A standard interoperable framework will allow novel clinical solutions to be safely and efficiently incorporated.

Interoperability will enable:

- Standards-based connectivity of medical devices to IT networks and streamlining equipment management and deployment.

- New medical sensors and actuators (manufactured by small vendors) that can be integrated with the existing infrastructure as they become available.

This chapter includes text excerpted from "Medical Device Interoperability," National Institute of Standards and Technology (NIST), April 4, 2017.

- Easily deployable protocols and treatment solutions that are driven by what the healthcare providers need instead of what a technology manufacturer can supply.

- Fewer transcription errors and a richer set of information with which clinicians can manage their patients.

- Synchronization, safety interlocks, and closed-loop device control for medical devices.

National Institute of Standards and Technology (NIST) researchers (in collaboration with experts from other agencies, industry, and academia) are currently working on efforts that promote standard-based medical device interoperability and communication.

Medical Device Interoperability Research

Medical Device Interoperability National Institute of Standards and Technology (NIST) researchers in collaboration with the Massachusetts General Hospital and the Center for Integration of Medicine & Innovative Technology are working to achieve the vision of interoperability by conducting research in clinical requirements as outlined by the American Society for Testing and Materials (ASTM) F2761 standard. This standard specifies requirements and characteristics necessary for the safe integration of medical devices in operating rooms, emergency rooms, and intensive care units. The research effort includes a gap analysis of the medical device communication standard IEEE 11073 versus use case scenarios outlined in the ASTM F2761 standard. NIST software engineers are also working with the ASTM F2761 Standards Committee to improve the functional architectures embodied in the standard, and with developers of reference implementations funded through National Institutes of Health (NIH) grants. This work will result in testable prototypes and improved standards documents for use by industry to develop improved medical devices.

Medical Device Communication

NIST researchers are collaborating with medical device vendors and domain experts to facilitate the development and adoption of standards for medical device communications throughout the healthcare enterprise as well as integrating it into the electronic health record. NIST researchers are actively developing medical device communication test methodologies, tools, and tests to provide a key tool set needed to enable consistent and correct communication between medical devices, device-gateways, and across the healthcare enterprise. This work serves to provide standards-based and rigorous validation of medical device communication through conformance leading to interoperability. Rigorous testing is essential to achieve multi-vendor and enterprise-wide interoperability and must be predicated on sufficiently specified medical device and enterprise-communication standards. To this end, NIST researchers are participating in key medical device standards working groups, special interest groups, and multi-vendor medical device integration consortiums.

NIST's medical device communication test team is developing and advancing software test tools to support device communication in point-of-care and personal health settings. These tools are derived and implemented to meet medical device-level communication requirements defined in the ISO/IEEE 11073-TM Medical Device Communication (x73) family of standards and enterprise/electronic health record level defined in the Health Level 7 (HL7) messaging standard. NIST researchers, in conjunction with medical device experts, work on meaningful medical device use cases to enable consistent and complete information exchange. NIST has developed and is advancing HL7 message validation in support of constraints applied by the Integrating the Healthcare Enterprise—Patient Care Device (IHE-PCD). This work targets syntactical and semantic message verification of device-derived data carried in electronic messages destined as electronic health records. NIST research is evolving a health information technology test infrastructure to develop tooling—enabling a higher level of rigor and thus providing the healthcare industry and certification entities an increased probability of interoperable systems.

Chapter 12

Clinical Decision Support

What Is Clinical Decision Support (CDS)?

Clinical decision support provides clinicians, staff, patients, or other individuals with knowledge and person-specific information, intelligently filtered or presented at appropriate times, to enhance health and healthcare. CDS encompasses a variety of tools to enhance decision-making in the clinical workflow. These tools include computerized alerts and reminders to care providers and patients; clinical guidelines; condition-specific order sets; focused patient data reports and summaries; documentation templates; diagnostic support, and contextually relevant reference information, among other tools.

Why CDS?

CDS has a number of important benefits, including:

- Increased quality of care and enhanced health outcomes

- Avoidance of errors and adverse events

- Improved efficiency, cost-benefit, and provider and patient satisfaction

This chapter includes text excerpted from "Clinical Decision Support (CDS)," HealthIT.gov, Office of the National Coordinator for Health Information Technology (ONC), January 15, 2013. Reviewed December 2017.

CDS is a sophisticated health IT component. It requires computable biomedical knowledge, person-specific data, and a reasoning or inferencing mechanism that combines knowledge and data to generate and present helpful information to clinicians as care is being delivered. This information must be filtered, organized, and presented in a way that supports the current workflow, allowing the user to make an informed decision quickly and take action. Different types of CDS may be ideal for different processes of care in different settings.

Health information technologies designed to improve clinical decision making are particularly attractive for their ability to address the growing information overload clinicians face, and to provide a platform for integrating evidence-based knowledge into care delivery. The majority of CDS applications operate as components of comprehensive EHR systems, although standalone CDS systems are also used.

CDS Activities

Significant Clinical Decision Support (CDS) Developments

The Office of the National Coordinator for Health Information Technology (ONC) is committed to promoting the advancement of clinical decision support (CDS). Over the course of several years, ONC has facilitated a variety of activities to catalyze progress in CDS development and deployment in support of enhanced health and care.

Some noteworthy activities include:

- The award of an "Advancing CDS" contract to accelerate the successful implementation and effective use of CDS interventions. The project is designed to:

  - Advance the widespread dissemination of successful CDS implementation practices to promote broad CDS adoption

  - Improve the acceptance and usability of medication CDS systems through the development of a clinically important drug-drug interaction list

  - Advance the practical sharing of effective CDS interventions across care settings

  - Identify CDS-related gaps and goals specific to a broad range of clinical specialties

- A two-day Clinical Decision Support (CDS) Workshop, sponsored by ONC, which brought together a large group of subject matter experts who shared their thoughts on a series of topics related to advancing the utility, usability, and meaningful use of CDS. Attendees represented a broad spectrum of expertise, including clinical informatics, quality improvement, patient advocacy, provider, payer, knowledge vendor, and EHR system vendor perspectives.

- The creation of CDS recommendations across five American Health Information Community (AHIC) workgroups, which focused on:

  - Improving healthcare quality through the effective use of CDS

  - Facilitating collaboration across CDS initiatives

  - Accelerating CDS development and adoption through federal government programs and collaborations

- The development of a Roadmap for National Action on Clinical Decision Support, which recommends a series of activities to improve CDS development, implementation, and use throughout the United States. The roadmap, crafted in 2006, identified three critical pillars for fully realizing the promise of CDS:

  - Making the best available clinical knowledge well-organized for CDS interventions

  - Promoting the high adoption and effective use of CDS tools

  - Continuously improving knowledge and CDS methods

- The Inventory of Federal Clinical Decision Support Activities, which is a compilation of project summaries, describing CDS activities that are either funded by the U.S. Federal government, or that are being executed by agencies of the government.

- The CDS Federal Collaboratory, which is a federal community of interest, was formed in 2008 to focus on CDS as a key health information technology component for improving the quality, safety, efficiency, and effectiveness of healthcare.

CDS Implementation

How-To Guides for Clinical Decision Support (CDS) Implementation

The guides below are intended for both clinical and technical staff who are defining CDS clinical goals; planning and leading CDS implementations; and maintaining and monitoring CDS interventions. To this end, Clinical Directors, Directors of Information Systems, Chief Medical Information Officers, and Directors of Medical Informatics, as well as other healthcare organization leaders, would benefit from reviewing the guides and associated resources.

The Guides are presented as five separate documents covering five major stages or phases in implementing CDS.

Guide 1—Start with a Strong Foundation for CDS: Provides steps and resources to help organizations decide whether or not to use CDS as part of a quality improvement initiative.

Guide 2—Assemble a CDS Implementation Team: Helps organizations understand the roles necessary to implement CDS and to begin planning for acquiring or developing and implementing CDS interventions.

Guide 3—Plan for Successful CDS Development, Design, and Deployment: Helps match CDS interventions to the work processes and goals of the organization.

Guide 4—Roll Out Effective CDS Interventions: Offers recommendations for roll-out planning and for training. These activities help to ensure a smooth transition between planning and roll-out, or going live.

Guide 5—Measure Effects and Refine CDS Interventions: Provides steps to ensure that the effects of interventions are appropriately measured and monitored. This includes measures reported to external agencies and feedback about usability from individual clinicians.

Key Lessons in Clinical Decision Support (CDS) Implementation

This technical report distills key lessons in CDS implementation based on a comprehensive literature review, interviews with CDS Implementers, and lessons identified by exemplary practices. Lessons are organized by implementation stages and by practice type and size such as small outpatient practices and large academic hospitals. Interesting, practical examples and engaging quotes highlight real-life lessons and success factors drawing from several types of CDS. This resource is designed to help new CDS implementers such as providers complying with Meaningful Use requirements learn from the experiences of CDC implementers in order to be more successful in their implementation.

This deliverable provides resources to support the design, implementation, and use of Clinical Decision Support. The parenthetical numbers next to some of the tools and worksheets correspond to the matching numbers contained in the zip file. Other tools and resources are hyperlinked to a website where they are freely available.

There are three main categories of tools:

1. **Tools and Figures:** These resources provide information in the form of tables, figures, or online tools. Examples include tables describing stakeholder roles, online tools and questionnaires to help assess readiness, or figures that describe the different types of CDS Interventions.

2. **HIMSS Worksheets:** These worksheets are adapted from the HIMSS CDS book Improving Outcomes with Clinical Decision Support: An Implementer's Guide, Second Edition. These worksheets will be partially filled out as an example of how to use them, but are provided as word documents so that modifications may be made as necessary.

3. **Literature:** Key studies including literature reviews are provided throughout this document. In each case, annotation is provided to describe the content and use of a particular study. Hyperlinks are available for each source.

Clinical Decision Support Starter Kit

The Clinical Decision Support Starter Kit is designed to help small practices take the first steps toward implementing CDS tools. This Starter Kit will help implementers become familiar with CDS, and it provides step-by-step examples of how to manage the implementation of a CDS rule. Users of the CDS Starter Kit will gain an understanding of:

1. CDS and the rationale for using it

2. Five types of commonly used CDS

3. The relationship between CDS and Meaningful Use goals

4. Examples of how to implement CDS rules that relate to Meaningful Use

This Starter Kit is designed for practices that have completed an EHR implementation and are now ready to implement CDS tools.

Strength in Numbers—Shared Resources for Implementing Clinical Decision Support in the Small Practice

This resource is designed to help small practices leverage shared resources nationally, regionally, and locally to overcome their inherent resource limitations to successfully implement and use CDS in their practices.

Profiles of Exemplary Sites

The ACDS project sought practices that were recognized for their implementation of CDS. Many of the practices within the compendium were winners of the HIMSS Davies Awards. The compendium of exemplary practices contains two related deliverables:

- An Excel spreadsheet providing contact information for the practices and an overview of the key lessons and type of decision support used.

- For each of the practices recognized, there is a profile summary that provides greater depth about the organization, the IT environment, CDS achievements, and lessons learned.

Reference Workflow Taxonomy

The Reference Taxonomy of Clinical Workflows provides a common set of terms to CDS designers and implementers to support communication about CDS and its use in clinical workflows.

- CDS designers can use the taxonomy to identify points in the workflow when CDS can be used and design a CDS tool to fit that context. Designers can then tag the CDS tools with terms from the taxonomy to inform practices about the intended use of the CDS.

- CDS repositories can create tags based on the taxonomy to enable workflow-related organization and searches.

- CDS implementers can refer to the taxonomy when developing maps of the workflows and can use the terms to improve communication with their CDS vendor.

Chapter 13

Big Data in the Age of Genomics

The term "Big Data" is used to describe massive volumes of both structured and unstructured data that is so large and complex it is difficult to process and analyze. Examples of big data include the following: diagnostic medical imaging, deoxyribonucleic acid (DNA) sequencing and other molecular technologies, environmental exposures, behavioral factors, financial transactions, geographic information, and social media information. It turns out that Big Data is all around us! Genome sequencing of humans and other organisms has been a leading contributor to Big Data, but other types of data are increasingly larger, more diverse, and more complex, exceeding the abilities of currently used approaches to store, manage, share, analyze, and interpret it effectively. We have all heard claims that Big Data will revolutionize everything, including health and healthcare.

Some scientists even claim that "the scientific method itself is becoming obsolete" as giant computers and data analytic software sift through the digital world to provide predictive models for health and disease based on the information available. Are these promises too good to be true?

This chapter includes text excerpted from "Public Health Approach to Big Data in the Age of Genomics: How Can We Separate Signal from Noise?" Centers for Disease Control and Prevention (CDC), August 7, 2017.

There are several promising applications of Big Data in improving health involving use of genome sequencing technologies. For example:

- Diagnosis of rare and mysterious diseases

- Improved classification of cancer based on tumor genomes rather than anatomic locations

- Genomically driven personalized cancer treatment (precision medicine)

- Using whole genome sequencing to improved public health detection and response to outbreaks of infectious diseases

Here is a highly pertinent example for public health. In the mid 19th century, a cholera outbreak swept through London. John Snow, now considered by many as the father of modern epidemiology, mapped his investigation on paper, indicating homes where cholera had struck. After long and laborious work, he implicated the Broad Street pump as the source of the outbreak, even before the cause of cholera (the Vibrio cholera bacterium) was known. "Today, Snow might have crunched GPS information and disease prevalence data and solved the problem within hours."

Big Data today is often more noise than signal! Sorting through all of the data to determine what is a real signal and what is noise does not always work as expected. For example, in 2013, when influenza hit the United States hard and early, Google attempted to monitor the outbreak using analysis of flu-related Internet searches, drastically overestimating peak flu levels, compared with traditional public health surveillance efforts. Even more problematic could be the potential for many false alarms by mindless examination, on a large scale, leading to putative associations between Big Data points and disease outcomes. This process may falsely infer causality and could potentially lead to ineffective or harmful interventions. The field of genomics has recognized this problem and addressed it by requiring replication of study findings and for signals to be much stronger to be picked. To appropriately analyze big data, the field of genomics requires use of epidemiologic studies, animal models, and other work in addition to big data analysis. Big Data's strength is in finding associations, but its weakness is in not showing whether these associations have meaning. Finding a signal is only the first step.

Recommendations to realize the potential of Big Data in the age of genomics to improve health and prevent disease:

1. **Epidemiologic Foundation:** We need a strong epidemiologic foundation for studying Big Data in health and disease. The associations found using Big Data need to be studied and replicated in ways that confirm the findings and make them generalizable. By that, the study of well-characterized and representative populations such as the National Cancer Institute (NCI) sponsored cohort consortium that has been collecting information on more than 4 million people over multiple decades. Big Data analysis is currently based on convenient samples of people or data available on the Internet. Both sources may be fraught with all sorts of biases such as selection, confounding and lack of generalizability.

2. **Knowledge Integration:** We need to develop a robust "knowledge integration" (KI) enterprise to make sense of Big Data. In a recent article titled "Knowledge Integration at the Center of Genomic Medicine" we have elaborated on the definition of KI and its three components: knowledge management, knowledge synthesis, and knowledge translation in genomics. A similar evidence-based knowledge integration process applies to all Big Data beyond genomics. We hope that the recently launched National Institutes of Health (NIH) Biomedical Data to Knowledge (BD2K) awards will support the development of new approaches, software, tools, and training programs to improve access, analysis, synthesis and interpretation of genomic Big Data and improve our ability to make and validate new discoveries.

3. **Evidence-based Medicine:** We should embrace (and not run away from) principles of evidence-based medicine and population screening. In a previous blog, we have elaborated on the relationship between genomic medicine and evidence-based medicine. Big Data is literally a hypothesis-generating machine that could lead to interesting, robust and predictive associations with health outcomes. However, even after these associations are established, evidence of utility (i.e., improved health outcomes and no evidence of harms) is still needed. Documenting health-related utility of genomics and Big Data information may necessitate the use of randomized clinical trials and other experimental designs.

4. **Translational Research:** As with genomic medicine, we need a robust translational research agenda for Big Data that goes

beyond the initial discovery (the bench to bedside model). In genomics, most published research is either basic scientific discoveries or preclinical research designed to develop health related tests and interventions. What happens after that is really the research "road less traveled." In fact, less than 1 percent of published research deals with validation, implementation, policy, communication, and outcomes in the real world. Reaping the benefits of using Big Data for genomics research will require a more expanded translational research agenda beyond the initial discoveries.

Chapter 14

Big Data for Infectious Disease Surveillance

Big data derived from electronic health records, social media, the Internet, and other digital sources have the potential to provide more timely and detailed information on infectious disease threats or outbreaks than traditional surveillance methods. A team of scientists led by the National Institutes of Health (NIH) reviewed the growing body of research on the subject and has published its analyses in a special issue of The Journal of Infectious Diseases.

Traditional infectious disease surveillance—typically based on laboratory tests and other data collected by public health institutions—is the gold standard. But, the authors note it can have time lags, is expensive to produce, and typically lacks the local resolution needed for accurate monitoring. Furthermore it can be cost-prohibitive in low-income countries. In contrast, big data streams from Internet queries, for example, are available in real time and can track disease activity locally, but have their own biases. Hybrid tools that combine traditional surveillance and big data sets may provide a way forward, the scientists suggest, serving to complement, rather than replace, existing methods.

"The ultimate goal is to be able to forecast the size, peak or trajectory of an outbreak weeks or months in advance in order to better

This chapter includes text excerpted from "NIH-Led Effort Examines Use of Big Data for Infectious Disease Surveillance," National Institutes of Health (NIH), November 14, 2016.

respond to infectious disease threats. Integrating big data in surveillance is a first step toward this long-term goal," says Cecile Viboud, Ph.D., coeditor of the supplement and a senior scientist at the NIH's Fogarty International Center. "Now that we have demonstrated proof of concept by comparing data sets in high-income countries, we can examine these models in low-resource settings where traditional surveillance is sparse."

Experts in epidemiology, computer science, and modeling collaborated on the supplement's 10 articles. They report on the opportunities and challenges associated with three types of data: medical encounter files, such as records from healthcare facilities and insurance claim forms; crowdsourced data collected from volunteers who self-report symptoms in near real time; and data generated by the use of social media, the Internet and mobile phones, which may include self-reporting of health, behavior, and travel information to help elucidate disease transmission.

But big data's potential must be tempered with caution, the authors say. Nontraditional data streams may lack key demographic identifiers such as age and sex, or provide information that underrepresents infants, children, the elderly and developing countries. Social media outlets may not be stable sources of data, as they can disappear if there is a loss of interest or financing. Most importantly, any novel data stream must be validated against established infectious disease surveillance data and systems, the authors said.

Each article features a promising example of the use of big data to monitor and model infectious diseases activity:

- In the United States, researchers found what they describe as "excellent alignment" between medical insurance claim data for flu-like illnesses and proven influenza activity reported by the Centers for Disease Control and Prevention (CDC).

- A European surveillance system that began collecting crowdsourced data on influenza as part of a research project is now considered an adjunct to existing surveillance activities. Influenzanet uses standardized online surveys to gather information from volunteers who self-report their symptoms on a weekly basis. A number of European Union member states are now using the tool and expanding it to include Zika, salmonella, and other diseases.

- An online platform, ResistanceOpen, was developed by U.S. and Canadian scientists to monitor antibiotic resistance at the regional level. The site takes advantage of publicly available, online data from community healthcare institutions as well as regional, national, and international bodies. An analysis showed online information compared favorably with traditional reporting systems in the two countries.

- Multiple studies have looked at social media and Internet health forums for information on drug use and to detect adverse drug reactions. While there are technical and ethical challenges, the authors suggest Internet search logs and social media posts can provide information more quickly than traditional physician-based reporting systems.

- In a comparison of the relatively new field of epidemic forecasting to the better-established one for weather forecasting, the authors note the former is much more difficult given that there is less observational data for disease, and because human behavior has the potential to rapidly alter the course of an epidemic.

- An examination of spatial data—including from insurance claims and social media posts—shows their potential for filling geographical information gaps but also presents technical, practical, and privacy challenges that must be addressed.

- With appropriate safeguards to ensure anonymity, call data records from mobile phones may provide "an unprecedented opportunity" to determine how travel affects disease transmission. Studies of malaria and rubella in Kenya showed call data improved the understanding of the spatial transmission of those diseases.

- Online news articles and health bulletins from public health agencies were manually extracted and modeled to elucidate transmission patterns for two recent outbreaks—the Ebola epidemic in West Africa and a Middle East Respiratory Syndrome outbreak in South Korea. Internet findings were in line with traditional data, providing a proof of concept that this approach can be generalized and automatized to a variety of online sources and generate information on disease transmission.

- Researchers also describe the benefits of a novel, publicly available epidemic simulation data management system, called epiDMS, which provides storage and indexing services for large data simulation sets, as well as search functionality and data analysis to aid decision makers during healthcare emergencies.

While the new hybrid models that combine traditional and digital disease surveillance methods show promise, the scientists agree there is still an overall scarcity of reliable surveillance information, especially compared to other fields such as climatology, where the data sets are huge. "To be able to produce accurate forecasts, we need better observational data that we just don't have in infectious diseases," notes Professor Shweta Bansal of Georgetown University, a coeditor of the supplement. "There's a magnitude of difference between what we need and what we have, so our hope is that big data will help us fill this gap."

Multi-disciplinary initiatives such as the NIH-led Big Data to Knowledge program will be instrumental in expanding the use of big data in research, as noted in the supplement.

Satellite Predicts Malaria Outbreaks

The Peruvian government and Duke University have collaborated with NASA to predict regions where Anopheles darlingi (mosquitoes that spread malaria) are commonly found by using information like precipitation, soil moisture, temperature, and vegetation.

(Source: "Using NASA Satellite Data to Predict Malaria Outbreaks," National Aeronautics and Space Administration (NASA).)

Chapter 15

Screening and Detection Technologies

Chapter Contents

Section 15.1—Advanced Molecular Detection (AMD)............... 116

Section 15.2—Cancer Screening in a Briefcase........................ 118

Section 15.3—DNA Microchip Technology 120

Section 15.4—Early Detection of Colorectal Cancer................. 122

Section 15.5—Genetic Testing 123

Section 15.6—Sensitive Stroke Detection 125

Section 15.7—Tool to Detect Cardiovascular
Disease Risk 126

Section 15.1

Advanced Molecular Detection (AMD)

This section includes text excerpted from "Advanced Molecular
Detection (AMD)," Centers for Disease Control and Prevention
(CDC), August 18, 2015.

Centers for Disease Control and Prevention's (CDC) Advanced
Molecular Detection (AMD) program introduces rapid technological
innovation to build bridges from trusted methods to new horizons in
disease detection. By increasing critical next generation sequencing
and bioinformatics capacities, CDC and state health departments
can take back the advantage in controlling infectious diseases. The
combined talents of experts in epidemiology, laboratory science, and
bioinformatics are applying innovation to real world problems to keep
us safe from new threats. Just as computerized tomography (CT) scans
help doctors find things that aren't visible in a physical exam, two
important tools give new insight into microbes:

- sequencing machines that can read the deoxyribonucleic acid
  (DNA) or ribonucleic acid (RNA) code of a microbe and

- supercomputers that have the capacity to manage massive
  amounts of information with the software to intelligently detect
  patterns

Many of these projects include state and local partners as well as
several CDC laboratories. The projects focus on a range of pathogens
and advance a variety of methods to protect public health.

CDC is transforming disease detection and response. Through
technological innovation, CDC continually advances safeguards for
America's health.

The Disease Threat

Highly resistant microbes in healthcare settings, disease organisms
that jump from animals to humans, and emerging dangerous pathogens create constant concerns.

- At least five microbes are resistant to nearly all available antibiotics.

- CDC estimates that 1 in 6 Americans—48 million people—get sick from contaminated food each year. This costs the United States $77 billion every year in healthcare treatment and workplace and other economic losses.

- Each year the flu costs businesses approximately $10.4 billion in direct costs for hospitalizations and outpatient visits for adults.

CDC continually introduces new technology and methods. But the rapid expansion of new threats calls for swift and broad application of new approaches.

The AMD Program

CDC's AMD program unlocks the promise of technology to protect Americans from microbial threats. AMD lets scientists see into microbes in ways and in detail that have never been possible before. This major enhancement of CDC's microbiology and bioinformatics capabilities helps scientists and public health professionals find and stop infectious disease outbreaks that threaten Americans every day.

AMD will transform how the U.S. public health system detects and responds to diseases by providing more precise and accurate means to:

- Diagnose known and emerging infections

- Find disease outbreaks we are missing now

- Understand and control antibiotic resistance

- Develop and target measures—like vaccines—to protect people's health

Using AMD, experts in laboratory science, epidemiology, and bioinformatics join forces to go from a hunch to certainty in record time to prevent illness and save lives.

Priority Areas for AMD

- Improve pathogen identification and characterization using whole genome sequencing and other advanced molecular technologies

- Adapt next-generation molecular diagnostics to meet evolving public health needs

- Build bioinformatics capacity at CDC and state public health laboratories

- Establish enhanced, sustainable, and integrated laboratory information systems

- Develop tools for prediction, modeling, and early recognition of emerging infections

Advantages of AMD

- The increasing availability and affordability of AMD technologies is rapidly changing the practice of microbiology. These technologies can deliver a greater level of detailed information on infectious pathogens while reducing reliance on more time-consuming and costly traditional diagnostic methods.

- When combined with enhanced laboratory and computing (i.e., bioinformatics) capacities, these new technologies are revolutionizing our ability to detect and respond to infectious disease threats.

- With AMD, CDC will be able to detect outbreaks sooner and respond more effectively, saving lives and reducing cost.

Section 15.2

Cancer Screening in a Briefcase

This section includes text excerpted from "Cancer Screening in a Briefcase," National Institutes of Health (NIH), August 20, 2015.

Optical imaging systems, suitable for use in low resource settings, have been developed to identify molecular signatures of oral cancer. At a time when the global incidence of cancer is rapidly increasing and many Americans lack health insurance, there's an urgent need for affordable tools to facilitate early detection and management of cancer.

A bioengineering group at Rice University, led by Rebecca Richards-Kortum, has developed both wide-field (macroscopic) and high-resolution (microscopic) optical imaging devices for screening and diagnosis of oral cancers. These low-cost, portable systems are suitable for targeting cancer screening and diagnosis in a wide range of settings.

Current procedures for cancer screening typically involve visually inspecting the entire tissue surface at risk. Unfortunately, the macroscopic appearance of precancerous lesions can be difficult to distinguish from many benign conditions. This situation can be improved by using specially filtered light (polarized) and fluorescence to detect disease.

With the new device, which recently received U.S. Food and Drug Administration (FDA) approval, health professionals can more easily inspect the oral cavity for cancer and its precursor lesions. Because of the low cost of the technology, it is feasible to deploy it in primary care settings like the dentist's office.

The National Institutes of Health (NIH)-supported team has also developed a portable system, contained within a briefcase and operated by a single 12-volt, rechargeable battery, to enable high-resolution evaluation of a patient's epithelial cells, such as those lining the mouth. After a fluorescent solution is applied inside a patient's mouth to make cell components visible, health professionals use a flexible fiber-optic bundle to image epithelial cells and look for changes that distinguish normal cells from precancerous or cancerous cells.

While these systems were initially developed to screen for oral cancer, researchers hope to adapt the technologies to screen for other types of cancer, such as cervical and esophageal.

Section 15.3

DNA Microchip Technology

This section includes text excerpted from "DNA Microchip Technology," National Human Genome Research Institute (NHGRI), April 20, 2014. Reviewed December 2017.

What Is a DNA Microchip?

Scientists know that a mutation—or alteration—in a particular gene's deoxyribonucleic acid (DNA) often results in a certain disease. However, it can be very difficult to develop a test to detect these mutations, because most large genes have many regions where mutations can occur. For example, researchers believe that mutations in the genes *BRCA1* and *BRCA2* cause as many as 60 percent of all cases of hereditary breast and ovarian cancers. But there is not one specific mutation responsible for all of these cases. Researchers have already discovered more than 800 different mutations in *BRCA1* alone.

The DNA microchip is a new tool used to identify mutations in genes like *BRCA1* and *BRCA2*. The chip, which consists of a small glass plate encased in plastic, is manufactured somewhat like a computer microchip. On the surface, each chip contains thousands of short, synthetic, single-stranded DNA sequences, which together add up to the normal gene in question.

What Is a DNA Microchip Used For?

Because chip technology is still relatively new, it is currently only a research tool. Scientists use it to conduct large-scale population studies—for example, to determine how often individuals with a particular mutation actually develop breast cancer.

As we gain more insight into the mutations that underlie various diseases, researchers will likely produce new chips to help assess individual risks for developing different cancers as well as heart disease, diabetes, and other diseases.

How Does a DNA Microchip Work?

To determine whether an individual possesses a mutation for *BRCA1* or *BRCA2*, a scientist first obtains a sample of DNA from the patient's blood as well as a control sample—one that does not contain a mutation in either gene.

The researcher then denatures the DNA in the samples—a process that separates the two complementary strands of DNA into single-stranded molecules. The next step is to cut the long strands of DNA into smaller, more manageable fragments and then to label each fragment by attaching a fluorescent dye. The individual's DNA is labeled with green dye and the control—or normal—DNA is labeled with red dye. Both sets of labeled DNA are then inserted into the chip and allowed to hybridize—or bind—to the synthetic *BRCA1* or *BRCA2* DNA on the chip. If the individual does not have a mutation for the gene, both the red and green samples will bind to the sequences on the chip.

If the individual does possess a mutation, the individual's DNA will not bind properly in the region where the mutation is located. The scientist can then examine this area more closely to confirm that a mutation is present.

Miniature Human Organ Systems

ORGANS-ON-CHIPS creates miniature human organ systems, or tissues, on micro-engineered chips about the size of an AA battery are being developed to accelerate the translation of basic discoveries into the clinic. These chip devices are designed to simulate the structure and function of human organs and help scientists gain a better understanding of the effects of medicines, vaccines, biological agents, chemicals, and other potentially harmful materials on the human body.

(Source: "About Tissue Chip," National Center for Advancing Translational Sciences (NCATS).)

Section 15.4

Early Detection of Colorectal Cancer

This section includes text excerpted from "Advances in
Colorectal Cancer Research," National Institutes of
Health (NIH), August 20, 2015.

Cancers of the colon and rectum, also known as colorectal cancers, are the third most commonly diagnosed cancers among men and
women in the United States and the second leading cause of cancer
death in this country. In 2010, it is estimated that more than 140,000
Americans will be diagnosed with colorectal cancer and more than
50,000 will die of the disease. Over the past several decades, researchers have learned a lot about colorectal cancer, but much more research
is needed to find ways to prevent the disease and to detect it earlier
and treat it more effectively should it occur.

At the National Institutes of Health (NIH), the research effort on
colorectal cancer is led by the National Cancer Institute (NCI). A vast
network of NCI-supported scientists, located on the NIH campus in
Bethesda, Md., and at research centers across the nation and around
the world, are exploring new ways to prevent, detect, and treat colorectal cancer. Many other NIH institutes and centers, including the
National Institute of Diabetes and Digestive and Kidney Diseases
(NIDDK), the National Institute of General Medical Sciences (NIGMS),
and the National Human Genome Research Institute (NHGRI), also
support colorectal cancer-related research.

Both basic and clinical research scientists are utilizing the latest
advances in technology in the effort to reduce the burden and toll of
colorectal cancer. In the area of cancer screening and early detection,
advances in computer-aided imaging, nanotechnology, and methods of
molecular analysis promise to enhance our ability to identify abnormal
growths in colorectal tissue that either are or could become cancerous.
Meanwhile, other researchers are investigating ways to ensure that
people adhere to current colorectal cancer screening recommendations.

In the area of cancer treatment, advances in DNA (deoxyribonucleic
acid) sequencing and genomic profiling methods should enable the
identification of the specific molecular defects in a person's cancer cells

and permit the development of therapies that target or take advantage of those defects. This genetic knowledge might also be exploited to help identify people who have an increased risk of colorectal cancer and to develop effective interventions to prevent the disease.

Section 15.5

Genetic Testing

This section includes text excerpted from "Is Genetic Testing Right for You?" MedlinePlus, National Institutes of Health (NIH), 2017.

What Is Genetic Testing?

Genetic testing looks at your genes. Genes are the deoxyribonucleic acid (DNA) instructions you receive from your mother and father. Genetic tests may identify risks of health problems. This can help people choose treatments or to understand how they may respond to treatments.

What Can I Learn from Testing?

Genetic testing tells you information about your DNA. Genetic test results can be hard to understand. Specialists like geneticists and genetic counselors can help explain information.

What Types of Genetic Tests Are There?

Diagnostic testing can identify the disease that is making a person sick. The results of a diagnostic test may help you make choices about your health.

Predictive and presymptomatic genetic tests find gene changes that increase a person's chance of developing diseases. This information could be useful in decisions about your lifestyle and healthcare.

Carrier testing is used to find people who carry a change in a gene that is linked to disease. Carriers may show no signs of the disease. However, they can pass on the gene change to their children, who may develop the disease or become carriers themselves.

Prenatal testing is offered during pregnancy to help identify fetuses that have certain diseases.

Newborn screening tests babies one or two days after birth to find out if they have certain diseases known to cause problems with health and development.

Pharmacogenomic testing gives information about how certain medicines are processed by an individual's body. This type of testing can help your healthcare provider choose the medicines that work best for you.

Research genetic testing is used to learn more about how genes affect health and disease.

What Are the Pros and Cons of Genetic Testing?

Benefits: Genetic testing may be helpful whether the test identifies a mutation or not. For some people, test results remove some of the uncertainty surrounding their health. These results may also help doctors and give people more information to make decisions about their health, as well as their family's health, allowing them to take steps to lower the chance of developing a disease.

Drawbacks: Genetic testing is relatively safe for your body. However, it can be hard to find out your results. Sometimes, testing can be costly.

Emotional: Learning that you or someone in your family has or is at risk for a disease can be scary. Some people also feel guilty, angry, anxious, or depressed when they learn their results.

Financial: Genetic testing can cost anywhere from less than $100 to more than $2,000. Health insurance companies may cover part or all the cost of testing.

Many people are worried about discrimination based on their genetic test results. In 2008, Congress enacted the Genetic Information Nondiscrimination Act to protect people from discrimination by their health insurance provider or employer.

How Do I Decide If I Should Be Tested?

There are many reasons why people might get genetic testing. A test could help doctors learn if you or your family have certain patterns of disease. You can decide if a genetic test will be helpful for you.

A geneticist or genetic counselor can help families decide if a particular genetic test will be helpful.

Genes against Diseases

Gene therapy uses genes to treat or prevent disease and allows doctors to insert a healthy copy of a gene into a patient's cells, inactivate a mutated gene, or introduce a new gene to help fight a disease. Although there is much hope for gene therapy, and researchers are testing it to treat certain inherited disorders, viral infections, and some types of cancer that have no other cures, the technique is still experimental and under study to make it safe and effective.

Source: "How Does Gene Therapy Work?" U.S. Department of Health and Human Services (HHS).)

Section 15.6

Sensitive Stroke Detection

This section includes text excerpted from "More Sensitive Stroke Detection," National Institutes of Health (NIH), August 20, 2015.

Researchers at the National Institute of Neurological Disorders and Stroke (NINDS) have found that magnetic resonance imaging (MRI) can provide a more sensitive diagnosis than computed tomography (CT) for the most common type of stroke, called ischemic stroke.

The researchers studied more than 350 patients who arrived in the emergency room with suspected strokes to determine whether MRI or CT was better for rapid diagnosis. Doctors face an urgent need to swiftly distinguish between acute ischemic stroke, which is caused by clots in blood vessels, and hemorrhagic stroke, which is caused by bleeding into the brain, because the two types of stroke are treated in very different ways.

Standard CT uses X-rays that are passed through the body at different angles and processed by a computer as cross-sectional images, or slices of the internal structure of the body or organ. Standard MRI uses computer-generated radio waves and a powerful magnet to produce detailed slices or three-dimensional images of body structures and nerves. A contrast dye may be used in both imaging techniques to enhance visibility of certain areas or tissues.

Results of the NINDS study showed that standard MRI is superior to standard CT in diagnosing acute stroke, particularly acute ischemic stroke. That is very good news for patients, says NINDS Deputy Director Walter J. Koroshetz, M.D., noting that brain injury from ischemic stroke often can be avoided if clot-busting therapy is administered within three hours of stroke onset.

Section 15.7

Tool to Detect Cardiovascular Disease Risk

This section includes text excerpted from "New NIST
Tool Aims to Improve Accuracy of Test to Determine
Cardiovascular Disease Risk," National Institute
Standards and Technology (NIST),
September 19, 2017.

Cardiovascular disease caused 1 out of 3 deaths in the United States in 2016, and for decades it has been the leading killer for both men and women. Hoping to reduce these numbers, researchers at the National Institute of Standards and Technology (NIST) have developed a new Standard Reference Material (SRM) that can improve the results of a common blood test used to assess a person's risk of heart disease.

The blood test measures C-reactive protein (CRP), which is a marker for inflammation in the body. While the precise relationship between slightly elevated CRP levels and cardiovascular disease is still being determined, research suggests that inflammation in arteries can lead to plaque buildup, and then to heart attacks and strokes. Some studies indicate (link is external) that high-sensitivity CRP (hsCRP) tests—which detect minute amounts of the protein in blood—may have advantages for predicting heart disease when cholesterol counts are normal.

The hsCRP test kits are made from antibodies that attach to CRP in a blood sample like a lock and key to provide an accurate count of the protein. However, depending on their source and quality, some of these antibodies attach better than others, leading to variable results between batches and kit makers.

"We began developing a reference material for the hsCRP test when we recognized that a patient's test results might depend on which test kit was used," said Eric Kilpatrick, a biologist who has specialized in protein measurement at NIST for more than a decade. "Repeatable, reliable results, no matter when or where the blood test is performed, are critical to health, and without them, it is difficult for doctors to use hsCRP to decide treatment options and to follow a patient's progress accurately," he said.

NIST's SRM 2924 C-Reactive Protein Solution provides a reference benchmark tool that manufacturers can use to ensure their kit test results are consistent from batch to batch by confirming that the antibodies going into the kits correctly bind CRP.

When the results of hsCRP tests can be traced to the NIST SRM, doctors can have greater trust in the test scores, and treat and advise their patients with confidence.

Researchers are continuing their quest for ultimate accuracy. "The gold standard for CRP will be an SRM in serum, the liquid component of blood," Kilpatrick said. That work will begin soon, and SRM 2924 is leading the way.

SRMs are among the most widely used NIST products. The institute prepares, analyzes and sells more than 1,200 carefully characterized materials used to check the accuracy of instruments and test procedures used in manufacturing, clinical chemistry, environmental monitoring, electronics, criminal forensics, and dozens of other fields.

Part Three

Diagnostic Technology

Chapter 16

Imaging Services

Chapter Contents

Section 16.1—Computed Tomography (CT) 132

Section 16.2—Electrocardiogram (ECG) 135

Section 16.3—Functional Near-Infrared
Spectroscopy (fNIRS) 137

Section 16.4—Magnetic Resonance Imaging (MRI)................. 139

Section 16.5—Mammogram 143

Section 16.6—Medical X-Ray Imaging 145

Section 16.7—Nuclear Medicine 148

Section 16.8—Optical Imaging.. 151

Section 16.9—Ultrasound... 154

Section 16.1

Computed Tomography (CT)

This section includes text excerpted from "Science Education—
Computed Tomography (CT)," National Institute of Biomedical
Imaging and Bioengineering (NIBIB), December 9, 2016.

What Is a Computed Tomography (CT) Scan?

The term "computed tomography," or CT, refers to a computerized
X-ray imaging procedure in which a narrow beam of X-rays is aimed
at a patient and quickly rotated around the body, producing signals
that are processed by the machine's computer to generate cross-sectional images—or "slices"—of the body. These slices are called tomographic images and contain more detailed information than conventional X-rays. Once a number of successive slices are collected by the
machine's computer, they can be digitally "stacked" together to form
a three-dimensional image of the patient that allows for easier identification and location of basic structures as well as possible tumors
or abnormalities.

How Does CT Work?

Unlike a conventional X-ray—which uses a fixed X-ray tube—a CT
scanner uses a motorized X-ray source that rotates around the circular
opening of a donut-shaped structure called a gantry. During a CT scan,
the patient lies on a bed that slowly moves through the gantry while
the X-ray tube rotates around the patient, shooting narrow beams
of X-rays through the body. Instead of film, CT scanners use special
digital X-ray detectors, which are located directly opposite the X-ray
source. As the X-rays leave the patient, they are picked up by the
detectors and transmitted to a computer.

Each time the X-ray source completes one full rotation, the CT
computer uses sophisticated mathematical techniques to construct a
2D image slice of the patient. The thickness of the tissue represented
in each image slice can vary depending on the CT machine used, but
usually ranges from 1–10 millimeters. When a full slice is completed,

the image is stored and the motorized bed is moved forward incrementally into the gantry. The X-ray scanning process is then repeated to produce another image slice. This process continues until the desired number of slices is collected.

Image slices can either be displayed individually or stacked together by the computer to generate a 3D image of the patient that shows the skeleton, organs, and tissues as well as any abnormalities the physician is trying to identify. This method has many advantages including the ability to rotate the 3D image in space or to view slices in succession, making it easier to find the exact place where a problem may be located.

When Would I Get a CT Scan?

CT scans can be used to identify disease or injury within various regions of the body. For example, CT has become a useful screening tool for detecting possible tumors or lesions within the abdomen. A CT scan of the heart may be ordered when various types of heart disease or abnormalities are suspected. CT can also be used to image the head in order to locate injuries, tumors, clots leading to stroke, hemorrhage, and other conditions. It can image the lungs in order to reveal the presence of tumors, pulmonary embolisms (blood clots), excess fluid, and other conditions such as emphysema or pneumonia. A CT scan is particularly useful when imaging complex bone fractures, severely eroded joints, or bone tumors since it usually produces more detail than would be possible with a conventional X-ray.

Are There Risks?

CT scans can diagnose possibly life-threatening conditions such as hemorrhage, blood clots, or cancer. An early diagnosis of these conditions could potentially be life-saving. However, CT scans use X-rays, and all X-rays produce ionizing radiation. Ionizing radiation has the potential to cause biological effects in living tissue. This is a risk that increases with the number of exposures added up over the life of an individual. However, the risk of developing cancer from radiation exposure is generally small.

A CT scan in a pregnant woman poses no known risks to the baby if the area of the body being imaged isn't the abdomen or pelvis. In general, if imaging of the abdomen and pelvis is needed, doctors prefer to use exams that do not use radiation, such as magnetic resonance imaging (MRI) or ultrasound. However, if neither of those can provide the answers needed, or there is an emergency or other time constraint, CT may be an acceptable alternative imaging option.

In some patients, contrast agents may cause allergic reactions, or in rare cases, temporary kidney failure. IV contrast agents should not be administered to patients with abnormal kidney function since they may induce a further reduction of kidney function, which may sometimes become permanent. Children are more sensitive to ionizing radiation and have a longer life expectancy and, thus, a higher relative risk for developing cancer than adults. Parents may want to ask the technologist or doctor if their machine settings have been adjusted for children.

What Is a CT Contrast Agent?

As with all X-rays, dense structures within the body—such as bone—are easily imaged, whereas soft tissues vary in their ability to stop X-rays and, thus, may be faint or difficult to see. For this reason, intravenous (IV) contrast agents have been developed that are highly visible in an X-ray or CT scan and are safe to use in patients. Contrast agents contain substances that are better at stopping X-rays and, thus, are more visible on an X-ray image. For example, to examine the circulatory system, a contrast agent based on iodine is injected into the bloodstream to help illuminate blood vessels. This type of test is used to look for possible obstructions in blood vessels, including those in the heart. Oral contrast agents, such as barium-based compounds, are used for imaging the digestive system, including the esophagus, stomach, and gastrointestinal tract (GI tract).

Section 16.2

Electrocardiogram (ECG)

This section contains text excerpted from the following sources:
Text in this section begins with excerpts from "Electrocardiogram,"
National Heart, Lung, and Blood Institute (NHLBI), December 9,
2016; Text under the heading "Understanding the Heart's Electrical
System and EKG Results" is excerpted from "Understanding the
Heart's Electrical System and EKG Results," National Heart, Lung,
and Blood Institute (NHLBI), July 9, 2012. Reviewed December 2017.

An electrocardiogram, also called an ECG or EKG, is a simple, painless test that detects and records your heart's electrical activity. An EKG can show how fast your heart is beating, whether the rhythm of your heartbeats is steady or irregular, and the strength and timing of the electrical impulses passing through each part of your heart. You may have an EKG as part of a routine exam to screen for heart disease. This test also is used to detect and study heart problems such as heart attacks, arrhythmia or irregular heartbeat, and heart failure. Results from this test also may suggest other heart disorders.

An EKG may be recorded in a doctor's office, an outpatient facility, in a hospital before major surgery, or as part of stress testing. For the test, you will lie still on a table. A nurse or technician will attach up to 12 electrodes to the skin on your chest, arms, and legs. Your skin may need to be shaved to help the electrodes stick. The electrodes are connected by wires to a machine that records your heart's electrical activity on graph paper or on a computer. After the test, the electrodes will be removed.

EKG has no serious risks. EKGs don't give off electrical charges such as shocks. You may develop a slight rash where the electrodes were attached to your skin. This rash usually goes away on its own without treatment.

Understanding the Heart's Electrical System and EKG Results

Doctors use a test called an EKG (electrocardiogram) to help diagnose heart block. This test detects and records the heart's electrical activity. An EKG records the strength and timing of electrical signals as they pass through the heart.

The data are recorded on a graph so your doctor can study your heart's electrical activity. Different parts of the graph show each step of an electrical signal's journey through the heart.

Each electrical signal begins in a group of cells called the sinus node or sinoatrial (SA) node. The SA node is located in the right atrium, which is the upper right chamber of the heart. (Your heart has two upper chambers and two lower chambers.)

In a healthy adult heart at rest, the SA node sends an electrical signal to begin a new heartbeat 60 to 100 times a minute.

From the SA node, the signal travels through the right and left atria. This causes the atria to contract, which helps move blood into the heart's lower chambers, the ventricles. The electrical signal moving through the atria is recorded as the P wave on the EKG.

The electrical signal passes between the atria and ventricles through a group of cells called the atrioventricular (AV) node. The signal slows down as it passes through the AV node. This slowing allows the ventricles enough time to finish filling with blood. On the EKG, this part of the process is the flat line between the end of the P wave and the beginning of the Q wave.

The electrical signal then leaves the AV node and travels along a pathway called the bundle of His. From there, the signal travels into the right and left bundle branches. The signal spreads quickly across your heart's ventricles, causing them to contract and pump blood to your lungs and the rest of your body. This process is recorded as the QRS waves on the EKG.

The ventricles then recover their normal electrical state (shown as the T wave on the EKG). The muscle stops contracting to allow the heart to refill with blood. This entire process continues over and over with each new heartbeat.

Section 16.3

Functional Near-Infrared Spectroscopy (fNIRS)

This section includes text excerpted from "Functional Near-Infrared Spectroscopy (fNIRS) Cognitive Brain Monitor," National Aeronautics and Space Administration (NASA), October 1, 2015.

New signal-processing techniques excludes motion artifacts to yield more accurate data.

Innovators at National Aeronautics and Space Administration's (NASA) Glenn Research Center have developed a Functional Near-Infrared Spectroscopy (fNIRS) Cognitive Brain Monitor with improved signal processing to obtain more accurate data. fNIRS has been used successfully to monitor cognitive states and activity, and Glenn's system can be used to continuously monitor brain function during safety-critical tasks, such as flying an airplane or driving a train. Using head-worn sensors, the technique employs near-infrared light and advanced signal processing to allow real-time, in-task monitoring. The system not only determines changes in cognitive state by tracking blood hemoglobin levels in the brain, but also filters nonrelevant artifacts, such as the probes' own motion, rendering the collected data even more accurate. Glenn's novel use and refinement of fNIRS signals stands to improve safety in a wide variety of applications and environments.

The Technology

Functional near-infrared spectroscopy (fNIRS) is an emerging hemodynamic neuroimaging brain-computer interface (BCI) technology that indirectly measures neuronal activity in the brain's cortex via neuro-vascular coupling. fNIRS works by quantifying hemoglobin-concentration changes in the brain based on optical intensity measurements, measuring the same hemodynamic changes as functional magnetic resonance imaging (fMRI). With enough probes in enough locations, fNIRS can detect these hemodynamic activations across the subject's entire head, thus allowing the determination of cognitive

137

state through the use of pattern classification. fNIRS systems offer low-power, low-cost, highly mobile alternatives for real-time monitoring in safety-critical situations.

Glenn's specific contribution to this field is the algorithms capable of removing motion artifacts (environment- or equipment-induced errors) from the device's head-worn optical sensors. In other words, Glenn's adaptive filter can determine the presence of a potential motion artifact based on a phase shift in the data measured; identify the artifact by examining the correlation between the phase shift and changes in hemoglobin concentration; and finally remove the artifact using Kalman filtering whenever changes in hemoglobin level and changes in the phase shift are not correlated. Glenn's breakthrough allows the advantages of fNIRS to be used for noninvasive real-time brain monitoring applications in motion-filled environments that could potentially save lives.

Benefits

- Improved safety: Continuous monitoring of brain activity during safety-critical tasks could prevent serious accidents

- High accuracy: Removing motion artifacts allows real-world data capture to approach laboratory quality

- Portability: The system features comfortable headworn sensors, and is compact enough to fit into smaller spaces

Applications

The technology has several potential applications:

- Safety simulations, training, and monitoring for airline pilots, train, and mass transit engineers, ship captains, truck drivers, crane, and other heavy-equipment operators, and air traffic controllers.

- Military simulations and training.

- In-home, real-time monitoring and feedback during patient rehabilitation for cognitive impairment or depression.

- Replacement for or supplement to functional brain imaging.

Section 16.4

Magnetic Resonance Imaging (MRI)

This section includes text excerpted from "MRI
(Magnetic Resonance Imaging)," U.S. Food and Drug
Administration (FDA), November 7, 2016.

Magnetic resonance imaging (MRI) is a medical imaging procedure for making images of the internal structures of the body. MRI scanners use strong magnetic fields and radio waves (radio frequency energy) to make images. The signal in an MR image comes mainly from the protons in fat and water molecules in the body.

During an MRI exam, an electric current is passed through coiled wires to create a temporary magnetic field in a patient's body. Radio waves are sent from and received by a transmitter/receiver in the machine, and these signals are used to make digital images of the scanned area of the body. A typical MRI scan lasts 20–90 minutes, depending on the part of the body being imaged.

For some MRI exams, intravenous (IV) drugs, such as gadolinium-based contrast agents (GBCAs) are used to change the contrast of the MR image. Gadolinium-based contrast agents are rare earth metals that are usually given through an IV in the arm.

Uses

MRI gives healthcare providers useful information about a variety of conditions and diagnostic procedures including:

- abnormalities of the brain and spinal cord

- abnormalities in various parts of the body such as breast, prostate, and liver

- injuries or abnormalities of the joints

- the structure and function of the heart (cardiac imaging)

- areas of activation within the brain (functional MRI or fMRI)

- blood flow through blood vessels and arteries (angiography)

139

- the chemical composition of tissues (spectroscopy)

In addition to these diagnostic uses, MRI may also be used to guide certain interventional procedures.

Benefits and Risks

Benefits

An MRI scanner can be used to take images of any part of the body (e.g., head, joints, abdomen, legs, etc.), in any imaging direction. MRI provides better soft tissue contrast than CT and can differentiate better between fat, water, muscle, and other soft tissue than CT (CT is usually better at imaging bones). These images provide information to physicians and can be useful in diagnosing a wide variety of diseases and conditions.

Risks

MR images are made without using any ionizing radiation, so patients are not exposed to the harmful effects of ionizing radiation. But while there are no known health hazards from temporary exposure to the MR environment, the MR environment involves a strong, static magnetic field, a magnetic field that changes with time (pulsed gradient field), and radiofrequency energy, each of which carry specific safety concerns:

- The strong, static magnetic field will attract magnetic objects (from small items such as keys and cell phones, to large, heavy items such as oxygen tanks and floor buffers) and may cause damage to the scanner or injury to the patient or medical professionals if those objects become projectiles. Careful screening of people and objects entering the MR environment is critical to ensure nothing enters the magnet area that may become a projectile.

- The magnetic fields that change with time create loud knocking noises which may harm hearing if adequate ear protection is not used. They may also cause peripheral muscle or nerve stimulation that may feel like a twitching sensation.

- The radiofrequency energy used during the MRI scan could lead to heating of the body. The potential for heating is greater during long MRI examinations.

The use of gadolinium-based contrast agents (GBCAs) also carries some risk, including side effects such as allergic reactions to the contrast agent.

Some patients find the inside of the MRI scanner to be uncomfortably small and may experience claustrophobia. Imaging in an open MRI scanner may be an option for some patients, but not all MRI systems can perform all examinations, so you should discuss these options with your doctor. Your doctor may also be able to prescribe medication to make the experience easier for you.

To produce good quality images, patients must generally remain very still throughout the entire MRI procedure. Infants, small children, and other patients who are unable to lay still may need to be sedated or anesthetized for the procedure. Sedation and anesthesia carry risks not specific to the MRI procedure, such as slowed or difficult breathing, and low blood pressure.

Patients with Implants, External, and Accessory Devices

The MR environment presents unique safety hazards for patients with implants, external devices and accessory medical devices. Examples of implanted devices include artificial joints, stents, cochlear implants, and pacemakers. An external device is a device that may touch the patient like an external insulin pump, a leg brace, or a wound dressing. An accessory device is a nonimplanted medical device (such as a ventilator, patient monitor) that is used to monitor or support the patient.

- The strong, static magnetic field of the MRI scanner will pull on magnetic materials and may cause unwanted movement of the medical device.

- The radiofrequency energy and magnetic fields that change with time may cause heating of the implanted medical device and the surrounding tissue, which could lead to burns.

- The magnetic fields and radiofrequency energy produced by an MRI scanner may also cause electrically active medical devices to malfunction, which can result in a failure of the device to deliver the intended therapy.

- The presence of the medical device will degrade the quality of the MR image, which may make the MRI scan uninformative or may lead to an inaccurate clinical diagnosis, potentially resulting in inappropriate medical treatment.

Therefore patients with implanted medical devices should not receive an MRI exam unless the implanted medical device has been positively identified as MR Safe or MR Conditional. An MR Safe device is nonmagnetic, contains no metal, does not conduct electricity and poses no known hazards in all MR environments. An MR Conditional device may be used safely only within an MR environment that matches its conditions of safe use. Any device with an unknown MRI safety status should be assumed to be MR Unsafe.

Adverse Events

Adverse events for MRI scans are very rare. Millions of MRI scans are performed in the United States every year, and the FDA receives around 300 adverse event reports for MRI scanners and coils each year from manufacturers, distributors, user facilities, and patients. The majority of these reports describe heating and/or burns (thermal injuries). Second degree burns are the most commonly reported patient problem. Other reported problems include injuries from projectile events (objects being drawn toward the MRI scanner), crushed and pinched fingers from the patient table, patient falls, and hearing loss or a ringing in the ear (tinnitus). The FDA has also received reports concerning the inadequate display or quality of the MR images.

Multimodal Imaging

Future research on imaging will focus on multimodal imaging technology that will use MRI as either a base or a complimentary technique. Multimodal imaging combines information from two or more imaging modalities such as MRI, computed tomography (CT), positron emission tomography (PET), and ultrasound (US).

(Source: "Multimodal Imaging," National Institutes of Health (NIH).)

Section 16.5

Mammogram

This section includes text excerpted from "Breast
Cancer—Basic Information—What Is a Mammogram?"
Centers for Disease Control and Prevention (CDC), July 25, 2017.

A mammogram is an X-ray picture of the breast. Doctors use a mammogram to look for early signs of breast cancer. Regular mammograms are the best tests doctors have to find breast cancer early, sometimes up to three years before it can be felt.

How Is a Mammogram Done?

You will stand in front of a special X-ray machine. A technologist will place your breast on a clear plastic plate. Another plate will firmly press your breast from above. The plates will flatten the breast, holding it still while the X-ray is being taken. You will feel some pressure. The steps are repeated to make a side view of the breast. The other breast will be X-rayed in the same way. You will then wait while the technologist checks the four X-rays to make sure the pictures do not need to be re-done. Keep in mind that the technologist cannot tell you the results of your mammogram. Each woman's mammogram may look a little different because all breasts are a little different.

What Does Having a Mammogram Feel Like?

Having a mammogram is uncomfortable for most women. Some women find it painful. A mammogram takes only a few moments, though, and the discomfort is over soon. What you feel depends on the skill of the technologist, the size of your breasts, and how much they need to be pressed. Your breasts may be more sensitive if you are about to get or have your period. A doctor with special training, called a radiologist, will read the mammogram. He or she will look at the X-ray for early signs of breast cancer or other problems.

Tips for Getting a Mammogram

Try not to have your mammogram the week before you get your period or during your period. Your breasts may be tender or swollen then.

- On the day of your mammogram, don't wear deodorant, perfume, or powder. These products can show up as white spots on the X-ray.

- Some women prefer to wear a top with a skirt or pants, instead of a dress. You will need to undress from your waist up for the mammogram.

When will I Get the Results of My Mammogram?

You will usually get the results within a few weeks, although it depends on the facility. A radiologist reads your mammogram and then reports the results to you or your doctor. If there is a concern, you will hear from the mammography facility earlier. Contact your healthcare provider or the mammography facility if you do not receive a report of your results within 30 days.

What Happens If My Mammogram Is Normal?

Continue to get mammograms according to recommended time intervals. Mammograms work best when they can be compared with previous ones. This allows the radiologist to compare them to look for changes in your breasts.

What Happens If My Mammogram Is Abnormal?

An abnormal mammogram does not always mean that there is cancer. But you will need to have additional mammograms, tests, or exams before the doctor can tell for sure. You may also be referred to a breast specialist or a surgeon. It does not necessarily mean you have cancer or need surgery. These doctors are experts in diagnosing breast problems. Doctors will do follow-up tests to diagnose breast cancer or to find that there is no cancer.

Where Can I Get a Mammogram and Who Can I Talk to If I Have Questions?

If you have a regular doctor, talk to him or her.

Call the National Cancer Institute's (NCI) Cancer Information Service (CIS) at 800-4-CANCER (800-422-6237). TTY: 800-332-8615.

For Medicare information, you can call 800-MEDICARE (800-633-4227) or visit The Centers for Medicare and Medicaid Services (CMS).

Section 16.6

Medical X-Ray Imaging

This section contains text excerpted from the following sources: Text under the heading "What Are Medical X-Rays?" is excerpted from "X-Rays," MedlinePlus, National Institutes of Health (NIH), March 4, 2016; Text beginning with the heading "How Do Medical X-Rays Work?" is excerpted from "Science Education—X-Rays," National Institute of Biomedical Imaging and Bioengineering (NIBIB), July 26, 2013. Reviewed December 2017.

What Are Medical X-Rays?

X-rays are a type of radiation called electromagnetic waves. X-ray imaging creates pictures of the inside of your body. The images show the parts of your body in different shades of black and white. This is because different tissues absorb different amounts of radiation. Calcium in bones absorbs X-rays the most, so bones look white. Fat and other soft tissues absorb less, and look gray. Air absorbs the least, so lungs look black.

The most familiar use of X-rays is checking for broken bones, but X-rays are also used in other ways. For example, chest X-rays can spot pneumonia. Mammograms use X-rays to look for breast cancer.

When you have an X-ray, you may wear a lead apron to protect certain parts of your body. The amount of radiation you get from an X-ray is small. For example, a chest X-ray gives out a radiation dose similar to the amount of radiation you're naturally exposed to from the environment over 10 days.

How Do Medical X-Rays Work?

To create a radiograph, a patient is positioned so that the part of the body being imaged is located between an X-ray source and an

X-ray detector. When the machine is turned on, X-rays travel through the body and are absorbed in different amounts by different tissues, depending on the radiological density of the tissues they pass through. Radiological density is determined by both the density and the atomic number (the number of protons in an atom's nucleus) of the materials being imaged. For example, structures such as bone contain calcium, which has a higher atomic number than most tissues. Because of this property, bones readily absorb X-rays and, thus, produce high contrast on the X-ray detector. As a result, bony structures appear whiter than other tissues against the black background of a radiograph. Conversely, X-rays travel more easily through less radiologically dense tissues such as fat and muscle, as well as through air-filled cavities such as the lungs. These structures are displayed in shades of gray on a radiograph.

When Are Medical X-Rays Used?

Listed below are examples of examinations and procedures that use X-ray technology to either diagnose or treat disease:

Diagnostic

X-ray radiography: Detects bone fractures, certain tumors and other abnormal masses, pneumonia, some types of injuries, calcifications, foreign objects, dental problems, etc.

Mammography: A radiograph of the breast that is used for cancer detection and diagnosis. Tumors tend to appear as regular or irregular-shaped masses that are somewhat brighter than the background on the radiograph (i.e., whiter on a black background or blacker on a white background). Mammograms can also detect tiny bits of calcium, called microcalcifications, which show up as very bright specks on a mammogram. While usually benign, microcalcifications may occasionally indicate the presence of a specific type of cancer.

Computed Tomography (CT): Combines traditional X-ray technology with computer processing to generate a series of cross-sectional images of the body that can later be combined to form a three-dimensional X-ray image. CT images are more detailed than plain radiographs and give doctors the ability to view structures within the body from many different angles.

Fluoroscopy: Uses X-rays and a fluorescent screen to obtain real-time images of movement within the body or to view diagnostic processes, such as following the path of an injected or swallowed contrast agent. For example, fluoroscopy is used to view the movement of the beating heart, and, with the aid of radiographic contrast agents, to view blood flow to the heart muscle as well as through blood vessels and organs. This technology is also used with a radiographic contrast agent to guide an internally threaded catheter during cardiac angioplasty, which is a minimally invasive procedure for opening clogged arteries that supply blood to the heart.

Therapeutic

Radiation therapy in cancer treatment: X-rays and other types of high-energy radiation can be used to destroy cancerous tumors and cells by damaging their deoxyribonucleic acid (DNA). The radiation dose used for treating cancer is much higher than the radiation dose used for diagnostic imaging. Therapeutic radiation can come from a machine outside of the body or from a radioactive material that is placed in the body, inside or near tumor cells, or injected into the bloodstream.

Are There Risks?

When used appropriately, the diagnostic benefits of X-ray scans significantly outweigh the risks. X-ray scans can diagnose possibly life-threatening conditions such as blocked blood vessels, bone cancer, and infections. However, X-rays produce ionizing radiation—a form of radiation that has the potential to harm living tissue. This is a risk that increases with the number of exposures added up over the life of the individual. However, the risk of developing cancer from radiation exposure is generally small.

An X-ray in a pregnant woman poses no known risks to the baby if the area of the body being imaged isn't the abdomen or pelvis. In general, if imaging of the abdomen and pelvis is needed, doctors prefer to use exams that do not use radiation, such as magnetic resonance imaging (MRI) or ultrasound. However, if neither of those can provide the answers needed, or there is an emergency or other time constraint, an X-ray may be an acceptable alternative imaging option.

Children are more sensitive to ionizing radiation and have a longer life expectancy and, thus, a higher relative risk for developing cancer than adults. Parents may want to ask the technologist or doctor if their machine settings have been adjusted for children.

Section 16.7

Nuclear Medicine

This section includes text excerpted from "Science Education—Nuclear Medicine," National Institute of Biomedical Imaging and Bioengineering (NIBIB), July 2016.

What Is Nuclear Medicine?

Nuclear medicine is a medical specialty that uses radioactive tracers (radiopharmaceuticals) to assess bodily functions and to diagnose and treat disease. Specially designed cameras allow doctors to track the path of these radioactive tracers. Single Photon Emission Computed Tomography or SPECT and Positron Emission Tomography or PET scans are the two most common imaging modalities in nuclear medicine.

What Are Radioactive Tracers?

Radioactive tracers are made up of carrier molecules that are bonded tightly to a radioactive atom. These carrier molecules vary greatly depending on the purpose of the scan. Some tracers employ molecules that interact with a specific protein or sugar in the body and can even employ the patient's own cells. For example, in cases where doctors need to know the exact source of intestinal bleeding, they may radiolabel (add radioactive atoms) to a sample of red blood cells taken from the patient. They then reinject the blood and use a SPECT scan to follow the path of the blood in the patient. Any accumulation of radioactivity in the intestines informs doctors of where the problem lies.

For most diagnostic studies in nuclear medicine, the radioactive tracer is administered to a patient by intravenous injection. However a radioactive tracer may also be administered by inhalation, by oral ingestion, or by direct injection into an organ. The mode of tracer administration will depend on the disease process that is to be studied.

Approved tracers are called radiopharmaceuticals since they must meet U.S. Food and Drug Administration's (FDA) exacting standards for safety and appropriate performance for the approved clinical use. The nuclear medicine physician will select the tracer that will provide the most specific and reliable information for a patient's particular problem. The tracer that is used determines whether the patient receives a SPECT or PET scan.

What Is Single Photon Emission Computed Tomography (SPECT)?

SPECT imaging instruments provide three-dimensional (tomographic) images of the distribution of radioactive tracer molecules that have been introduced into the patient's body. The 3D images are computer generated from a large number of projection images of the body recorded at different angles. SPECT imagers have gamma camera detectors that can detect the gamma ray emissions from the tracers that have been injected into the patient. Gamma rays are a form of light that moves at a different wavelength than visible light. The cameras are mounted on a rotating gantry that allows the detectors to be moved in a tight circle around a patient who is lying motionless on a pallet.

What Is Positron Emission Tomography (PET)?

PET scans also use radiopharmaceuticals to create three-dimensional images. The main difference between SPECT and PET scans is the type of radiotracers used. While SPECT scans measure gamma rays, the decay of the radiotracers used with PET scans produce small particles called positrons. A positron is a particle with roughly the same mass as an electron but oppositely charged. These react with electrons in the body and when these two particles combine they annihilate each other. This annihilation produces a small amount of energy in the form of two photons that shoot off in opposite directions. The detectors in the PET scanner measure these photons and use this information to create images of internal organs.

What Are Nuclear Medicine Scans Used For?

SPECT scans are primarily used to diagnose and track the progression of heart disease, such as blocked coronary arteries. There are also radiotracers to detect disorders in bone, gall bladder disease and intestinal bleeding. SPECT agents have recently become available for aiding in the diagnosis of Parkinson disease in the brain, and distinguishing this malady from other anatomically related movement disorders and dementias.

The major purpose of PET scans is to detect cancer and monitor its progression, response to treatment, and to detect metastases. Glucose utilization depends on the intensity of cellular and tissue activity so it is greatly increased in rapidly dividing cancer cells. In fact, the degree of aggressiveness for most cancers is roughly paralleled by their rate of glucose utilization. In the last 15 years, slightly modified radiolabeled glucose molecules (F-18 labeled deoxyglucose or FDG) have been shown to be the best available tracer for detecting cancer and its metastatic spread in the body.

A combination instrument that produces both PET and CT scans of the same body regions in one examination (PET/CT scanner) has become the primary imaging tool for the staging of most cancers worldwide.

Recently, a PET probe was approved by the U.S. Food and Drug Administration (FDA) to aid in the accurate diagnosis of Alzheimer disease, which previously could be diagnosed with accuracy only after a patient's death. In the absence of this PET imaging test, Alzheimer disease can be difficult to distinguish from vascular dementia or other forms of dementia that affect older people.

Are There Risks?

The total radiation dose conferred to patients by the majority of radiopharmaceuticals used in diagnostic nuclear medicine studies is no more than what is conferred during routine chest X-rays or computed tomography (CT) exams. There are legitimate concerns about possible cancer induction even by low levels of radiation exposure from cumulative medical imaging examinations, but this risk is accepted to be quite small in contrast to the expected benefit derived from a medically needed diagnostic imaging study.

Like radiologists, nuclear medicine physicians are strongly committed to keeping radiation exposure to patients as low as possible, giving the least amount of radiotracer needed to provide a diagnostically useful examination.

Section 16.8

Optical Imaging

This section includes text excerpted from "Science
Education—Optical Imaging," National Institute of Biomedical
Imaging and Bioengineering (NIBIB), May 2016.

What Is Optical Imaging?

Optical imaging is a technique for noninvasively looking inside the
body, as is done with X-rays. But, unlike X-rays, which use ionizing
radiation, optical imaging uses visible light and the special properties
of photons to obtain detailed images of organs and tissues as well as
smaller structures including cells and molecules. These images are
used by scientists for research and by clinicians for disease diagnosis
and treatment.

What Are the Advantages of Optical Imaging?

Optical imaging offers a number of advantages over other radiological imaging techniques:

- Optical imaging significantly reduces patient exposure to harmful radiation by using nonionizing radiation, which includes
  visible, ultraviolet, and infrared light. These types of light
  generate images by exciting electrons without causing the damage that can occur with ionizing radiation used in some other
  imaging techniques. Because it is much safer for patients, and
  significantly faster, optical imaging can be used for lengthy and
  repeated procedures over time to monitor the progression of disease or the results of treatment.

- Optical imaging is particularly useful for visualizing soft tissues.
  Soft tissues can be easily distinguished from one another due
  to the wide variety of ways different tissues absorb and scatter
  light.

- Because it can obtain images of structures across a wide range
  of sizes and types, optical imaging can be combined with other

imaging techniques, such as magnetic resonance imaging (MRI) or X-rays, to provide enhanced information for doctors monitoring complex diseases or researchers working on intricate experiments.

- Optical imaging takes advantage of the various colors of light in order to see and measure many different properties of an organ or tissue at the same time. Other imaging techniques are limited to just one or two measurements.

What Types of Optical Imaging Are There and What Are They Used For?

Optical imaging includes a variety of techniques that use light to obtain images from inside the body, tissues or cells.

Endoscopy

The simplest and most widely recognized type of optical imaging is endoscopy. An endoscope consists of a flexible tube with a system to deliver light to illuminate an organ or tissue. For example, a physician can insert an endoscope through a patient's mouth to see the digestive cavity to find the cause of symptoms such as abdominal pain, difficulty swallowing, or gastrointestinal bleeding. Endoscopes are also used for minimally invasive robotic surgery to allow a surgeon to see inside the patient's body while remotely manipulating the thin robotic arms that perform the procedure.

Optical Coherence Tomography (OCT)

Optical coherence tomography (OCT) is a technique for obtaining subsurface images such as diseased tissue just below the skin. OCT is a well-developed technology with commercially available systems now in use in a variety of applications, including art conservation and diagnostic medicine. For example, ophthalmologists use OCT to obtain detailed images from within the retina. Cardiologists also use it to help diagnose coronary artery disease.

Photoacoustic Imaging

During photoacoustic imaging, laser pulses are delivered to a patient's tissues; the pulses generate heat, expanding the tissues and enabling their structure to be imaged. The technique can be used for a number of clinical applications including monitoring blood vessel growth in tumors, detecting skin melanomas, and tracking blood oxygenation in tissues.

Diffuse Optical Tomography (DOT)

Diffuse optical tomography (DOT) can be used to obtain information about brain activity. A laser that uses near-infrared light is positioned on the scalp. The light goes through the scalp and harmlessly traverses the brain. The absorption of light reveals information about chemical concentrations in the brain. The scattering of the light reflects physiological characteristics such as the swelling of a neuron upon activation to pass on a neural signal.

Raman Spectroscopy

This technique relies on what is known as Raman scattering of visible, near-infrared, or near-ultraviolet light that is delivered by a laser. The laser light interacts with molecular vibrations in the material being examined, and shifts in energy are measured that reveal information about the properties of the material. The technique has a wide variety of applications including identifying chemical compounds and characterizing the structure of materials and crystals. In medicine, Raman gas analyzers are used to monitor anesthetic gas mixtures during surgery.

Super-Resolution Microscopy

This form of light microscopy encompasses a number of techniques used in research to obtain very high-resolution images of individual cells at a level of detail not feasible using normal microscopy. One example is a technique called photoactivated localization microscopy (PALM), which uses fluorescent markers to pinpoint single molecules. PALM can be performed sequentially to create a super-resolution image from the series of molecules isolated in the sample tissue.

Terahertz Tomography

This relatively new, experimental technique involves sectional imaging using terahertz radiation. Terahertz radiation consists of electromagnetic waves, which are found on the spectrum between microwaves and infrared light waves. They are of great interest to scientists because terahertz radiation can "see" what visible and infrared light cannot, and holds great promise for detecting unique information unavailable via other optical imaging methods.

Section 16.9

Ultrasound

This section includes text excerpted from "Ultrasound,"
National Institute of Biomedical Imaging and
Bioengineering (NIBIB), July 2016.

What Is Medical Ultrasound?

Medical ultrasound falls into two distinct categories: diagnostic and therapeutic.

Diagnostic ultrasound is a noninvasive diagnostic technique used to image inside the body. Ultrasound probes, called transducers, produce sound waves that have frequencies above the threshold of human hearing (above 20KHz), but most transducers in current use operate at much higher frequencies (in the megahertz (MHz) range). Most diagnostic ultrasound probes are placed on the skin. However, to optimize image quality, probes may be placed inside the body via the gastrointestinal tract, vagina, or blood vessels. In addition, ultrasound is sometimes used during surgery by placing a sterile probe into the area being operated on.

Diagnostic ultrasound can be further sub-divided into anatomical and functional ultrasound. Anatomical ultrasound produces images of internal organs or other structures. Functional ultrasound combines information such as the movement and velocity of tissue or blood, softness or hardness of tissue, and other physical characteristics, with anatomical images to create "information maps." These maps help doctors visualize changes/differences in function within a structure or organ.

Therapeutic ultrasound also uses sound waves above the range of human hearing but does not produce images. Its purpose is to interact with tissues in the body such that they are either modified or destroyed. Among the modifications possible are: moving or pushing tissue, heating tissue, dissolving blood clots, or delivering drugs to specific locations in the body. These destructive, or ablative, functions are made possible by use of very high-intensity beams that can destroy diseased or abnormal tissues such as tumors. The advantage of using ultrasound therapies is that, in most cases, they are noninvasive. No incisions or cuts need to be made to the skin, leaving no wounds or scars.

How Does It Work?

Ultrasound waves are produced by a transducer, which can both emit ultrasound waves, as well as detect the ultrasound echoes reflected back. In most cases, the active elements in ultrasound transducers are made of special ceramic crystal materials called piezoelectrics. These materials are able to produce sound waves when an electric field is applied to them, but can also work in reverse, producing an electric field when a sound wave hits them. When used in an ultrasound scanner, the transducer sends out a beam of sound waves into the body. The sound waves are reflected back to the transducer by boundaries between tissues in the path of the beam (e.g., the boundary between fluid and soft tissue or tissue and bone). When these echoes hit the transducer, they generate electrical signals that are sent to the ultrasound scanner. Using the speed of sound and the time of each echo's return, the scanner calculates the distance from the transducer to the tissue boundary. These distances are then used to generate two-dimensional images of tissues and organs.

During an ultrasound exam, the technician will apply a gel to the skin. This keeps air pockets from forming between the transducer and the skin, which can block ultrasound waves from passing into the body.

What Is Ultrasound Used For?

Diagnostic ultrasound. Diagnostic ultrasound is able to noninvasively image internal organs within the body. However, it is not good for imaging bones or any tissues that contain air, like the lungs. Under some conditions, ultrasound can image bones (such as in a fetus or in small babies) or the lungs and lining around the lungs, when they are filled or partially filled with fluid. One of the most common uses of ultrasound is during pregnancy, to monitor the growth and development of the fetus, but there are many other uses, including imaging the heart, blood vessels, eyes, thyroid, brain, breast, abdominal organs, skin, and muscles. Ultrasound images are displayed in either 2D, 3D, or 4D (which is 3D in motion).

Functional ultrasound. Functional ultrasound applications include Doppler and color Doppler ultrasound for measuring and visualizing blood flow in vessels within the body or in the heart. It can also measure the speed of the blood flow and direction of movement. This is done using color-coded maps called color Doppler imaging. Doppler ultrasound is commonly used to determine whether plaque buildup inside the carotid arteries is blocking blood flow to the brain.

Another functional form of ultrasound is elastography, a method for measuring and displaying the relative stiffness of tissues, which can be used to differentiate tumors from healthy tissue. This information can be displayed as either color-coded maps of the relative stiffness; black-and-white maps that display high-contrast images of tumors compared with anatomical images; or color-coded maps that are overlaid on the anatomical image. Elastography can be used to test for liver fibrosis, a condition in which excessive scar tissue builds up in the liver due to inflammation.

Ultrasound is also an important method for imaging interventions in the body. For example, ultrasound-guided needle biopsy helps physicians see the position of a needle while it is being guided to a selected target, such as a mass or a tumor in the breast. Also, ultrasound is used for real-time imaging of the location of the tip of a catheter as it is inserted in a blood vessel and guided along the length of the vessel. It can also be used for minimally invasive surgery to guide the surgeon with real-time images of the inside of the body.

Therapeutic or interventional ultrasound. Therapeutic ultrasound produces high levels of acoustic output that can be focused on specific targets for the purpose of heating, ablating, or breaking up tissue. One type of therapeutic ultrasound uses high-intensity beams of sound that are highly targeted, and is called High Intensity Focused Ultrasound (HIFU). HIFU is being investigated as a method for modifying or destroying diseased or abnormal tissues inside the body (e.g., tumors) without having to open or tear the skin or cause damage to the surrounding tissue. Either ultrasound or MRI is used to identify and target the tissue to be treated, guide and control the treatment in real time, and confirm the effectiveness of the treatment. HIFU is currently U.S. Food and Drug Administration (FDA)-approved for the treatment of uterine fibroids, to alleviate pain from bone metastases, and most recently for the ablation of prostate tissue. HIFU is also being investigated as a way to close wounds and stop bleeding, to break up clots in blood vessels, and to temporarily open the blood brain barrier so that medications can pass through.

Are There Risks?

Diagnostic ultrasound is generally regarded as safe and does not produce ionizing radiation like that produced by X-rays. Still, ultrasound is capable of producing some biological effects in the body under specific settings and conditions. For this reason, the FDA requires that diagnostic ultrasound devices operate within acceptable limits. The FDA, as well as many professional societies, discourage the casual use of ultrasound (e.g., for keepsake videos) and recommend that it be used only when there is a true medical need.

Chapter 17

Advances in Imaging

Chapter Contents

Section 17.1—Magnetic Resonance Electrography 160

Section 17.2—Neuroimaging Technique to Predict
                Autism among High-Risk Infants 161

Section 17.3—Metal-Free MRI Contrast Agent 162

Section 17.4—Virtual Colonoscopy 165

Section 17.5—Advanced Magnetic Imaging Methods 167

Section 17.1

Magnetic Resonance Electrography

This section includes text excerpted from
"Bye-Bye Biopsies?" National Institutes of
Health (NIH), August 20, 2015.

Nearly 200,000 Americans are hospitalized each year for chronic liver disease. Typically, a biopsy is used to diagnose and evaluate the liver for signs of stiffening, or fibrosis. For a biopsy, the doctor uses a needle to take a tiny sample of liver tissue and then examines it under the microscope for scarring or other signs of disease.

As an alternative to liver biopsies, National Institutes of Health (NIH)-funded investigators led by Richard Ehman at the Mayo Clinic have developed magnetic resonance (MR) elastography, a noninvasive magnetic resonance imaging (MRI) approach that can measure the amount of stiffness in a very small amount of tissue. The noninvasive detection of fibrosis by MR elastography offers patients multiple advantages over biopsy examination, including less discomfort, a much lower risk of complications, and a decrease in expense.

According to Dr. Ehman, MR elastography has already made a substantial difference in patient care. One example is a patient with hemophilia who previously contracted hepatitis C from a blood transfusion. Liver biopsy was contraindicated because of the hemophilia, but MR elastography was used to determine if there was fibrosis associated with the hepatitis. In this case, the results showed fibrosis and the individual was started on antiviral therapy.

Early results show this same technique might also be used to improve the detection of breast cancer and help distinguish a benign mass, such as fibrocystic disease, from cancer.

Section 17.2

Neuroimaging Technique to Predict Autism among High-Risk Infants

This section includes text excerpted from "Neuroimaging Technique
May Help Predict Autism among High-Risk Infants," National
Institutes of Health (NIH), June 7, 2017.

Functional connectivity magnetic resonance imaging (fcMRI) may
predict which high-risk, 6-month-old infants will develop autism
spectrum disorder by age 2 years, according to a study funded by
the *Eunice Kennedy Shriver* National Institute of Child Health and
Human Development (NICIID) and the National Institute of Mental
Health (NIMH), two components of the National Institutes of Health
(NIH). The study is published in the June 7, 2017, issue of Science
Translational Medicine.

Autism affects roughly 1 out of every 68 children in the United
States. Siblings of children diagnosed with autism are at higher risk
of developing the disorder. Although early diagnosis and intervention
can help improve outcomes for children with autism, there currently
is no method to diagnose the disease before children show symptoms.

"Previous findings suggest that brain-related changes occur in
autism before behavioral symptoms emerge," said Diana Bianchi,
M.D., NICHD Director. "If future studies confirm these results, detecting brain differences may enable physicians to diagnose and treat
autism earlier than they do today."

In the current study, a research team led by NIH-funded investigators at the University of North Carolina at Chapel Hill and Washington University School of Medicine in St. Louis focused on the brain's
functional connectivity—how regions of the brain work together during
different tasks and during rest. Using fcMRI, the researchers scanned
59 high-risk, 6-month-old infants while they slept naturally. The children were deemed high-risk because they have older siblings with
autism. At age 2 years, 11 of the 59 infants in this group were diagnosed with autism.

The researchers used a computer-based technology called machine
learning, which trains itself to look for differences that can separate

the neuroimaging results into two groups—autism or nonautism—and predict future diagnoses. One analysis predicted each infant's future diagnosis by using the other 58 infants' data to train the computer program. This method identified 82 percent of the infants who would go on to have autism (9 out of 11), and it correctly identified all of the infants who did not develop autism. In another analysis that tested how well the results could apply to other cases, the computer program predicted diagnoses for groups of 10 infants, at an accuracy rate of 93 percent.

"Although the findings are early-stage, the study suggests that in the future, neuroimaging may be a useful tool to diagnose autism or help healthcare providers evaluate a child's risk of developing the disorder," said Joshua Gordon, M.D., Ph.D., NIMH Director.

Overall, the team found 974 functional connections in the brains of 6-month-olds that were associated with autism-related behaviors. The authors propose that a single neuroimaging scan may accurately predict autism among high-risk infants, but caution that the findings need to be replicated in a larger group.

Section 17.3

Metal-Free MRI Contrast Agent

This section includes text excerpted from "NIH-Funded Researchers Develop Metal-Free MRIContrast Agent," National Institute of Biomedical Imaging and Bioengineering (NIBIB), October 6, 2017.

A team led by National Institutes of Health-funded researchers at the Massachusetts Institute of Technology (MIT) and the University of Nebraska has developed a method to enhance a magnetic resonance imaging (MRI) contrast agent with safe-to-use, metal-free compounds. The researchers used organic molecules carried by synthetic nanoparticles. The nanoparticles illuminated tumor tissue in mice just as well as metal-based contrast agents.

Metal-free magnetic resonance imaging (MRI) agents could overcome the toxicity associated with metal-based agents in some patient populations and enable new modes of functional MRI. The unique nanoparticle architecture of a metal-free contrast agent produces enhanced MRI contrast while remaining stable in the blood of mice and not causing toxicity. Left in the image is the chemical structure of nitroxide, an organic radical compound carried by the brush-arm star polymer, middle, to produce contrast in mouse tumor. Source: Johnson lab, MIT.

"The ability to diagnose and monitor many diseases using MRI can be greatly enhanced with the use of contrast agents," said Shumin Wang, Ph.D., program director of the National Institute of Biomedical Imaging and Bioengineering program in Magnetic Resonance Imaging. "The new metal-free contrast agents on the horizon are an exciting prospect that may be helpful for people who cannot tolerate metal-based MRI contrast agents, which are currently the only clinically available option for patients."

As with X-ray imaging, MRI is a noninvasive way to scan internal anatomy. While X-rays make bone visible, MRI scans mainly depict the soft tissues of the body. The MRI machine creates a magnetic field, pulling and then releasing spinning protons in the water molecules in the body. This releases energy that MRI sensors can detect and translate into an image of the tissue.

MRI contrast agents change the magnetic properties of water molecules and cause spinning protons to respond differently to the magnetic field created by an MRI magnet. These differences affect how different tissues appear on the MRI scans and can make certain tissues, like tumors, more visible. Tumor tissue tends to draw in certain contrast agents so that it accumulates there, temporarily making it possible for physicians to see the tumor clearly and monitor the disease progression.

All current MRI contrast agents are metal-based and have been used by radiologists for more than 30 years. Currently, gadolinium is the most commonly used metal in MRI contrast agents. Existing gadolinium agents are small molecules that, after a time, are cleared from the body relatively quickly through the kidneys. However, radiologists cannot use it with certain high-risk groups, primarily patients with kidney disease and those who have allergic reactions to it. While recent studies have shown that gadolinium from MRI procedures can be found in brain and bone tissue years after its application, at this time the U.S. Food and Drug Administration (FDA) says the agent has not been proven to be harmful based on existing studies.

In their study, published July 12, 2017 in ACS Central Science, the researchers who developed this new organic-based contrast agent contend that a nonmetal alternative would most benefit patients who cannot currently tolerate the metal-based agents but its use could be broadened to all patients needing MRI contrast agents. This approach would minimize concerns about contrast agent accumulation as clinically viable, nanoparticle-based MRI contrast agents are developed.

The researchers developed the metal-free agent through a collaboration among research labs. The team from University of Nebraska, who design and produce a variety of organic radical molecules, shared their organic compound with MIT researchers who specialize in the synthesis of complex polymer architectures. Polymers are made from various types of molecules that assemble into shapes that affect how they interact within biological systems.

Jeremiah Johnson, Ph.D., is the Firmenich Career Development Associate Professor of Chemistry at MIT and senior author of the study. His team designed a polymer shape they call the bottle brush because of its resemblance to the kitchen tool. By configuring multiple bottle-brush polymers into a spherical shape, they produced a variation on the bottle brush polymer they called a brush-arm star polymer, or BASP.

"This BASP nanostructure has useful features, including excellent scalability," Johnson said. Johnson's team previously published studies in which they described how BASPs can be designed with attached drug molecules and contrast agents, including the organic radical compound, nitroxide. "We had already been making our polymers with nitroxide attached," he said, "but this is the first time we were able to attach this new nitroxide molecule that works much better as an MRI contrast agent." The molecule was developed in the laboratory of coauthor Andrzej Rajca, Ph.D., the Charles Bessey Professor of Chemistry at the University of Nebraska, Lincoln.

The BASP polymer structure plays a key role in how the organic compound enhances imaging for tumor tissue and then is eliminated from the body. Nitroxides are normally broken down by chemicals in living systems before they can help to create MRI images. Putting them on BASP polymers protected them, allowing them to circulate in the bloodstream long enough to accumulate in mouse tumors, and to generate contrast in MRI scans. The researchers found that the nitroxide BASP nanoparticles are stable enough to last for up to 20 hours in mice, where they accumulated in the mouse tumors. They also showed that the particles are not harmful to mice, even at high doses.

"There's a need right now for good, safe MRI contrast agents," Johnson said. "We think the best could be an entirely organic one that has no metal and therefore no potential metal-induced toxicity." While there are many types of cancer and tumor types, their research has not yet focused on how to target specific tumors. "We're working right now on the fundamentals, asking how we get enough contrast from these agents but in the future plan to test ways to target specific tumor types."

Section 17.4

Virtual Colonoscopy

This section includes text excerpted from "Virtual Colonoscopy,"
National Cancer Institute (NCI), December 22, 2016.

Virtual colonoscopy (VC) (or computerized tomographic colonography (CTC)) uses X-rays and computers to produce two- and three-dimensional images of the colon (large intestine) from the lowest part, the rectum, all the way to the lower end of the small intestine and display them on a screen. The procedure is used to diagnose colon and bowel disease, including polyps, diverticulosis, and cancer. VC can be performed with computed tomography (CT), sometimes called a CAT scan, or with magnetic resonance imaging (MRI).

Virtual Colonoscopy Procedure

While preparations for VC vary, you will usually be asked to take laxatives or other oral agents at home the day before the procedure to clear stool from your colon. You may also be asked to use a suppository to cleanse your rectum of any remaining fecal matter.

VC takes place in the radiology department of a hospital or medical center. The examination takes about 10 minutes and does not require sedatives. During the procedure:

- The doctor will ask you to lie on your back on a table.

- A thin tube will be inserted into your rectum, and air will be pumped through the tube to inflate the colon for better viewing.

- The table moves through the scanner to produce a series of two-dimensional cross-sections along the length of the colon.

A computer program puts these images together to create a three-dimensional picture that can be viewed on the video screen.

• You will be asked to hold your breath during the scan to avoid distortion on the images.

• The scanning procedure is then repeated with you lying on your stomach.

After the examination, the information from the scanner must be processed to create the computer picture or image of your colon. A radiologist evaluates the results to identify any abnormalities.

You may resume normal activity after the procedure, although your doctor may ask you to wait while the test results are analyzed. If abnormalities are found and you need a conventional colonoscopy, it may be performed the same day.

In a conventional colonoscopy, the doctor inserts a colonoscope—a long, flexible, lighted tube—into the patient's rectum and slowly guides it up through the colon. Pain medication and a mild sedative help the patient stay relaxed and comfortable during the 30- to 60-minute procedure. A tiny camera in the scope transmits an image of the lining of the colon, so the doctor can examine it on a video monitor. If an abnormality is detected, the doctor can remove it or take tissue samples using tiny instruments passed through the scope.

Advantages of Virtual Colonoscopy

VC is more comfortable than a conventional colonoscopy for some people because it does not use a colonoscope. As a result, no sedation is needed, and you can return to your usual activities or go home after the procedure without the aid of another person. VC provides clearer, more detailed images than a conventional X-ray using a barium enema, sometimes called a lower gastrointestinal (GI) series. It also takes less time than either a conventional colonoscopy or a lower GI series.

Disadvantages of Virtual Colonoscopy

The doctor cannot take tissue samples or remove polyps during VC, so a conventional colonoscopy must be performed if abnormalities are found. Also, VC does not show as much detail as a conventional colonoscopy, so polyps smaller than 10 millimeters in diameter may not show up on the images.

Section 17.5

Advanced Magnetic Imaging Methods

This section includes text excerpted from "Advanced
Magnetic Imaging Methods," National Institute
Standards and Technology (NIST), July 13, 2017.

The scope of MRI is expanding with the development of both ultra-high field (14 T) and ultra-low field (0.1 mT) scanners not only for biomedical applications but for in situ materials characterization. In addition, entirely new types of magnetic imaging modalities are being developed, including magnetic particle imaging (MPI), EPR-enhanced MRI, and micro fabricated sensors and contrast agents visible in an MRI, to name a few examples. These advances will enable the development of new types of magnetic imaging agents that are useful not only for image enhancement but may have molecular and functional imaging capabilities, as well. The program focuses on techniques that challenge the current methodology of MRI to improve sensitivity, resolution, affordability, and portability.

Description

Ultra-low field (ULF) MRI

MRI systems are widely used for clinical diagnostics where imaging is typically done in high-field magnets ranging from 1.5 T to 7 T to achieve a manageable signal-to-noise ratio needed for short imaging times (few minutes) and high resolution (1 mm or less). Ultra-low field (ULF) MRI (100 μT) has several potential advantages: (a) narrower instrumentation line widths; (b) greater T1 contrast; (c) minimal susceptibility artifacts due to metallic implants or the presence of air; (d) air core B0, B1, Gx, Gy and Gz coils with relaxed uniformity and power requirements (100 ppm versus 0.1 ppm, less than1 kW versus 10 kW or more).

Dynamic Nuclear Polarization (DNP) enhanced MRI at low fields

Since its discovery in 1953, dynamic nuclear polarization (DNP) has provided a powerful means for enhancing the proton resonance signal.

The majority of recent research effort has focused on high magnetic fields, leading to many transformative experiments. Initial research into solution DNP in low magnetic fields has also been very exciting, especially in light of models predicting the magnitude of DNP enhancement at very low magnetic fields could be an order of magnitude greater than $\gamma e/\gamma H = 658x$ theoretical limit at high magnetic fields.

Portable low-field NMR

There are many instances where use of high magnetic field NMR is either unnecessary or impractical due to cost and large instrument footprint. Low magnetic field NMR instruments are considerably less expensive to build or purchase, and can be made portable for application to a greater variety of materials in a wide variety of environments. In many cases, simple electromagnets or small permanent magnets are sufficient to generate the required fields. Magnetic fields less than 100 mT (4.26 MHz) are optimally suited for extremely heterogeneous mixtures containing both liquids and solids. Internal gradients created by differences in liquid/solid susceptibility scale with main field strength, and are smaller in the low field regime.

Magnetic Particle Imaging (MPI)

Scientists are developing compact AC susceptometers for real-time monitoring of the conversion of precursors to magnetic nanoparticles in batch or continuous flow reactors. The goal is to rapidly assess specific magnetic performance parameters that are relevant to the final intended use of the magnetic particle solution. Ideally measurements on small sample aliquots (less than 1 μL) that are broadband and take a short time to perform (less than 1 s) are needed. Also, the physics package should be easily adaptable to the reactor as well as typical micro pumps or syringes for fluid control.

Chapter 18

Advanced Imaging in Laboratory Technology

Chapter Contents

Section 18.1—Live Cell Imaging 170

Section 18.2—Non-Linear Optical Imaging 172

Section 18.3—Surface Plasmon Resonance Imaging 174

169

Section 18.1

Live Cell Imaging

This section includes text excerpted from "Live Cell Imaging of Induced Pluripotent Stem Cell Populations," National Institute of Standards and Technology (NIST), November 23, 2016.

Induced pluripotent stem cell (iPSC) populations are complex, dynamic, and heterogeneous. Individual cells within a population are constantly changing, while maintaining the capacity to differentiate in numerous possible cell types. Sophisticated measurement tools are required to adequately describe and develop predictive models for complex cellular systems such as these. The technology to record live cell images from cellular populations has been available for some time, but only recently has it become routine to derive quantitative data from these image sets using image analysis. NIST has focused on developing live cell imaging tools to monitor large numbers of single cells and to quantify changes in morphology and gene expression using fluorescence protein reporters.

Description

Our live cell image program supports the advancement of iPSC technology in three ways:

1. **Identification of process control measurements:** A critical component to the translation of iPSCs into therapeutic applications is to design principles for predictably and reproducibly culturing cells and efficiently differentiating them into cell types of interest. Live cell imaging provides "high-resolution" measurements in the sense that NIST collects time-dependent data from large numbers of individual cells. Scientists then use this data to discover lower-resolution measurements, such as the activity of a biomarker at a single point in time, that can serve as critical process control points during processing of pluripotent stem cells.

2. **Interpreting biomarkers:** Cells are stochastic and dynamic and may interconvert between states and the expression of

biomarkers can change over time. The predictive power of a biomarker or a set of biomarkers the indicate the differentiated state of a cell can be evaluated by examining the history of that cell by tracking forward and backward in time through a time lapse image set.

3. **Predictive modeling:** NIST has shown that fluctuations in promoter activity can be used in combination with appropriate models to predict rates of state change in cell populations. Similar mathematical models that can inform bioprocessing decisions during scale-up will be critical to obtaining iPSC populations with a desired set of characteristics.

Over the past several years, NIST has developed tools for measuring parameters related to size, shape, and intensity from single cells over time. NIST has also developed modeling tools for using the temporal information to model the stochastic and deterministic components of gene expression.

NIST scientists are now applying these live cell imaging tools to the study of stem cell pluripotency and differentiation. Induced pluripotent stem cell technologies are a powerful new tool for biomedical research and have the potential to revolutionize medicine.

Additional Technical Details

Scientists at NIST use optical imaging to provide "high content" information about the size, shape, edge character, and internal structure of the cells and cell colonies under study in our laboratory. Here are shown images of H9 pluripotent stem cells in Zernike phase contrast (left) and fluorescence (right). The fluorescence is generated by a fluorescence protein reporter protein produced by a cell line that has been genetically engineered. The expression level of the fluorescent reporter provides information about the activity of a biochemical pathway. There's a need to identify critical attributes to measure during iPS processing schedules that can facilitate reaching the desired cellular product. Imaging is essential because cells are dynamic, heterogeneous, and spatial context is important. Optical microscopy is the only technique that allows to directly measure dynamic, spatially resolved information at the single cell level.

Section 18.2

Non-Linear Optical Imaging

This section includes text excerpted from "Non-Linear Optical Imaging," National Institute of Standards and Technology (NIST), July 13, 2017.

The traditional chemical labeling used in optical microscopy can alter cells and materials, thus impeding determination of their true structure, function, and response. Scientists are developing broadband coherent anti-Stokes Raman (BCARS) microscopy with the goal of producing a technique that allows label-free and noninvasive functional imaging of materials, cells, and tissues. On the materials side, scientists seek to image statics and dynamics of chemically heterogeneous and structured materials. For biological materials such as cells and tissues, scientists seek to attain near video-rate acquisition of high-resolution images that contain contrast from chemical processes occurring during cellular processes such as proliferation and differentiation, in order to discriminate normal and abnormal cell behaviors and differentiation states.

Description

Impact

There is a need for label-free chemical microscopy in medicine, biology and materials science. Most of the current methods use chemical labels that often disturb the distribution and nature of chemical components being investigated. The method scientists are developing enables noninvasive and rapid collection of Raman spectra for imaging.

BCARS can be used to track cell signaling processes and can provide functional readouts of cell differentiation, allowing researchers to obtain cell responses to biomaterials in real time and on a cell-by-cell basis.

BCARS can be used to acquire high-resolution chemical maps of pharmaceutical tablets, including information on morphology of active ingredients, 10 to 100 times faster than spontaneous Raman scattering.

All researchers who use Raman imaging methods will benefit from our work, including biomedical researchers (and, potentially, clinicians), pharmaceutical industry scientists, geologists and others. Additionally, laser manufacturers have been influenced by our work; PolarOnyx, Toptica, Time-Bandwidth and Spectra Physics Laser have all developed and are marketing laser sources to enable BCARS.

Approach

CARS provides a signal that contains the Raman response of interest for performing label-free chemically sensitive microscopy. In CARS, a vibrational coherence is generated when a pair of photons (pump and Stokes) interact with the sample to excite a vibrationally resonant Raman mode at frequency $\omega_{vib} = \omega_{pump} - \omega_{Stokes}$. A third (probe) photon is inelastically scattered off this coherent excitation, and anti-Stokes light ($\omega_{as} = \omega_{pump} - \omega_{Stokes} + \omega_{probe}$) is emitted from the sample.

The CARS signal has a frequency-independent nonresonant component and a frequency-dependent resonant component. The nonresonant component is entirely in phase with the driving field of the laser and gives no information about the chemical nature of the sample. The resonant component contains the chemical information and has a frequency-dependent amplitude. It is out of phase with respect to the driving electric field of the laser. The resonant component contains elements with the same bandshape as the spontaneous Raman signal.

Scientists obtain a broadband vibrational spectrum at each laser shot by using broadband Stokes light. The Stokes light contains 3000 cm-1 of bandwidth.

Section 18.3

Surface Plasmon Resonance Imaging

This section includes text excerpted from "Label-Free Imaging of Cells and Their Extracellular Matrix by SPR Imaging," National Institute of Standards and Technology (NIST), April 28, 2017.

Cellular remodeling of their neighboring environment, extracellular matrix (ECM), is an important biological process from development biology, to wound healing, to diseases and cancers this is a challenging process to measure and quantify.

Surface plasmon resonance imaging (SPRI) has been developed as a quantitative, label-free microscopy to image real-time observation of live cell engagement with the surface, and protein deposition and remodeling. The SPRI technique is an alternative to the commonly used fluorescence microscopy for examining cell-matrix interactions. This technique removes the requirement for modified biological molecules and transfected cells.

Researchers here have improved upon the spatial resolution of SPRI enabling the ability to visualize subcellular structures near the sensor surface. Along with quantitative interpretation of the images, essentially refractive index measurements, dry mass values of subcellular components can now be measured. For example, a smooth muscle cell has been measured to have focal adhesion dry mass of 980 ng/cm2 and can deposit up to 120 ng/cm2 of protein around it's periphery under normal growth condition.

Accomplishments have been:

1. Measurement of ECM, protein deposition, and cell phenotype with SPRI.

   - Surface plasmon resonance imaging of cells and surface-associated fibronectin

2. Quantification of cell areas, dynamic changes in cell-substrate, and changes in surface protein density over time.

174

- Using surface plasmon resonance imaging to probe dynamic interactions between cells and extracellular matrix

3. Improvement of spatial resolution to visualize subcellular components

    - High resolution surface plasmon resonance imaging for single cells

4. Calibration and correction strategy for quantitative analysis by optical modeling

    - Surface plasmon resonance microscopy: achieving a quantitative optical response

Research here is underway to develop SPRI as an imaging biosensor that can visualize dry mass changes down to a single bacterium that is part of a bacterial biofilm. Measuring antibiotic drug response at an individual cell level in addition to the biofilm as a whole can provide insight and understanding of how biofilms contribute to antibiotic drug resistance.

NIST has submitted a patent for this technology and is looking for collaborations with industry to commercialize this measurement technique.

Chapter 19

Point-of-Care Diagnostic Testing

Point-of-care testing allows patient diagnoses in the physician's office, an ambulance, the home, the field, or in the hospital. The results of care are timely, and allow rapid treatment to the patient. Empowering clinicians to make decisions at the "point-of-care" has the potential to significantly impact healthcare delivery and to address the challenges of health disparities. The success of a potential shift from curative medicine to predictive, personalized, and preemptive medicine could rely on the development of portable diagnostic and monitoring devices for point-of-care testing.

Yesterday

- In the earliest days of medicine, healthcare was similar to point-of-care in that it was delivered in the patient's home through physician house visits.

- As medical discoveries were made and new technologies developed, care then shifted to specialized hospitals with an emphasis on curative medicine.

- Large centralized laboratories were established, with cost-savings realized through the development of automated systems for analysis of patient samples.

This chapter includes text excerpted from "Point-of-Care Diagnostic Testing," National Institutes of Health (NIH), March 29, 2013. Reviewed December 2017.

- Point-of-care devices were used on a limited basis in the hospital for rapid analysis in intensive care units and for simple home testing, such as with pregnancy test kits.

Today

- The emphasis of care is shifting toward prevention and early detection of disease, as well as management of multiple chronic conditions.

- Point-of-care testing gives immediate results in nonlaboratory settings to support more patient-centered approaches to health-care delivery.

- The NIH supports the development of sensor and microsystem and low-cost imaging technologies for point-of-care testing. These instruments combine multiple analytical functions into self-contained, portable devices that can be used by nonspecialists to detect and diagnose disease, and can enable the selection of optimal therapies through patient screening and monitoring of a patient's response to a chosen treatment.

- Sensor technologies enable the rapid analysis of blood samples for several critical care assays, including blood chemistry, electrolytes, blood gases, and hematology.

- Biosensors are used clinically for toxicology and drug screens, measurement of blood cells and blood coagulations, bedside diagnosis of heart disease through detection of cardiac markers in the blood, and glucose self-testing.

- Current developments in point-of-care testing are addressing the challenges of diagnosis and treatment of cancer, stroke, and cardiac patients.

- Circulating tumor cells (CTCs) that spread, or metastasize, from a primary malignant tumor to distant organs are responsible for 90 percent of cancer-related deaths, a number that exceeds 500,000 every year in the United States alone. Early detection of cancer might be possible through capture and analysis of CTCs. In addition, the ability to capture and analyze CTCs in peripheral blood may be used in the development of therapeutic strategies that can be tailored to the individual patient and monitor an individual's responses to cancer therapies.

- Researchers supported by NIBIB have developed a unique microfluidic device capable of efficient separation of CTCs from whole blood. This technology has broad implications both for advancing cancer biology research and for the clinical management of cancer, including detection, diagnosis, and monitoring.

Tomorrow

- With the development of miniaturized devices and wireless communication, the way in which doctors care for patients will change dramatically and the role patients take in their own healthcare will increase. Healthcare will become more personalized through tailoring of interventions to individual patients.

- The next decade will bring a new realm of precision and efficiency to the way information is transmitted and interpreted and thus the way medicine is practiced. In the future, clinicians may be able to improve the regulation of diet in infants with inborn errors of metabolism through bedside monitoring. Currently, management of such diseases requires complex testing in a hospital setting. However, researchers are developing a chemical sensor, using a small sample of blood from a finger stick, which changes color in response to metabolic irregularities. When such abnormalities are found, the diet of the infant can be adjusted immediately to prevent adverse effects such as mental retardation.

- Low-cost diagnostic imaging devices can be used at the point-of-patient care for disadvantaged and under-served populations in the U.S. as well as in the developing world. The development of low-cost imaging devices could make affordable diagnostic imaging more widely available, particularly in remote or rural communities and small hospitals that do not have ready access to these technologies.

- A new method using an optical probe for cervical cancer detection and treatment could significantly lower the mortality rate worldwide. Combining a small optical imaging device with a treatment modality could provide both diagnosis and treatment of cervical cancer at the same time.

Chapter 20

Precision Medicine for Cancer Diagnostics

The conventional approach to medicine is rapidly changing to a data-driven strategy in which therapies are targeted to individual patients based on their unique genome, physiology, environment, and lifestyle. This approach is revolutionizing healthcare—especially in the treatment of cancer—but its success depends on the availability of reliable bioanalytical measurements, which can have many biases and uncertainties. For precision medicine to fulfill its promise, a measurement infrastructure is needed to assure the quality and reproducibility of diagnostic measurements.

National Institute of Standards and Technology (NIST) contributes to this effort by working with stakeholders in the cancer community to:

1. develop cancer biomarker reference materials to improve measurements in basic research and in the clinic,

2. evaluate data and assays to ensure confidence in discovery, and

3. conduct interlaboratory comparison studies to improve the accuracy and reliability of the measurements of new biomarkers.

This chapter includes text excerpted from "Precision Medicine for Cancer Diagnostics," National Institute Standards and Technology (NIST), July 13, 2017.

Description

A cancer biomarker is a biological molecule found in blood, other body fluids, or tissues that is indicative of the presence of cancer. Biomarkers can be used for cancer risk assessment, diagnosis, prognosis of disease, and prediction of response to treatment. Many candidate markers for cancer diagnosis and treatment are identified, but very few prove useful when translated into the clinic. To focus valuable resources on the development of useful biomarkers, it is necessary to ensure that a rigorous system of quality assurance is in place in laboratories. NIST can play a critical role in helping labs to achieve a high degree of such quality assurance by providing reference materials, interlaboratory testing, and working with the labs to establish analytical validation of their measurement processes.

NIST Cancer Biomarker Reference Materials

NIST develops reference materials for cancer biomarkers that can be used to improve measurements for the measurement assurance of assays used in basic research and for clinical measurements. The reference materials are developed in consultation with cancer experts from industry, academic, and government laboratories. Scientists have developed a Standard Reference Material (SRM) for Human Epidermal Growth Factor Receptor 2 (HER2), a gene that is frequently amplified in breast cancer. The standard consists of purified genomic DNA from five breast cancer cell lines with different amounts of HER2 gene amplification. This reference material is available from NIST as SRM 2373.

Scientists are also currently preparing a reference material for measurements of the genes for MET Proto-Oncogene (MET) and Epidermal Growth Factor Receptor (EGFR). Mutations or amplification of the genes for MET and EGFR can cause increased cellular signaling for cell growth or mobilization resulting in cancer. This new standard, when completed, will be available as Reference Material 8366. The standard consists of purified genomic DNA from six different cancer cell lines.

Chapter 21

Food Allergy Lab Fits on Your Keychain

More than 50 million Americans have food allergies, and often just trace amounts of allergens can trigger life-threatening reactions. Now, National Institute of Biomedical Imaging and Bioengineering (NIBIB)-funded researchers at Harvard Medical School have developed a $40 device that fits on a keychain and can accurately test for allergens, like gluten or nuts, in a restaurant meal in less than 10 minutes.

Food allergies are extremely common. Those fortunate enough not to be affected are likely to have a friend or family member who struggles to avoid dangerous reactions to food allergens every day. In the United States, Federal regulations require packaged foods to disclose the presence of some of the most common allergens such as gluten, nuts, and milk products, which is helpful but not always accurate.

When it comes to eating out, people with allergies have had to rely on their knowledge of what ingredients contain the allergens they must avoid, and on the efforts of the restaurant to provide dishes that eliminate allergens; and they must work to avoid cross-contamination between different ingredients in the kitchen. All in all, this approach generally leaves those with allergies with little choice but to completely avoid any foods that have the chance of containing an allergen, either

This chapter includes text excerpted from "Food Allergy Lab Fits on Your Keychain," National Institute of Biomedical Imaging and Bioengineering (NIBIB), October 25, 2017.

in the natural ingredients, or because of contact with other foods containing allergens during preparation in a restaurant kitchen.

Recognizing this widespread public health problem, researchers at Harvard Medical School in Boston have developed a system called integrated exogenous antigen testing (iEAT). The purpose of the iEAT system is to give those who suffer from food allergies a rapid, accurate device that allows them to personally test foods in less than 10 minutes.

Development of the iEAT system was led by cosenior team leaders Ralph Weissleder, M.D., Ph.D., the Thrall Professor of Radiology, Professor of Systems Biology at Harvard, and Director of the Center for Systems Biology (CSB) at Massachusetts General Hospital (MGH); and Hakho Lee, Ph.D., Associate Professor in Radiology at Harvard, Hostetter MGH Research Scholar, and Director of the Biomedical Engineering Program at the CSB, MGH. The work, is published in the August 2017 issue of ACS Nano.

"This invention is a fortuitous combination of the interests and expertise of Drs. Weissleder and Lee in developing tools for early disease detection, magnetic sensors, and point-of-care diagnostics," said Shumin Wang, Ph.D., director of the NIBIB program in Biomagnetic and Bioelectric Devices. "They have taken technologies they developed for other medical problems, such as early cancer detection from blood samples, and applied them to solving the daily, potentially life-threatening difficulties of people with food allergies—a highly significant public health problem that incurs 25 billion dollars in annual costs in the U.S. alone."

The device consists of three components. A small plastic test tube is used to dissolve a small sample of the food being tested and to add the magnetic beads that capture the food allergen of interest, such as gluten. A bit of that solution is then dropped onto electrode strips on a small module that is then inserted into the electronic keychain reader. The keychain reader has a small display that indicates whether the allergen is present and, if so, in what concentration. Testing showed that measurements of the concentration of the allergen is extremely accurate.

The high level of accuracy is very important. For example, even though Federal standards say that a food is considered gluten free if it has a concentration of less than 20 mg per kg of gluten, everyone's sensitivity is different, and many people would have a reaction at much lower gluten concentrations. Extensive testing of iEAT revealed that the system could detect levels of gluten that were 200 times lower than the Federal standard.

"High accuracy built into a compact system were the key goals of the project," says Weissleder. "Users can be confident that even if they are sensitive to very low levels, iEAT will be able to give them exact concentrations. Armed with accurate concentration levels they will not have to completely avoid potentially problematic foods, but will know whether an allergen is at a dangerous level for them or a concentration that is safe for them to eat."

Beyond obtaining the information they need in about 10 minutes using iEAT, a novel addition to the system was the development of a cell phone app, which offers the possibility of addressing food allergies at the community level. Using the app, users can compile and store the data they collect as they test different foods for various allergens at different restaurants and even in packaged foods. The app is set up to share this information online with both time and location stamps indicating when, where, and in what food or dish an allergen reading was taken. With the app, people will eventually have a personal record of levels that trigger a reaction. Others with the app will be able to find restaurants with foods they like to eat that consistently have no or low levels that are below the individual's triggering concentration.

"Although we believed iEAT could address a significant public health problem, we were surprised at the amount of interest the device has generated. We are receiving calls from people asking if we can adapt iEAT to test for other substances such as MSG or even pesticides," said Hakho Lee, cosenior leader of the project. "The good news is that we definitely can adapt the device to test for just about any allergen or substance."

Toward that end, the research team has granted a license to a local startup company to make iEAT commercially available. The company plans to merge the three components into a single module to make it even easier and more convenient to use. Production on a larger scale is also expected to reduce the price of the unit considerably.

In addition to contributing to food safety at the individual and community levels in the United States, the inventors point out that the device would be very valuable for travelers in countries where there are no specific requirements for food labels. Another use of the system would be to trace the source of food contamination with bacteria such as E. Coli or Salmonella to a specific food-processing site by testing DNA in the samples to potentially identify and contain an outbreak more quickly.

Chapter 22

Wireless Patient Monitoring

Why It's Needed

Paramedics and other emergency medical services (EMS) providers often operate in confined spaces and/or mobile environments. They are required to manage multiple tasks, including the monitoring of a patient's vital signs. Currently, emergency medical responders must attach numerous wires and instruments to a patient to monitor vital signs. While the information received from these instruments is displayed on one screen, the entanglement of wires and the process of connecting and disconnecting the patient can be overwhelming and take up precious time and space in confined ambulatory transports (i.e., the back of an ambulance or an aircraft). EMS personnel need a hands-free, wireless technology that monitors all required patient vital signs from one location, and the ViSi Mobile® device meets this need by providing continuous, noninvasive blood pressure (cNIBP) monitoring.

How It Works

In late 2012, the U.S. Department of Homeland Security Science and Technology Directorate (DHS S&T) partnered with Sotera Wireless, Inc. to develop a ViSi Mobile® device that can monitor

This chapter includes text excerpted from "Wireless Patient Monitoring," U.S. Department of Homeland Security (DHS), June 15, 2016.

vital signs without connecting wired sensors from the patient to other equipment. The device monitors blood pressure, 12-lead electrocardiograms, temperature, and respiration. The system works with existing devices, including traditional sensor patches attached to a patient that transmit data wirelessly back to a central monitor. The system is capable of operating in confined and "on the go" spaces (e.g., when a distressed patient is moved from the scene of an incident into an ambulance) and uses a single monitor that is lightweight and easier to transport than existing models on the market.

The Value

This technology provides paramedics, clinicians, and other medical personnel with a hands-free, wireless device to monitor a patient's vital signs, creating a safer environment for both EMS personnel and patients. No longer will first responders have to worry about entangled wires and a heavy monitor to transport with the patient. If patients require movement downstairs or through tight doorways, this wireless monitoring device poses fewer snag hazards and saves valuable time and space when connecting a patient to the ViSi sensors. Reducing snag hazards with just one device and a lightweight monitor will allow paramedics to respond to emergency incidents and perform daily operations more seamlessly and effectively. The technology also allows end-to-end, real-time connectivity between the emergency medical technician in the field and the emergency room. Data can be forwarded through a remote system from the ambulance to the hospital to give doctors, nurses, and other staff better situational awareness prior to the patient's arrival.

Rapid Prototype Development to Transition

In keeping with its mission of providing first responders with solutions to fill critical technology gaps, DHS S&T's R-Tech program worked with Sotera Wireless to address the technology requirements identified by EMS subject-matter experts with backgrounds in patient transport and vital sign monitoring. The continuous surveillance monitoring capabilities developed were tested during an operational field assessment (OFA) with EMS participants in San Diego, California in December 2013. Technological and operational feedback from this OFA has supported transitioning this device to the emergency medical response community.

Since transitioning the product to the commercial market, Sotera Wireless has targeted the device for use in a hospital-based setting. The U.S. Food and Drug Administration (FDA) has approved the ViSi Mobile® device for continuous, noninvasive blood pressure (cNIBP) monitoring.

Part Four

Role of Technology in Treatment

Chapter 23

Medical Treatment Technology (MTT)

Chapter Contents

Section 23.1—Genomic Medicine 194

Section 23.2—Personalized Medicine 198

Section 23.3—Nanomedicine 200

Section 23.4—Drug Delivery Systems 202

Section 23.5—Artificial Pancreas Device System 205

Section 23.1

Genomic Medicine

This section includes text excerpted from "What is
Genomic Medicine?" National Human Genome Research
Institute (NHGRI), July 21, 2016.

National Human Genome Research Institute (NHGRI) defines
genomic medicine as "an emerging medical discipline that involves
using genomic information about an individual as part of their clinical
care (e.g., for diagnostic or therapeutic decision-making) and the health
outcomes and policy implications of that clinical use." Already, genomic
medicine is making an impact in the fields of oncology, pharmacology,
rare and undiagnosed diseases, and infectious disease.

The nation's investment in the Human Genome Project (HGP) was
grounded in the expectation that knowledge generated as a result of
that extraordinary research effort would be used to advance the understanding of biology and disease and to improve health. In the years
since the HGP's completion there has been much excitement about
the potential for so-called "personalized medicine" to reach the clinic.
More recently, a report from the National Academy of Sciences (NAS)
has called for the adoption of "precision medicine," where genomics,
epigenomics, environmental exposure, and other data would be used
to more accurately guide individual diagnosis. Genomic medicine, as
defined above, can be considered a subset of precision medicine.

The translation of new discoveries to use in patient care takes many
years. Based on discoveries over the past 5–10 years, genomic medicine is beginning to fuel new approaches in certain medical specialties. Oncology, in particular, is at the leading edge of incorporating
genomics, as diagnostics for genetic and genomic markers are increasingly included in cancer screening, and to guide tailored treatment
strategies.

How Do We Get There?

It has often been estimated that it takes, on average, 17 years to
translate a novel research finding into routine clinical practice. This

time lag is due to a combination of factors, including the need to validate research findings, the fact that clinical trials are complex and take time to conduct and then analyze, and because disseminating information and educating healthcare workers about a new advance is not an overnight process.

Once sufficient evidence has been generated to demonstrate a benefit to patients, or "clinical utility," professional societies and clinical standards groups will use that evidence to determine whether to incorporate the new test into clinical practice guidelines. This determination will also factor in any potential ethical and legal issues, as well economic factors such as cost-benefit ratios.

The NHGRI Genomic Medicine Working Group (GMWG) has been gathering expert stakeholders in a series of genomic medicine meetings to discuss issues surrounding the adoption of genomic medicine. Particularly, the GMWG draws expertise from researchers at the cutting edge of this new medical toolset, with the aim of better informing future translational research at NHGRI. Additionally the working group provides guidance to the National Advisory Council on Human Genome Research (NACIIGR) and NIIGRI in other areas of genomic medicine implementation, such as outlining infrastructural needs for adoption of genomic medicine, identifying related efforts for future collaborations, and reviewing progress overall in genomic medicine implementation.

Examples of Genomic Medicine

Translational

- The causes of intellectual disability are often unknown, but a team in The Netherlands has used diagnostic exome sequencing of 100 affected individuals and their unaffected parents in order to uncover novel candidate genes and mutations that cause severe intellectual disability.

- Colorectal cancers with a particular mutation can benefit from treatment with aspirin post-diagnosis. Aspirin (and other non-steroidal anti-inflammatory drugs (NSAIDs)) decrease the activity of a signaling pathway called PI3K. Between 15 and 20 percent of colorectal cancer patients have a mutation in a gene called PIK3CA that makes a protein that's part of the PI3K pathway, and it has been discovered that regular aspirin treatment is associated with increased survival compared to colorectal cancer patients who have the nonmutated version of PIK3CA.

- Currently, every baby born in the United States is tested at birth for between 29 and 50 severe, inherited, treatable genetic diseases through a public health program called newborn screening. Whole genome sequencing would enable clinicians to look for mutations across the entire genome simultaneously for a much larger number of diseases or conditions. Rapid whole genome sequencing has been shown to provide a useful differential diagnosis within 50 hours for children in the neonatal intensive care unit.

- Researchers at Stanford University in California have been developing a new test to detect when a transplanted heart may be rejected by the recipient. Currently, the only way to detect the onset of rejection is by performing an invasive tissue biopsy. This novel approach only requires blood samples, and detects the levels of cell-free circulating deoxyribonucleic acid (DNA) from the donor organ in the recipient's blood stream. This circulating DNA from the donor can be elevated for up to five months before rejection can be detected by biopsy, and the level of DNA correlates with the severity of the rejection event (i.e., more circulating DNA signals a more severe event).

- Cell-free circulating DNA is also being explored as a biomarker for cancers. As tumor cells die they release fragments of their mutated DNA into the bloodstream. Sequencing this DNA can give insights into the tumor and possible treatments, and even be used to monitor tumor progression (as an alternative to invasive biopsies).

Clinical

- Pharmacogenomics involves using an individual's genome to determine whether or not a particular therapy, or dose of therapy, will be effective. Currently, more than 100 U.S. Food and Drug Administration (FDA)-approved drugs have pharmacogenomics information in their labels, in diverse fields such as analgesics, antivirals, cardiovascular drugs, and anti-cancer therapeutics.

- FDA has also cleared or approved 45 human genetic tests, and more than 100 nucleic acid-based tests for microbial pathogens.

- DNA sequencing is being used to investigate infectious disease outbreaks, including Ebola virus, drug-resistant strains of

Staphylococcus aureas and Klebsiella pneumoniae, as well as food poisoning following contamination with Escherichia coli. Sequencing has also recently been used to diagnose bacterial meningoencephalitis, rapidly identifying the correct therapeutic agent for the patient.

- Cystic fibrosis is one of the most common genetic diseases, caused by mutations in a gene called *CTFR*. More than 900 different CTFR mutations that cause cystic fibrosis have been identified to date. Approximately four percent of cases are caused by a mutation known as G551D, and now a drug called ivacaftor has been developed that is extraordinarily effective at treating this disease in individuals with this particular mutation.

- Whole genome sequencing or whole exome sequencing (where only the protein-coding exons within genes, rather than the entire genome, are sequenced), has been used to help doctors diagnose and, in some extraordinary cases, identify available treatments in rare disease cases. For example, Alexis and Noah Beery, a pair of Californian twins, were misdiagnosed with cerebral palsy, but DNA sequencing pointed to a new diagnosis, as well as a treatment, to which both children are responding well. Another patient who was misdiagnosed (for 30 years) with cerebral palsy was also found to have a treatable dopa-responsive dystonia thanks to whole exome sequencing. In another case, a young boy in Wisconsin, Nic Volker, was able to be cured of an extreme form of inflammatory bowel disease after his genome sequence revealed that a bone marrow transplant would likely be life-saving.

- The translation of new genomic medicine discoveries is already making a difference to patient care.

Section 23.2

Personalized Medicine

This section includes text excerpted from "FDA
Continues to Lead in Precision Medicine," U.S. Food and
Drug Administration (FDA), March 23, 2015.

Everyone knows that different people don't respond the same way to medications, and that "one size does not fit all." U.S. Food and Drug Administration (FDA) has been pushing for targeted drug therapies, sometimes called "personalized medicines" or "precision medicines," for a long time.

Targeted therapies make use of blood tests, images of the body, or other technologies to measure individual factors called "biomarkers." These biomarkers can then be used to determine who is most likely to benefit from a treatment, who is at higher risk of a side effect, or who needs a different dose. Targeting therapy can improve drug safety, and make sure that only people likely to have a good response get put on a drug.

Targeted therapies have gained public attention since President Obama announced a Precision Medicine Initiative in a State of the Union address. This initiative will reinforce their work at FDA, where development of targeted drug therapies has been a priority since the 1990s. In 1998, FDA approved the targeted therapy, Herceptin (trastuzumab), offering new hope for many patients with breast cancer. High levels of a biomarker, known as "HER-2," identified breast tumors that were more likely to be susceptible to this drug.

Since the approval of Herceptin, the development of targeted therapies has grown rapidly. FDA's Center for Drug Evaluation and Research (CDER) approved 30 targeted therapies since 2012, including Kalydeco (ivacaftor), a targeted drug for cystic fibrosis. In 2014 alone, eight of the 41 novel drugs approved were targeted, including:

1. **Lynparza** (olaparib) for the treatment of advanced ovarian cancer.

2. **Blincyto** (blinatumomab) for the treatment of B-cell precursor acute lymphoblastic leukemia (ALL).

3. **Harvoni** (ledipasvir and sofosbuvir) to treat patients with chronic hepatitis C infection.

4. **Viekira Pak** (ombitasvir, paritaprevir, dasabuvir and ritonavir) for the treatment of chronic hepatitis C infection.

5. **Cardelga** (eliglustat) for the long-term treatment of Gaucher disease type 1.

6. **Beleodaq** (belinostat) for the treatment of peripheral T-cell lymphoma.

7. **Zykadia** (ceritinib) to treat patients with nonsmall cell lung cancer (NSCLC).

8. **Vimizim** (elosulfase alpha) for the treatment of Mucopolysaccharidosis Type IV (Morquio Syndrome).

Since the 1990s, FDA has also been working on personalized drug dosing. People differ in how they eliminate a drug—some eliminate it much more slowly than most other people and are susceptible to overdosing, and others eliminate it much faster, and may not get any effect. There are biomarkers to identify people who have these unusual results, and CDER has been actively working for more than 15 years to put these findings into drug labels, so that each patient gets the correct dose, particularly for highly toxic or critically important drugs.

Personalized drug safety has also gotten attention. Often, one person experiences a serious side effect that does not affect thousands of others. Science is beginning to unlock the reasons for these rare toxicities, and the labels of some medicines advise screening people to make sure they are not at high risk for a severe side effect. This can make drugs much safer.

CDER has been recognized with awards from the Personalized Medicine Coalition and the Personalized Medicine World Conference for its longstanding work in this area.

CDER uses a lot of flexibility when reviewing applications for targeted drugs. Targeting people with a good chance of response means fewer people are eligible for a drug. CDER has adapted to the resulting small development programs. For example, among the targeted therapies approved in recent years, almost 60 percent were approved on the basis of one main clinical trial along with supporting evidence. In addition, 90 percent used one or more of FDA's expedited programs such as Breakthrough, Fast Track, Priority Review and Accelerated Approval.

It is still hard to develop targeted therapies for many diseases, because there isn't enough scientific understanding of why the disease occurs and what biomarkers would be useful. For many common illnesses, much more research is needed to reveal the individual differences that would enable development of targeted therapies.

Section 23.3

Nanomedicine

This section includes text excerpted from "Nanomedicine," National Human Genome Research Institute (NHGRI), January 22, 2014. Reviewed December 2017.

What if doctors had tiny tools that could search out and destroy the very first cancer cells of a tumor developing in the body? What if a cell's broken part could be removed and replaced with a functioning miniature biological machine? Or what if molecule-sized pumps could be implanted in sick people to deliver life-saving medicines precisely where they are needed? These scenarios may sound unbelievable, but they are the ultimate goals of nanomedicine, a cutting-edge area of biomedical research that seeks to use nanotechnology tools to improve human health.

What Is a Nanometer?

A lot of things are small in today's high-tech world of biomedical tools and therapies. But when it comes to nanomedicine, researchers are talking very, very small. A nanometer is one-billionth of a meter, too small even to be seen with a conventional lab microscope.

What Is Nanotechnology?

Nanotechnology is the broad scientific field that encompasses nanomedicine. It involves the creation and use of materials and devices at the level of molecules and atoms, which are the parts of matter that combine to make molecules. Nonmedical applications of nanotechnology now under development include tiny semiconductor chips made out of strings of single molecules and miniature computers made out of DNA, the material of our genes. Federally supported research in this area, conducted under the rubric of the National Nanotechnology Initiative, is ongoing with coordinated support from several agencies.

What Is Being Done to Advance Nanomedicine?

For hundreds of years, microscopes have offered scientists a window inside cells. Researchers have used ever more powerful visualization tools to extensively categorize the parts and sub-parts of cells in vivid detail. Yet, what scientists have not been able to do is to exhaustively inventory cells, cell parts, and molecules within cell parts to answer questions such as, "How many?" "How big?" and "How fast?" Obtaining thorough, reliable measures of quantity is the vital first step of nanomedicine.

As part of the National Institutes of Health (NIH) Common Fund Do we normally keep web addresses in the print editions? has established a handful of nanomedicine centers. These centers are staffed by a highly interdisciplinary scientific crew, including biologists, physicians, mathematicians, engineers, and computer scientists. Research conducted over the first few years was spent gathering extensive information about how molecular machines are built.

Once researchers had catalogued the interactions between and within molecules, they turned toward using that information to manipulate those molecular machines to treat specific diseases. For example, one center is trying to return at least limited vision to people who have lost their sight. Others are trying to develop treatments for severe neurological disorders, cancer, and a serious blood disorder.

The availability of innovative, body-friendly nanotools that depend on precise knowledge of how the body's molecular machines work, will help scientists figure out how to build synthetic biological and biochemical devices that can help the cells in our bodies work the way they were meant to, returning the body to a healthier state.

Section 23.4

Drug Delivery Systems

This section includes text excerpted from "Science
Education—Drug Delivery Systems: Getting Drugs to Their Targets
in a Controlled Manner," National Institute of Biomedical
Imaging and Bioengineering (NIBIB), October 2016.

What Are Drug Delivery Systems?

Drug delivery systems are engineered technologies for the targeted delivery and/or controlled release of therapeutic agents.

Drugs have long been used to improve health and extend lives. The practice of drug delivery has changed dramatically in the past few decades and even greater changes are anticipated in the near future. Biomedical engineers have contributed substantially to our understanding of the physiological barriers to efficient drug delivery, such as transport in the circulatory system and drug movement through cells and tissues; they have also contributed to the development several new modes of drug delivery that have entered clinical practice.

Yet, with all of this progress, many drugs, even those discovered using the most advanced molecular biology strategies, have unacceptable side effects due to the drug interacting with healthy tissues that are not the target of the drug. Side effects limit our ability to design optimal medications for many diseases such as cancer, neurodegenerative diseases, and infectious diseases.

Drug delivery systems control the rate at which a drug is released and the location in the body where it is released. Some systems can control both.

How Are Drug Delivery Systems Used in Current Medical Practice?

Clinicians historically have attempted to direct their interventions to areas of the body at risk or affected by a disease. Depending on the medication, the way it is delivered, and how our bodies respond, side effects sometimes occur. These side effects can vary greatly from person to person in type and severity. For example, an oral drug for seasonal allergies may cause unwanted drowsiness or an upset stomach.

Administering drugs locally rather than systemically (affecting the whole body) is a common way to decrease side effects and drug toxicity while maximizing a treatment's impact. A topical (used on the skin) antibacterial ointment for a localized infection or a cortisone injection of a painful joint can avoid some of the systemic side effects of these medications. There are other ways to achieve targeted drug delivery, but some medications can only be given systemically.

What Are Some Important Areas for Future Research in Drug Delivery Systems?

As scientists study how diseases develop and progress, they are also learning more about the different ways our bodies respond to illness and the influence of specific environmental or genetic cues. Coupled with advances in technology, this increased understanding suggests new approaches for drug delivery research. Key areas for future research include:

Crossing the Blood-Brain Barrier (BBB) in Brain Diseases and Disorders

When working properly, the various cells that comprise the BBB constantly regulate the transfer of essential substances between the bloodstream and the central nervous system as well as recognize and block entry of substances that may harm the brain. Delivering drugs into the brain is critical to the successful treatment of certain diseases such as brain tumors, Alzheimer disease, and Parkinson disease, but better methods are needed to cross or bypass the BBB. One method currently under study uses advanced ultrasound techniques that disrupt the BBB briefly and safely so medications can target brain tumors directly, with no surgery required.

Enhancing Targeted Intracellular Delivery

Just as the immune system defends the body against disease, each cell also has internal processes to recognize and get rid of potentially harmful substances and foreign objects. These foreign agents may include drugs enclosed in targeted delivery vehicles. So as researchers work to develop reliable methods of delivering treatments to targeted cells, further engineering is still needed to ensure the treatments reach the correct structures inside cells. Ideally, future healthcare will incorporate smart delivery systems that can bypass cellular defenses, transport drugs to targeted intracellular sites, and release the drugs in response to specific molecular signals.

Combining Diagnosis and Treatment

The full potential of drug delivery systems extends beyond treatment. By using advanced imaging technologies with targeted delivery, doctors may someday be able to diagnose and treat diseases in one step, a new strategy called theranostics.

Nanosized Treatment for Cancer

Nanoparticles can encapsulate or otherwise help to deliver medication directly to cancer cells and dramatically reduce the toxic effects of chemotherapy. Gold nanoparticles are being clinically investigated for application as probes for the detection of targeted sequences of nucleic acids and as potential treatments for cancer and other diseases.

(Source: "Benefits and Applications," U.S. National Nanotechnology Initiative.)

Section 23.5

Artificial Pancreas Device System

This section includes text excerpted from "Artificial Pancreas Device System," U.S. Food and Drug Administration (FDA), February 2, 2017.

What Is the Pancreas?

The pancreas is an organ in the body that secretes several hormones, including insulin and glucagon, as well as digestive enzymes that help break down food. Insulin helps cells in the body take up glucose (sugar) from the blood to use for energy, which lowers blood glucose levels. Glucagon causes the liver to release stored glucose, which raises blood glucose levels.

Type 1 diabetes occurs when the pancreas produces little or none of the insulin needed to regulate blood glucose. Type 2 diabetes occurs when the pancreas does not produce enough insulin or the body becomes resistant to the insulin that is present. Patients with type 1 diabetes and some patients with type 2 diabetes inject insulin, and occasionally glucagon, to regulate their blood glucose, which is critical to lower their risk of long-term complications such as blindness, kidney failure and cardiovascular disease.

When managing diabetes, many patients must vigilantly test blood glucose with a glucose meter, calculate insulin doses, and administer necessary insulin doses with a needle or insulin infusion pump to lower blood glucose. Glucagon may be injected in an emergency to treat severe low blood glucose. Some patients benefit from additional monitoring with a continuous glucose monitoring system.

What Is an Artificial Pancreas Device System (APDS)?

The Artificial Pancreas Device System (APDS) is a system of devices that closely mimics the glucose regulating function of a healthy pancreas.

Most APDS consists of devices already familiar to many people with diabetes: a continuous glucose monitoring system (CGM) and an insulin infusion pump. A blood glucose device (such as a glucose meter) is used to calibrate the CGM.

A computer-controlled algorithm connects the CGM and insulin infusion pump to allow continuous communication between the two devices. Sometimes an artificial pancreas device system is referred to as a "closed-loop" system, an "automated insulin delivery" system, or an "autonomous system for glycemic control."

An Artificial Pancreas Device System will not only monitors glucose levels in the body but also automatically adjusts the delivery of insulin to reduce high blood glucose levels (hyperglycemia) and minimize the incidence of low blood glucose (hypoglycemia) with little or no input from the patient.

The U.S. Food and Drug Administration (FDA) is collaborating with diabetes patient groups, diabetes care providers, medical device manufacturers, researchers, and academic investigators to foster innovation by clarifying agency expectations for clinical studies and product approvals. These efforts have accelerated the development of the first hybrid closed loop system, the Medtronic's MiniMed 670G System.

The FDA's guidance, The Content of Investigational Device Exemption (IDE) and Premarket Approval (PMA) Applications for Artificial Pancreas Device Systems, addresses requirements for clinical studies and premarket approval applications for and artificial pancreas device system, and provided a flexible regulatory approach to support the rapid, safe, and effective development of artificial pancreas device systems.

Types of Artificial Pancreas Device Systems

Researchers and manufacturers are developing three main categories of Artificial Pancreas Delivery System. They differ in how the insulin pump acts on readings from the continuous glucose monitoring system.

- Threshold Suspend Device System

- Insulin Only System

- Bi-Hormonal Control System

Threshold Suspend Device System

Threshold Suspend Device System The goal of a threshold suspend device system is to help reverse a dangerous drop in blood glucose level (hypoglycemia) or reduce its severity by temporarily suspending insulin delivery when the glucose level falls to or approaches a low glucose threshold. These are sometimes referred to as "low glucose suspend systems." This kind of system serves as a potential back-up when a patient is unable to respond to a low blood sugar (hypoglycemic) event. Patients using this system will still need to be active partners in managing their blood glucose levels by periodically checking their blood glucose levels and by giving themselves insulin or eating.

Insulin-Only System

An insulin-only system achieves a target glucose level by automatically increasing or decreasing the amount of insulin infused based on the CGM values. These systems could be hybrid systems that only automatically adjust basal insulin with the user manually delivering bolus insulin to cover meals, or could be fully closed loop systems, where the system can automatically adjust basal insulin and provide insulin for meals.

Bi-Hormonal Control System

A bi-hormonal control system achieves a target glucose level by using two algorithms to instruct an infusion pump to deliver two different hormones one hormone (insulin) to lower glucose levels and another (such as glucagon) to increase blood glucose levels. The bad word break here monal system mimics the glucose-regulating function of a healthy pancreas more closely than an insulin-only system.

The Artificial Pancreas System (An Autonomous System for Glycemic Control)

This image shows the parts of a type of artificial pancreas device system and describes how they work together.

1. **Continuous Glucose Monitor (CGM).** A CGM provides a steady stream of information that reflects the patient's blood glucose levels. A sensor placed under the patient's skin (subcutaneously) measures the glucose in the fluid around the cells (interstitial fluid) which is associated with blood glucose levels. A small transmitter sends information to a receiver. A CGM continuously displays both an estimate of blood glucose levels and their direction and rate of change of these estimates.

   - **Blood Glucose Device (BGD).** Currently, to get the most accurate estimates of blood glucose possible from a CGM,

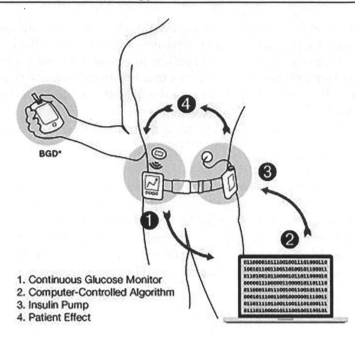

1. Continuous Glucose Monitor
2. Computer-Controlled Algorithm
3. Insulin Pump
4. Patient Effect

Figure 23.1. *Artificial Pancreas Device System*

the patient needs to periodically calibrate the CGM using a blood glucose measurement from a BGD; therefore, the BGD still plays a critical role in the proper management of patients with an APDS. However, over time, we anticipate that improved CGM performance may do away with the need for periodic blood glucose checks with a BGD.

2. **Control algorithm.** A control algorithm is software embedded in an external processor (controller) that receives information from the CGM and performs a series of mathematical calculations. Based on these calculations, the controller sends dosing instructions to the infusion pump. The control algorithm can be run on any number of devices including an insulin pump, computer or cellular phone. The FDA does not require the control algorithm to reside on the insulin pump.

3. **Insulin pump.** Based on the instructions sent by the controller, an infusion pump adjusts the insulin delivery to the tissue under the skin.

4. **The patient.** The patient is an important part of Artificial
   Pancreas Delivery System. The concentration of glucose circulating in the patient's blood is constantly changing. It is
   affected by the patient's diet, activity level, and how his or her
   body metabolizes insulin and other substances.

The Miracle of an Artificial Pancreas

This is going to be a life-changing technology for people with type 1
diabetes. To effectively manage type 1 diabetes requires a constant
monitoring of blood glucose levels, delivering the right amount of
insulin considering the diet, amount of physical activity and other
activities of daily living.

*(Source: "The Miracle of an Artificial Pancreas," National Institutes
of Health (NIH).)*

Chapter 24

Surgical Treatment Technology (STT)

Chapter Contents

Section 24.1—Surgical Robots for Tumor Treatment 212

Section 24.2—Robotic-Assisted Surgery (RAS) 214

Section 24.3—Computer-Assisted Surgical Systems 220

Section 24.4—Technologies Enhance Tumor Surgery 222

Section 24.5—Smart Operating Rooms of the Future 225

Section 24.1

Surgical Robots for Tumor Treatment

This section includes text excerpted from "From Orbit to Operating Rooms, Space Station Technology Translates to Tumor Treatment," National Aeronautics and Space Administration (NASA), November 22, 2013. Reviewed December 2017.

People commonly use rocket science or brain surgery to refer to something incredibly complex and difficult. No wonder, then, that combining the two could result in something wonderful.

Powerful robotic arms developed by the Canadian Space Agency (CSA) for the space shuttle and International Space Station—Canadarm and Canadarm2—and a delicate surgical tool, dubbed neuroArm, are examples of the "wonderful things" that can happen when experts from different disciplines work together, says Garnette Sutherland, MD.

Sutherland, a neurosurgery professor at the University of Calgary in Canada, used the first-generation neuroArm to conduct a clinical trial on 50 patients. That work, the subject of a paper published in the Journal of Neurosurgery, concluded that surgical robots such as this one improve precision and accuracy during brain surgery.

"A machine is inherently more precise and accurate than a human, as it can move in increments of microns while humans move in increments of millimeters," said Sutherland. "The registration parameter of a robotic machine can be set to a specific patient and so is very accurate. It can do motion scaling, meaning if you move your hand an inch the machine might move one-twentieth of an inch, according to the scale you set. It moves much less and so is more precise." Robotics also can filter out the tremors and shakiness that everyone has in their hands, further increasing the precision of the tool.

The surgical robotic arm was designed to work in conjunction with a magnetic resonance imaging (MRI) machine, as well as actually inside an MRI. This gives surgeons the ability to continually monitor their progress through detailed, three-dimensional images. A surgeon operates from a remote workstation that recreates the sight, sound and touch of surgery.

"When the tool tip hits tissue, it sends force back to the hand controller so the surgeon can feel what is touched," Sutherland said, somewhat like the vibration players feel in a videogame joystick, only much more realistic.

The robotic sense of touch also allows surgeons to create a defined area within the body so that the tool encounters resistance if it reaches the edges of that area. The surgeon can see the operation through high-resolution, three-dimensional screens and hear it through a headset. Theoretically, the machine can even give surgeons the ability to see what they normally could not through the use of fluorescent markers and feel what they cannot normally feel, as the robotic arm can detect forces smaller than those normally appreciated by humans. In essence, the robot amplifies the surgeon's innate abilities.

The surgeon remains a critical part of the process, according to Sutherland. In between the hand controller and the surgical robotic arm is a computer. Computers are linear processors, needing all the data before they can execute a motion independently, and they can't rely on past experience. A surgeon, based on past experience, can anticipate or guess what might happen during surgery. "Computers can't guess and humans can," he adds. "The human brain is a parallel processing unit, capable of responding to incomplete data, resulting in fast and smooth motion. A machine is slower, but more certain." Another benefit of collaboration.

The leap from a large and powerful robotic arm in space to a small, precise one in the operating room wasn't as great of a stretch as it might seem at first, said Sutherland. "Many years ago, MacDonald, Dettwiler and Associates Ltd. (MDA) received the contract to build Canadarm and (the Canadian Special Purpose Dexterous Manipulator) Dextre on the (space station). They hired a pile of engineers to go through the process of building these robots. When we had the idea to use a robot for neurosurgery, we gave MDA the requirements, and those same engineers with decades of experience building robots for space began to translate that work into this one."

Similarities between the Canadarms and neuroArm include the control mechanism and the joint architecture, albeit on a smaller scale. The surgery tool incorporates other features of its larger counterparts, such as the strong, lightweight materials developed for the space station, including nonmagnetic polymers, because materials used inside an MRI must be nonmagnetic.

In July, Sutherland was recognized at the second annual International Space Station Research and Development Conference for Advancing Neurosurgery through Space Technology, with neuroArm named a Top Medical Application from the International Space Station for 2012. The award recognizes the translation of technology developed specifically for one field—space—into an unrelated field in a unique and practical fashion. Looking toward the future, Sutherland notes that this robot/human collaboration potentially can benefit any kind of operation requiring precision. "It's built for micro-surgery, whatever that might be." Either way, it's still rocket science.

Section 24.2

Robotic-Assisted Surgery (RAS)

This section includes text excerpted from "Robotic Surgery: Risks vs. Rewards," Agency for Healthcare Research and Quality (AHRQ), U.S. Department of Health and Human Services (HHS), February 2016.

Background and Prevalence of Robotics in Surgery

The use of robotic assistance in surgery has expanded exponentially since it was first approved in 2000. It is estimated that, worldwide, more than 570,000 procedures were performed with the da Vinci robotic surgical system in 2014, with this figure growing almost 10 percent each year. Robotic-assisted surgery (RAS) has found its way into almost every surgical subspecialty and now has approved uses in urology, gynecology, cardiothoracic surgery, general surgery, and otolaryngology. RAS is most commonly used in urology and gynecology; more than 75 percent of robotic procedures performed are within these two specialties. Robotic surgical systems have the potential to improve surgical technique and outcomes, but they also create a unique set of risks and patient safety concerns.

RAS is a derivative of standard laparoscopic surgery and was developed to overcome the limitations of standard laparoscopy. Like traditional laparoscopy, RAS uses small incisions and insufflation of the anatomical operative space with carbon dioxide. The robotic camera and various instruments are placed through the ports into the body and can be manipulated by the surgeon performing the operation. In the case of RAS, though, the surgeon, seated at a computer console in the operating room, uses robot assistance to utilize the tools (instead of doing it himself or herself directly at the bedside). In RAS, a bedside assistant exchanges the instruments and performs manual tasks like retraction and suction. The da Vinci robotic surgical system, made by Intuitive Surgical, Inc., is the only robotic system on the market today. There are three major components of the system including:

- The robot, which is a mobile tower with four arms, including a camera arm and three instrument arms.

- The bedside cart, consisting of the image processing equipment and light source, which is transmitted to monitors in the operating suite and sends the image to the surgeon console.

- The console, at which the surgeon sits to operate; there are two binocular lenses that magnify and create a three-dimensional image for the surgeon. Two handpieces transmit the surgeon's hand movements to the instruments within the patient, manipulating the surgical instruments to perform the operation. A built-in motion filtration system minimizes tremor, and foot pedals at the console control different types of energy and also allow for movement of the different robotic components within the patient.

Benefits of Robotic-Assisted Surgery

In theory, RAS marries the benefits of laparoscopic surgery with that of open techniques by combining a minimally invasive approach with the additional benefit of a three-dimensional, magnified image. In addition, RAS offers improved ergonomics and dexterity compared to traditional laparoscopy, and these advantages may lead to a shorter learning curve for surgeons. The purported benefits of RAS also include smaller incisions, decreased blood loss, shorter hospital stays, faster return to work, improved cosmesis, and lower incidence of some surgical complications.

Most of these benefits are short term and limited to the acute perioperative period. In fact, there is little evidence demonstrating that robotic surgery provides any long-term benefits over open techniques. Taking the above case as an example, robotic-assisted laparoscopic prostatectomy (RALP) has been one of the most commonly adopted robotic procedures; more than 85 percent of all prostatectomies are now performed with robotic assistance in the United States. Multiple, well-validated studies have shown that RALP has significantly less blood loss, with much lower transfusion rates, and shorter hospital stays than with open approaches. In addition, the rates of some complications—deep vein thrombosis, wound infections, lymphoceles and hematomas, anastomotic leaks, and ureteral injuries—appear to be slightly lower than with open approaches. RALP appears to have similar advantages over laparoscopic prostatectomy, although the difference is less pronounced. When compared to standard laparoscopic prostatectomy, robotic assistance has been shown to have decreased blood loss, lower rates of blood transfusion, and slightly shorter hospital stays. Like with robotic assistance, pure laparoscopic techniques share a significant learning curve. While some studies have also suggested that robotic surgery may be more effective at total removal of cancerous tissue in prostate surgery (i.e., lower positive surgical margin rates) than with open and pure laparoscopic procedures, large systematic reviews and well-validated meta-analyses have shown similar rates of oncologic control.

Interestingly, the proponents of RALP frequently boast improved urinary continence and sexual function after surgery (or at least equivalent rates) when compared to open prostatectomy. The data has generally been equivocal in this area; standardized, comparable, long-term data are lacking. A study using surveillance, epidemiology, and end results Medicare claims data compared open to minimally invasive prostatectomy (laparoscopic and robotic). Their results supported previous findings of lower transfusion rates, shorter hospital stays, similar oncologic control, and fewer miscellaneous complications. On the other hand, they discovered that men who had undergone robotic prostatectomy had higher rates of postprostatectomy incontinence and erectile dysfunction than men who had an open procedure. It may be a matter of experience: many of RALP proponents have performed thousands of procedures, which may lead to improved outcomes in their hands but may not be generalized to other, less experienced, urologists.

Risks of Robotic-Assisted Surgery

RAS shares the same risks of open and laparoscopic surgery, including the potential for infection, bleeding, and the cardiopulmonary risks of anesthesia. On top of that, there are additional risks that are unique to the robotic system. Not only is there potential for human error in operating the robotic technology, but an added risk of mechanical failure is also introduced. Multiple components of the system can malfunction, including the camera, binocular lenses, robotic tower, robotic arms, and instruments. The energy source, which is prone to electric arcing, can cause unintended internal burn injuries from the cautery device. Arcing occurs when electrical current from the robotic instrument leaves the robotic arm and is misdirected to surrounding tissue. This can cause sparks and burns leading to tissue damage which may not always be immediately recognized. There is a small risk of temporary, and even permanent, nerve palsies from the extreme body positioning needed to dock the robot and access the pelvis adequately to perform RALP. Direct nerve compression from the robotic arms can also lead to nerve palsies. RAS has also been shown to take significantly longer than nonrobotic procedures when performed at centers with lower robotic volume and by surgeons with less experience, and, overall, it is more expensive than open surgery.

As mentioned earlier, the outcomes in RAS seem to correlate with individual surgeon experience. For example, in cancer surgery, surgeons with more experience are more likely to have clean margins. Other studies have documented lower complication rates with an increasing number of procedures. These findings of practice makes perfect are not specific to robotic surgery; such findings have been seen in many procedures. There are varying reports of exactly how many cases are required to master the robotic learning curve, and the number varies by surgical procedure. For RALP, the range has been reported from as low as 40 to as many as 250. For hysterectomies, the literature reports a range of 20–50 cases to master the operation and reports that less experienced surgeons have significantly longer operative times.

Notwithstanding the concerns, RAS has been accepted as generally safe. RALP has reported complication rates (including all grades of perioperative complications, from minor to life-threatening) of around 10 percent. Multiple risk factors can increase the possibility of complications and errors: patient factors (i.e., obesity or underlying comorbidities), surgeon factors (training and experience), and robotic factors (i.e., mechanical malfunction). The reported complication rate related directly to robotic malfunction is very low (approximately 0.1%–0.5%). However, when robotic errors do occur, the rates of permanent injury have been reported anywhere from 4.8 percent–46.6 percent, and this literature may suffer from underreporting. Although fewer than 800 complications directly attributable to the robotic operating system have been reported to the U.S. Food and Drug Administration (FDA) over the past 10 years, in a web-based survey among urologists performing RALP, almost 57 percent of respondents had experienced an irrecoverable intraoperative malfunction of the robot. The most common areas of complications were malfunction of the robotic arms, joint setup and camera, followed by power error, instrument malfunction, and breakage of the handpiece.

Preventing Complications of Robotic-Assisted Surgery

Standardized Credentialing and Training

Currently, there are no universal standard guidelines on appropriate training or credentialing for robotic surgery. Some organizations have made progress in this area. The American Urological Association (AUA) has made recommendations for training and credentialing procedures consisting of specific online curriculum, testing, caseload requirements, and also recommendations that all physicians complete the da Vinci online robotic safety training course on set-up, draping, specific safety features, and troubleshooting. Training in robotics is still a relatively new field, and there is not a strong body of evidence to support a specific training and credentialing model. Various authors have developed different curriculums and simulation models, but an ideal model has yet to be found, as this is a new and developing field. Until well-validated credentialing and training models can be developed, hospitals should require a basic robotic safety curriculum, such as provided by the AUA, for any surgeons using the surgical robot, and require case logs be supplied or case proctoring prior to granting robotic privileges.

Stricter Reporting Guidelines

Developing a more uniform system of error reporting and tougher penalties for noncompliance may potentially help capture a more accurate representation of the true incidence of adverse events. It is important to determine the true incidence of different complications and the surrounding circumstances. The goal should be to identify key risk factors for errors and complications with a focus on those that are modifiable. This ideally would lead to improved outcomes and fewer complications. There are clearly gaps with the current FDA device tracking system, as many more robotic errors are experienced than are ever reported to the FDA. There needs to be a more rigorous reporting effort by individual hospitals to capture the true incidence of robotic malfunction. These institutional reports can be submitted to the FDA so that recurrent mechanical problems can be more easily and rapidly recognized and addressed by the manufacturer.

Appropriate Risk Disclosure to Patients

The idea of robotic surgery is very enticing to patients and has influenced the growth of robotics in the United States. However, Schroeck and colleagues found that men undergoing robotic prostatectomy were more likely to express "regret" and "dissatisfaction" than men undergoing open surgery, which was attributed to unrealistic patient expectations associated with the robot. Kaushik and colleagues found that less than 70 percent of patients were appropriately counseled preoperatively on the potential risks specific to robotic surgery, including possible robotic malfunction or potential conversion to an open procedure. The direct-to-consumer marketing phenomenon could be used to improve safety in robotics by appropriately educating patients. Institutions should ensure appropriate patient counseling and informed consent for RAS is happening consistently. This tracking could be accomplished through auditing of informed consent materials as well as intermittent patient interviews.

While RAS has many potential benefits for patients and providers, the case above clearly demonstrates that the technology itself may place patients at risk. National organizations and individual institutions should ensure appropriate training and credentialing, accurate and timely error reporting, and consistent informed consent for patients. Discussions about robotic surgery—both with individual patients and at the policy level—should appropriately balance the advantages and potential with the real risks and limited evidence of major advantages in terms of long-term outcomes.

Take-Home Points

- Robotic surgery is a rapidly expanding technology that has found a niche in multiple different surgical specialties worldwide.

- Although robotic-assisted surgery shows some short-term benefits surrounding the direct perioperative period, it has fairly equivalent long-term outcomes when compared to open surgery.

- Robotic surgery is generally safe with low overall complication rates, but adding the robot to the surgical equation inserts another potential entry point for error into an already complex and risk-fraught arena.

- In general, surgical outcomes are ultimately a direct manifestation of the skill and experience of the surgeon, not the technology or approach used.

- Potential areas for improvement and reduction of error in robotic surgery include more standardized training and credentialing practices, improved reporting systems for robotic-associated adverse events, and enhanced patient education.

Section 24.3

Computer-Assisted Surgical Systems

This section includes text excerpted from "Medical Devices—Computer-Assisted Surgical Systems," U.S. Food and Drug Administration (FDA), July 29, 2015.

What Are Computer-Assisted Surgical Systems?

Different types of computer-assisted surgical systems can be used for preoperative planning, surgical navigation and to assist in performing surgical procedures. Robotically-assisted surgical (RAS) devices are one type of computer-assisted surgical system. Sometimes referred to as robotic surgery, RAS devices enable the surgeon to use computer and software technology to control and move surgical instruments through one or more tiny incisions in the patient's body (minimally invasive) for a variety of surgical procedures.

The benefits of a RAS device may include its ability to facilitate minimally invasive surgery and assist with complex tasks in confined areas of the body. The device is not actually a robot because it cannot perform surgery without direct human control.

RAS devices generally have several components, which may include:

- A console, where the surgeon sits during surgery. The console is the control center of the device and allows the surgeon to view the surgical field through a 3D endoscope and control movement of the surgical instruments;

- The bedside cart that includes three or four hinged mechanical arms, camera (endoscope) and surgical instruments that the surgeon controls during surgical procedures; and

- A separate cart that contains supporting hardware and software components, such as an electrosurgical unit (ESU), suction/irrigation pumps, and light source for the endoscope.

Most surgeons use multiple surgical instruments and accessories with the RAS device, such as scalpels, forceps, graspers, dissectors, cautery, scissors, retractors and suction irrigators.

Common Uses of Robotically-Assisted Surgical (RAS) Devices

The U.S. Food and Drug Administration (FDA) has cleared RAS devices for use by trained physicians in an operating room environment for laparoscopic surgical procedures in general surgery cardiac, colorectal, gynecologic, head and neck, thoracic and urologic surgical procedures. Some common procedures that may involve RAS devices are gall-bladder removal, hysterectomy and prostatectomy (removal of the prostate).

Recommendations for Patients and Healthcare Providers about Robotically-Assisted Surgery

Patients: Robotically-assisted surgery is an important treatment option but may not be appropriate in all situations. Talk to your physician about the risks and benefits of robotically-assisted surgeries, as well as the risks and benefits of other treatment options.

Patients who are considering treatment with robotically-assisted surgeries should discuss the options for these devices with their healthcare provider, and feel free to inquire about their surgeon's training and experience with these devices.

Healthcare Providers: Robotically-assisted surgery is an important treatment option that is safe and effective when used appropriately and with proper training. The FDA does not regulate the practice of medicine and therefore does not supervise or provide accreditation for physician training nor does it oversee training and education related to legally marketed medical devices. Instead, training development and implementation is the responsibility of the manufacturer, physicians, and healthcare facilities. In some cases, professional societies and specialty board certification organizations may also develop and support training for their specialty physicians. Specialty boards also maintain certification status of their specialty physicians.

Physicians, hospitals and facilities that use RAS devices should ensure that proper training is completed and that surgeons have appropriate credentials to perform surgical procedures with these devices. Device users should ensure they maintain their credentialing.

Hospitals and facilities should also ensure that other surgical staff that use these devices complete proper training.

Users of the device should realize that there are several different models of robotically-assisted surgical devices. Each model may operate differently and may not have the same functions. Users should know the differences between the models and make sure to get appropriate training on each model.

If you suspect a problem or complications associated with the use of RAS devices, the FDA encourages you to file a voluntary report through MedWatch, the FDA Safety Information and Adverse Event Reporting program. Healthcare personnel employed by facilities that are subject to FDA's user facility reporting requirements should follow the reporting procedures established by their facilities.

Section 24.4

Technologies Enhance Tumor Surgery

This section includes text excerpted from "Technologies Enhance Tumor Surgery," *NIH News in Health*, National Institutes of Health (NIH), February 2016.

Helping Surgeons Spot and Remove Cancer

For surgeons, removing a tumor is a balancing act. Cut out too much and you risk removing healthy tissues that have important functions. Remove too little and you may leave behind cancer cells that could grow back into a tumor over time.

National Institutes of Health (NIH)-funded researchers are developing new technologies to help surgeons determine exactly where tumors end and healthy tissue begins. Their ultimate goal is to make surgery for cancer patients safer and more effective.

"Currently, surgeons view magnetic resonance imaging (MRI) and Computed Tomography (CT) scans taken prior to an operation to establish where a tumor is located and to plan a surgical approach that will minimize damage to healthy tissues," says Dr. Steven Krosnick, an NIH expert in image-guided surgery. "But once the operation has begun, surgeons generally rely only on their eyes and sense of touch to distinguish tumor from healthy tissue."

Surgeons go through many years of training to understand the subtle cues that can distinguish tumor from normal surroundings. Sometimes the tumor is a slightly different color than healthy tissue, or it feels different. It might also bleed more readily or could contain calcium deposits. Even with these cues, however, surgeons don't always get it right.

"In a lot of cases, we leave tumor behind that could be safely removed if only we were able to better visualize it," says Dr. Daniel Orringer, a neurosurgeon at the University of Michigan.

In today's operating rooms, pathologists can often help surgeons determine if all of a tumor has been taken out. A pathologist may view the edges of the tissue under a microscope and look for cancer cells. If they're found, the surgeon will remove more tissue from the patient and send these again to the pathologist for review. This process can occur repeatedly while the patient remains on the operating table and continue until no cancer cells are detected.

"Each time a pathologist analyzes tissue during an operation, it can take up to 30 minutes because the tissue has to be frozen, thinly sliced, and stained so it can be viewed under the microscope," Krosnick says. "If multiple rounds of tissue are taken, it can greatly increase the length of the surgery."

In the days following an operation, the pathologist conducts a more thorough review of the tissue. If cancer cells are found at the margins, the patient may undergo a second surgery to remove cancer that was left behind.

Orringer is part of a research team that's testing a new technology that could help surgeons tell the difference between a tumor and healthy brain tissue during surgery. The team developed a special microscope with NIH support that shoots a pair of low-energy lasers at the tissue. That causes the chemical bonds in the tissue's molecules to vibrate. The vibrations are then analyzed by a computer and used to create detailed images of the tissue.

From a molecular point of view, the components of a tumor differ from those in healthy tissue. This specialized microscope can reveal differences between the tissues that can't be seen with the naked eye.

"Our technology enables us to get a microscopic view of human tissues without taking them out of the body," Orringer says. "We can see cells, blood vessels, the connections between brain cells, all of the microscopic components that make up the brain."

Orringer and colleagues developed a computer program that can quickly analyze the images and assess whether or not cancer cells are present. This type of analysis could help surgeons decide whether all of a tumor has been cut out. To date, Orringer has used the specialized microscope to help remove cancer tissue in nearly 100 patients with brain tumors.

Other researchers are taking different approaches. For example, Dr. Quyen Nguyen—a head and neck surgeon at the University of California, San Diego—has developed a fluorescent molecule that's currently being tested in clinical trials. The patient receives an injection of the molecules before surgery. When exposed to certain types of light, these molecules cause cancer cells to glow, making them easier to spot and remove. The surgeon then uses a near-infrared camera to visualize the glowing tumor cells while operating.

Nguyen is also developing a fluorescent molecule to light up nerves. Accidental nerve injury during surgery can leave patients with loss of movement or feeling. In some cases, sexual function may be impaired.

"Nerves are really, really small, and they're often buried in soft tissue or encased within bone. When we have to do cancer surgery, they can be encased in the cancer itself," Nguyen says. The fluorescent molecule could help surgeons detect hard-to-spot nerves, so they can be protected. The nerve-tagging molecule is now being tested in animal studies.

Other NIH-funded researchers are focusing on ways to speed up cancer surgeries. Dr. Milind Rajadhyaksha, a researcher at Memorial Sloan Kettering Cancer Center, has developed a microscope technique to reduce the amount of time it takes to perform a common surgery for removing nonmelanoma skin cancers.

Each year about 2 million people in the U.S. undergo Mohs surgery, in which a doctor successively removes suspicious areas until the surrounding skin tissue is free of cancer. The procedure can take several hours, because each time more tissue is removed, it has to be prepared and reviewed under a microscope to determine if cancer cells remain. This step can take up to 30 minutes.

The technique developed by Rajadhyaksha shortens the time for assessing removed tissue to less than 5 minutes, which greatly reduces the overall length of the procedure. Tissue is mounted in a specialized microscope that uses a focused laser line to do multiple scans of the tissue. The resulting image "strips" are then combined, like a mosaic, into a complete microscopic image of the tissue.

About 1,000 specialized skin surgeries have already been performed guided by this technique. Rajadhyaksha is currently developing an approach that would allow doctors to use the technology directly on a patient's skin, before any tissue has been removed. This would allow doctors to identify the edges of tumors before the start of surgery and reduce the need for several pre-surgical "margin-mapping" biopsies.

There are many types of cancer surgeries, and researchers continue to work hard to develop better techniques.

Mini-Heat Pipes Wick Away Heat in Brain Surgery

In any brain surgery, the neurosurgeon must have precise and reliable tools for procedures. One important tool is bipolar forceps. It uses electricity to cut and cauterize tissues. This process produces enormous heat and can burn healthy tissues.

(Source: "Mini Heat Pipes Wick Away Heat in Brain Surgery," National Aeronautics and Space Administration (NASA).)

Section 24.5

Smart Operating Rooms of the Future

This section includes text excerpted from "Pillars of a Smart, Safe Operating Room," Agency for Healthcare Research and Quality (AHRQ), U.S. Department of Health and Human Services (HHS), August 2008. Reviewed December 2017.

The state of the art in operating room (OR) safety, while always evolving, can be revolutionized through smart application of technology and knowledge. Recent advances in technology have moved us from a traditional surgical suite toward one that is more efficient and safe. That evolution continues in the operating rooms of future (ORF), where research seeks to identify and address novel approaches to an array of domains often overlooked in the safety literature.

Cognitive Simulation

As new surgical technologies and techniques emerge, patients are often torn between wanting to avail themselves of the latest therapeutic options, yet wanting to be reassured that their surgeon is adequately trained and has already ascended the requisite learning curve. Surgical educators have been hesitant to mandate simulators for the training of surgical novices even as they recognize the need to separate surgical trainee learning from direct patient contact. The cautious approach to acceptance of simulation training was based, in part, on the initial lack of robust scientific evidence to support the use of medical simulation for skills training and also on the lack of knowledge of how to effectively apply simulation to a surgical skills training program. Fortunately, the acceptance of simulation training by boards and certifying agencies is on the rise.

Smart Imaging

Medical practice is considered among the most complex and difficult fields. That no two patients are exactly alike is one of the challenges that makes it so. Anatomic and physiologic differences make each case unique. In surgery, these variations can complicate an operation; the discovery of unexpected anatomical variations often requires a surgeon to stray from standard, well-practiced techniques to attempt a novel approach to the procedure. With novelty comes a reduced margin of safety. This situation is exacerbated by a trend toward further physical separation between the patient and interventionalists (e.g., surgeons, endoscopists, radiologists) and a greater dependence on an image of the patient's (target) anatomy to effect therapy or establish a diagnosis.

Informatics

The manager of a well run OR suite should maintain an awareness of the surgeons, anesthetists, nurses, patients, and major pieces of equipment that are present. The harsh reality in current medical practice is that most commercial warehouses and supermarkets track their assets and inventories in a far more sophisticated way than it's done in the perioperative environment.

Smart Environments

In the future, smart environments would guide the training of medical care providers by tracking their progress, providing feedback, and assuring proper credentialing. Smart environments would also speed training and improve safety. In the operative environment, this same type of tracking would augment human vigilance, further preventing adverse outcomes through automated, context aware safety checks.

Future Vision of the Operating Room Environment

Well-trained care providers, who have reached a level of proficiency on realistically simulated patients, are supported by an array of smart technology enabling surgical procedures to be performed in an ever safer environment. Cases start on time with all team members informed of the goals and possible trouble spots of each operation. Contingency plans are in place for dealing with anticipated complications. The smart environment checks that all required equipment and people are present and cross-checks drugs and blood products brought into the room, ensuring patient compatibility in terms of allergies and blood type. Surgeons do not have to fight fatigue and discomfort during surgery, as the layout of the surgical workspace is ergonomically correct. Thus, the time and effort needed to perform surgery is minimized and improvement of both technique and outcomes is realized.

Chapter 25

Technology and the Future of Mental Health Treatment

Technology has opened a new frontier in mental health support and data collection. Mobile devices like cell phones, smartphones, and tablets are giving the public, doctors, and researchers new ways to access help, monitor progress, and increase understanding of mental well-being.

Mobile mental health support can be very simple but effective. For example, anyone with the ability to send a text message can contact a crisis center. New technology can also be packaged into an extremely sophisticated app for smartphones or tablets. Such apps might use the device's built-in sensors to collect information on a user's typical behavior patterns. If the app detects a change in behavior, it may provide a signal that help is needed before a crisis occurs. Some apps are stand-alone programs that promise to improve memory or thinking skills. Others help the user connect to a peer counselor or to a healthcare professional.

Excitement about the huge range of opportunities has led to a burst of app development. There are thousands of mental health apps available in iTunes and Android app stores, and the number is growing

This chapter includes text excerpted from "Technology and the Future of Mental Health Treatment," National Institute of Mental Health (NIMH), February 2017.

every year. However, this new technology frontier includes a lot of uncertainty. There is very little industry regulation and very little information on app effectiveness, which can lead consumers to wonder which apps they should trust.

Before focusing on the state of the science and where it may lead, it's important to look at the advantages and disadvantages of expanding mental health treatment and research into a mobile world.

The Pros and Cons of Mental Health Apps

Experts believe that technology has a lot of potential for clients and clinicians alike. A few of the advantages of mobile care include:

Convenience: Treatment can take place anytime and anywhere (e.g., at home in the middle of the night or on a bus on the way to work) and may be ideal for those who have trouble with in-person appointments.

Anonymity: Clients can seek treatment options without involving other people.

An introduction to care: Technology may be a good first step for those who have avoided mental healthcare in the past.

Lower cost: Some apps are free or cost less than traditional care.

Service to more people: Technology can help mental health providers offer treatment to people in remote areas or to many people in times of sudden need (for example, following a natural disaster or terror attack).

Interest: Some technologies might be more appealing than traditional treatment methods, which may encourage clients to continue therapy.

24-hour service: Technology can provide round-the-clock monitoring or intervention support.

Consistency: Technology can offer the same treatment program to all users.

Support: Technology can complement traditional therapy by extending an in-person session, reinforcing new skills, and providing support and monitoring.

This new era of mental health technology offers great opportunities but also raises a number of concerns. Tackling potential problems will be an important part of making sure new apps provide benefits without causing harm. That is why the mental health community and software developers are focusing on:

Effectiveness: The biggest concern with technological interventions is obtaining scientific evidence that they work and that they work as well as traditional methods.

For whom and for what: Another concern is understanding if apps work for all people and for all mental health conditions.

Guidance: There are no industry-wide standards to help consumers know if an app or other mobile technology is proven effective.

Privacy: Apps deal with very sensitive personal information so app makers need to be able to guarantee privacy for app users.

Regulation: The question of who will or should regulate mental health technology and the data it generates needs to be answered.

Overselling: There is some concern that if an app or program promises more than it delivers, consumers may turn away from other, more effective therapies.

Current Trends in App Development

Creative research and engineering teams are combining their skills to address a wide range of mental health concerns. Some popular areas of app development include:

Self-Management Apps

"Self-management" means that the user puts information into the app so that the app can provide feedback. For example, the user might set up medication reminders, or use the app to develop tools for managing stress, anxiety, or sleep problems. Some software can use additional equipment to track heart rate, breathing patterns, blood pressure, etc. and may help the user track progress and receive feedback.

Apps for Improving Thinking Skills

Apps that help the user with cognitive remediation (improved thinking skills) are promising. These apps are often targeted toward people with serious mental illnesses.

Skill-Training Apps

Skill-training apps may feel more like games than other mental health apps as they help users learn new coping or thinking skills. The user might watch an educational video about anxiety management or the importance of social support. Next, the user might pick some new strategies to try and then use the app to track how often those new skills are practiced.

Illness Management, Supported Care

This type of app technology adds additional support by allowing the user to interact with another human being. The app may help the user connect with peer support or may send information to a trained healthcare provider who can offer guidance and therapy options. Researchers are working to learn how much human interaction people need for app-based treatments to be effective.

Passive Symptom Tracking

A lot of effort is going into developing apps that can collect data using the sensors built into smartphones. These sensors can record movement patterns, social interactions (such as the number of texts and phone calls), behavior at different times of the day, vocal tone and speed, and more. In the future, apps may be able to analyze these data to determine the user's real-time state of mind. Such apps may be able to recognize changes in behavior patterns that signal a mood episode such as mania, depression, or psychosis before it occurs. An app may not replace a mental health professional, but it may be able to alert caregivers when a client needs additional attention. The goal is to create apps that support a range of users, including those with serious mental illnesses.

Data Collection

Data collection apps can gather data without any help from the user. Receiving information from a large number of individuals at the same time can increase researchers' understanding of mental health and help them develop better interventions.

Research via Smartphone

Dr. Patricia Areán's pioneering BRIGHTEN study, showed that research via smartphone app is already a reality. The BRIGHTEN study was remarkable because it used technology to both deliver treatment interventions and also to actually conduct the research trial. In other words, the research team used technology to recruit, screen, enroll, treat, and assess participants. BRIGHTEN was especially exciting because the study showed that technology can be an efficient way to pilot test promising new treatments, and that those treatments need to be engaging.

Evaluating Apps

There are no review boards, checklists, or widely accepted rules for choosing a mental health app. Most apps do not have peer-reviewed research to support their claims, and it is unlikely that every mental health app will go through a randomized, controlled research trial to test effectiveness. One reason is that testing is a slow process and technology evolves quickly. By the time an app has been put through rigorous scientific testing, the original technology may be outdated.

Currently, there are no national standards for evaluating the effectiveness of the hundreds of mental health apps that are available. Consumers should be cautious about trusting a program. However, there are a few suggestions for finding an app that may work for you:

- Ask a trusted healthcare provider for a recommendation. Some larger providers may offer several apps and collect data on their use.

- Check to see if the app offers recommendations for what to do if symptoms get worse or if there is a psychiatric emergency.

- Decide if you want an app that is completely automated or an app that offers opportunities for contact with a trained person.

- Search for information on the app developer. Can you find helpful information about his or her credentials and experience?

- Beware of misleading logos. The National Institute of Mental Health (NIMH) has not developed and does not endorse any apps. However, some app developers have unlawfully used the NIMH logo to market their products.

- If there is no information about a particular app, check to see if it is based on a treatment that has been tested. For example, research has shown that Internet-based cognitive behavior therapy (CBT) is as effective as conventional CBT for disorders that respond well to CBT, like depression, anxiety, social phobia, and panic disorder.

- Try it. If you're interested in an app, test it for a few days and decide if it's easy to use, holds your attention, and if you want to continue using it. An app is only effective if keeps users engaged for weeks or months.

What Is NIMH's Role in Mental Health Intervention Technology?

Between FY2009 and FY2015, NIMH awarded 404 grants totaling 445 million for technology-enhanced mental health intervention grants. These grants were for studies of computer-based interventions designed to prevent or treat mental health disorders.

NIMH staff actively review and evaluate research grants related to technology. In recent years, these grants focused on:

- Feasibility, efficacy, and effectiveness research

- Technology for disorders such as schizophrenia, HIV, depression, anxiety, autism, suicide, and trauma

- More interventions for cognitive issues, illness management, behavior, and health communication

- Fewer interventions for a personal computer and more interventions for mobile devices

- More engaging ways to deliver therapies or skill development (for example, interactive formats or game-like approaches)

- Real-time (users exchanging information with peers or professionals as needed)

- Active and passive mobile assessment/monitoring

The Future: What Types of Research Does NIMH Expect in the Future?

Recently, there has been increased interest in:

- Using mobile technology for a wider range of disorders, from mild depression or anxiety to schizophrenia, autism, and suicide prevention

- Developing and refining new interventions, instead of adapting existing interventions to work with new technologies

- Developing technologies that work on any device

- Incorporating face-to-face contact or remote counseling (phone or online) to provide a balance between technology and the "human touch"

Chapter 26

New Technology to Optimize Cancer Therapy

A team of bioengineers, molecular biologists, and clinicians used a novel rare cell-sorter to isolate breast cancer cells from the blood of patients, with the aim of identifying the most effective drugs to treat each individual tumor. Circulating tumor cells (CTCs) were isolated and grown in the laboratory for extensive genetic analysis, which enabled the identification and testing of the most effective cancer-killing drugs for those tumors. The ability to perform such genetic analysis in the laboratory paves the way for providing the most effective treatment, not only initially, but throughout the course of the disease, as mutating tumors become resistant to certain drugs, but susceptible to others.

CTCs are tumor cells that are shed from primary tumors in the body and are carried through the circulation. For a number of years now, researchers have worked to develop technologies to capture and perform genetic analysis on these cells to learn about their growth characteristics and molecular evolution. Led by senior authors Daniel Haber, MD, PhD, and Shyamala Maheswaran, PhD, of Massachusetts General Hospital Cancer Center at Harvard Medical School; and Mehmet Toner, PhD, Harvard Center for Bioengineering in Medicine,

---

This chapter includes text excerpted from "New Technology Isolates Tumor Cells from Blood to Optimize Cancer Therapy," National Institute of Biomedical Imaging and Bioengineering (NIBIB), October 2, 2014. Reviewed December 2017.

237

the research team, who developed a microfluidic chip called the CTC-iChip, used it to isolate the minute numbers of tumor cells circulating in the blood.

The study design incorporated several crucial technologies necessary for successfully using CTCs to gain accurate information about the tumors from which they originated. The CTC-iChip is unique in that it does not use cancer cell markers on the surface of the CTCs to identify cells for capture. This is important because these markers change as the cancer progresses, so that captured cells obtained by using such markers may only represent a subset of cells shed by the tumor. Instead the iChip efficiently removes the normal blood cells, leaving behind viable CTCs that represent cells shed from both the primary tumor as well as metastatic tumor deposits—tumor nodules arising in distant organs due to the deposition of CTCs.

The other key advance in the study was the development of a cell culture system that allowed the CTCs to successfully grow in the laboratory. The expansion of the CTCs in cell culture is critical for having enough cells for genetic analysis and subsequent testing of anticancer drugs and drug combinations that target the newly evolved mutations. After much trial and error the group found that the cells could be successfully grown and expanded when cultured as suspended spheres of cells rather than when attached as a monolayer to the bottom of the cell culture plate. Importantly, with this new culture technique, the cells did not mutate over time while in culture—a common problem when growing cells in the laboratory.

The researchers used the iChip to isolate CTCs from the blood of 36 breast cancer patients. Cell lines were successfully established from the CTCs of six of these patients. Genetic analysis of the cell lines were compared with biopsies from the parent tumor to determine whether the metastatic tumors had evolved over time. Cultures derived from the same patient at multiple time points were compared to verify that culture conditions did not result in genetic changes in the CTCs. Standard care at Massachusetts General Hospital involves screening for a variety of mutations in just 25 genes. In contrast, the CTC cell lines enabled a far more extensive mutational analysis, including screening for mutations in 1,000 cancer genes.

Armed with such a comprehensive genetic analysis, the researchers then tested CTC lines for sensitivity to panels of single medications and medication combinations, based on knowledge of the susceptibility of various cancer mutations to certain drugs. The aim of these experiments was to identify which medications worked best on the tumor cells of each individual patient.

The test results indicated that tumors from several patients responded to therapy with medications commonly used for tumors carrying the mutations identified with the standard 25-gene analysis. However, several of the tumor samples did not respond to such treatments, but were responsive to different combinations of medications identified through the more extensive 1,000 gene screening made possible by isolation of the CTCs. Therefore, this proof of concept study successfully demonstrated that this approach has the potential to identify a wider range of genetic mutations, enabling treatments that successfully target the specific mutations in each patient's tumor.

The work is a significant first step toward "precision medicine" in oncology where treatments are tailored to the drug sensitivity patterns in individual patients. Furthermore, the system offers the opportunity to adjust treatments throughout the course of disease based on evolving tumor mutation profiles. By repeated sampling of CTCs throughout the course of a patient's disease, medications can be adjusted as individual tumors become resistant to certain medications but susceptible to others.

Tiffani Lash, PhD., the National Institute of Biomedical Imaging and Bioengineering (NIBIB) Program Director for Micro- and Nano-System Technologies, elaborates on the significance of the research. "With the hope of improving cancer therapies, NIBIB has supported the development of the sophisticated technologies necessary to capture and analyze CTCs. The ability to grow the CTCs in the laboratory and test them for cancer drug susceptibility is a major step towards providing targeted therapies with the real potential to significantly improve patient outcomes."

Chapter 27

Nutrigenomics

The importance of diet and nutrition in the etiology of a number of metabolic and autoimmune diseases affecting mortality and morbidity is well recognized. However, the exact nature of how diet impacts health and disease is not clearly understood. Several studies involving children of famine cohorts clearly demonstrate that nutrition is not only important at every stage in life of an individual but also plays a critical role in the health and disease from in utero to old age, thus providing a broad window of opportunity for nutrition in disease prevention.

In addition, nutrients and dietary components alter gene expression, modulate protein, and metabolite levels in target tissues, modify cellular and metabolic pathways, affect epigenetic phenomena, and modify response to drugs. These nutrient-host interactions thus influence an individual's predisposition to disease and potential therapeutic response. However, the exact nature of these interactions and underlying causal mechanisms are poorly understood. Current nutritional research methodologies often fail to explore nutrient-host interactions beyond associations. For this reason, there exists a critical need for novel approaches and methodologies employed in nutrition research that allow for the characterization of nutrient host interactions and how they play a critical role in health and disease.

This chapter includes text excerpted from "Nutrigenetics and Nutrigenomics Approaches for Nutrition Research," National Institutes of Health (NIH), May 10, 2017.

In the genomic era, the high throughput omic technologies are emerging as reliable technical platforms for generating high dimensional biological data, for studying the impact of environmental exposures such as diet, on multiple biological pathways affecting human health and disease in ways that complement conventional scientific approaches. In the recent years, there is a lot of enthusiasm for the application of these methodologies to nutrition research. Specifically, the field of nutrigenetics explores the impact of genetic variants on nutrient metabolism whereas nutrigenomics explores the gene expression, function and regulation in response to nutrient intake and collectively comprises the approaches namely transcriptomics, proteomics, epigenomics and metabolomics that enable analysis of multiple mRNA species, proteins and metabolites respectively. Such approaches can be targeted to a defined set of analytes, or untargeted allowing the analysis of global molecular species. The molecular signatures from these approaches can provide valuable insights into pathophysiological processes and yield potentially clinically relevant markers of diseases.

While the field is still in its initial stages, the application of these omic approaches to well-designed animal and human nutritional intervention studies and disease models holds great promise for understanding the impact of nutrients and dietary constituents on host metabolism and allow for identification of unique metabolic signatures critical for patho-physiological processes, in response to multiple, cumulative nutrient exposures. When applied to various transgenic and disease models and target tissues, these approaches have the ability to yield mechanistic information on the role of nutrients in the etiology and provide temporal changes associated with the disease process. The initial literature in this area already indicates a great promise on how omic approaches can be successfully applied to nutrition research to unravel nutrient-gene interactions both at the basic and population level.

The goal of this funding opportunity announcement is to foster collaborative research between nutrition researchers and experts in omics technologies and encourages applications that employ nutrigenetics and/or nutrigenomics approaches to basic, translational and clinical nutrition research. Collaboration between investigators with demonstrated expertise in nutrition research and omics techniques is highly encouraged. For the purposes of this funding opportunity, both hypothesis-driven and hypothesis-generating nutrigenomic studies targeted to specific nutrient metabolic pathways are appropriate.

Examples of the application of nutrigenetics and nutrigenomics approaches to nutrition research include but are not limited to:

- Impact of genetic polymorphisms on nutrient absorption, transport, and metabolism

- Impact of nutrients and dietary components on gene expression that affect nutrient absorption, transport, and metabolism in target tissues and relevant bio-specimens in health and diseases relevance to participating NIH Institutes

- Mechanisms by which specific nutrients/dietary components modulate intestinal physiology (transporters), barrier function, inflammation, and/or microbiome composition

- Mechanisms by which nutrient sensing in the gut is transduced to extra-intestinal organs and tissues

- Studies that explore the interaction/competition between various nutrients for their absorption, transport, metabolism, and elimination

- Studies that explore the interaction/competition between various nutrients and drugs for their absorption, transport, metabolism, and elimination

- Impact of nutrient excess and deficiency in health and diseases relevant to participating NIH Institutes

- Mechanism of action of prebiotics and resistant starches on intestinal function and host metabolism, and

- Mechanism of action of probiotics and secreted probiotic factors on intestinal function and host metabolism

Potential applicants to National Cancer Institute (NCI) and National Center for Complementary and Integrative Health (NCCIH) are also encouraged to read the following information on IC-specific research interests.

The National Cancer Institute (NCI)

The National Cancer Institute (NCI) has multiple interests in nutrigenetic and nutrigenomic-based mechanistic studies including vitamins, minerals, and other nutritive agents present in food that reduce the risk of cancer. Genetic variations present in individuals may alter their susceptibility to cancer. Specific interests include strategies to facilitate precision medicine using nutrition-focused interventions to reduce cancer risks in various populations including those mediated by host-microbiome interactions.

National Center for Complementary and Integrative Health (NCCIH)

The National Center for Complementary and Integrative Health (NCCIH) is particularly interested in nutrigenetic and nutrigenomic-based mechanistic studies of interaction and competition between nutrient-nutrient, nutrient-drug, dietary supplements, and probiotics/prebiotics on host-microbial metabolism, immunologic/inflammatory signaling, neuro-hormonal pathways and target tissues (including bioavailability, absorption, transport, metabolism, and excretion studies) that impact the basic fundamentals that will eventually lead to a better understanding of the gut brain function in health promotion and disease prevention. NCCIH is also interested in the impact of (selected) nutrient, dietary supplements, the ketogenic diet, and probiotic/prebiotic modulation of specific conditions including pain. In addition, NCCIH is interested in studying mechanisms for how botanical products, fish oil and other dietary supplements, and prebiotics in helping to identify their relationship to pain and inflammation.

Chapter 28

Nanotechnology

Chapter Contents

Section 28.1—Nanotechnology Research at NIH...................... 246

Section 28.2—Benefits of Nanotechnology 249

Section 28.3—Nanotechnology in Cancer................................... 254

Section 28.1

Nanotechnology Research at NIH

This section includes text excerpted from "Nanotechnology at the National Institutes of Health," National Institutes of Health (NIH), March 6, 2009. Reviewed December 2017.

What Is Nanotechnology?

Nanotechnology is defined as the understanding and control of matter at dimensions of roughly 1 to 100 nanometers, where the nanoscale, the physical, chemical, and biological properties of materials differ from the properties of individual atoms and molecules, or of bulk matter. Nanotechnology involves imaging, measuring, modeling, and manipulating matter at this scale.

Nanotechnology is advancing quickly. In 1996, the Nobel Prize in Chemistry was awarded for the discovery of fullerenes, a highly ordered, specific arrangement of carbon atoms at the nanoscale with unique properties attributable to their structure. More recently, in 2007, the Nobel Prize in Physics was awarded for the discovery of giant magnetoresistance, a quantum mechanical effect that appears only at the nanoscale.

This work already has had enormous practical benefit, leading to radical improvements in storage capacities in computer hard drives and other electronic devices. Novel nanomaterial properties similarly provide tremendous promise for biomedicine. The National Institutes of Health (NIH) funds a wide array of projects and programs focusing on two broad goals: manipulating and understanding biological structures and processes at the nanoscale and utilizing the unique properties of materials at the nanoscale to develop new diagnostics, therapeutics, biological interfaces, drug delivery systems, and other applications.

NIH Nanotechnology Activities

The NIH is the nation's medical research agency, comprising 27 institutes and centers that fund biomedical research across the United

States and around the world to improve human health. For more than seven years, the NIH has recognized the tremendous potential of nanotechnology as a scientific focus that could transform our current understanding of biology and our ability to prevent and treat disease. The NIH sponsored a national symposium to evaluate the state of the science in this area and to increase awareness of the NIH's interest in funding applications of nanotechnology to biomedical problems.

Most nanotechnology research at the NIH is funded by individual institutes with disease-specific, technology driven, or basic research missions. The NIH invests over $200 million per year on nanotechnology research, and many of the institute-specific programs are noted below.

Nano Task Force

The NIH Nano Task Force, established in 2006, consists of several working groups charged with addressing a range of issues including developing an overarching scientific vision for nanotechnology at the NIH; communicating to the public and scientific communities; understanding the health and safety implications of nanomaterials; exploring ethical, legal, and societal issues; and analyzing the NIH nanoscience research portfolio. Members also represent the NIH on federal interagency matters and at international meetings and activities related to nanotechnology.

Nanotechnology in Biology and Medicine

Novel materials are being developed with unique utility for ultra-sensitive detection of biomolecules, for targeted delivery of therapeutic agents directly to affected cells and tissues in the body, and as a tissue scaffold to promote healing. Novel diagnostic methods and treatments are emerging from our increasing ability to control the synthesis of materials such as quantum dots, dendrimers, and nanotubes, and to develop methods for optimizing the properties of these materials in living biological systems.

Major NIH Programs

Although the majority of NIH funding in nanotechnology is awarded using investigator-initiated grant mechanisms, three major NIH programs complement those efforts. All NIH institutes and centers participate in supporting a network of Nanomedicine Development Centers that represent a unique approach to translational biomedical research.

The centers were challenged to develop a deep understanding of a fundamental biological system and gradually move the research to apply this basic knowledge to improve our understanding, diagnosis, and treatment of one or more diseases. This requires a multidisciplinary effort in which teams of scientists and clinicians are working together to improve health.

The National Heart, Lung, and Blood Institute (NHLBI) supports a unique Program of Excellence in Nanotechnology (PEN). This program brings together bioengineers, materials scientists, biologists, and physicians who also work in interdisciplinary teams. This research is expected to spur the development of novel technologies to diagnose and treat heart, lung, blood, and sleep disorders.

The National Cancer Institute (NCI) has created the NCI Alliance for Nanotechnology in Cancer. This comprehensive program consists of four major components: Nanotechnology Platform Partnerships focused on developing new technologies and novel products for cancer diagnosis and treatment; Cancer Centers of Nanotechnology Excellence (CCNE) that complement existing cancer research centers to integrate nanotechnology into basic and applied research; a Nanotechnology Characterization Lab to facilitate product safety and regulatory approval; and training opportunities in relevant multidisciplinary sciences.

National Nanotechnology Initiative (NNI)

The NIH participates in the National Nanotechnology Initiative (NNI), a federal R&D program established to coordinate multi-agency efforts in nanoscale science, engineering, and technology. Twenty-six federal agencies currently participate in the NNI by funding or conducting studies, applying results from federally funded R&D efforts, or through collaborations with other agencies. The NNI is managed within the framework of the National Science and Technology Council (NSTC), the Cabinet-level council by which the U.S. President coordinates science, space, and technology policies across the federal government. The Nanoscale Science Engineering and Technology (NSET) Subcommittee of the NSTC coordinates planning, budgeting, program implementation, and review to ensure a balanced and comprehensive initiative. The NSET Subcommittee is comprised of representatives from each of the agencies participating in the NNI.

Section 28.2

Benefits of Nanotechnology

This section includes text excerpted from "Benefits of
Nanotechnology for Cancer," National Cancer
Institute (NCI), August 8, 2017.

Nanoscale devices are 100 to 10,000 times smaller than human
cells. They are similar in size to large biological molecules ("biomolecules") such as enzymes and receptors. As an example, hemoglobin,
the molecule that carries oxygen in red blood cells, is approximately 5
nanometers in diameter. Nanoscale devices smaller than 50 nanometers can easily enter most cells, while those smaller than 20 nanometers can move out of blood vessels as they circulate through the body.
Because of their small size, nanoscale devices can readily interact with
biomolecules on both the surface and inside cells. By gaining access to
so many areas of the body, they have the potential to detect disease
and deliver treatment in ways unimagined before now.

Biological processes, including ones necessary for life and those that
lead to cancer, occur at the nanoscale. Thus, in fact, we are composed
of a multitude of biological nano-machines. Nanotechnology provides
researchers with the opportunity to study and manipulate macromolecules in real time and during the earliest stages of cancer progression.
Nanotechnology can provide rapid and sensitive detection of cancer-related molecules, enabling scientists to detect molecular changes even
when they occur only in a small percentage of cells. Nanotechnology
also has the potential to generate entirely novel and highly effective
therapeutic agents.

Ultimately and uniquely, the use of nanoscale materials for cancer
comes down to its ability to be readily functionalized and easily tuned;
its ability to deliver and/or act as the therapeutic, diagnostic, or both;
and its ability to passively accumulate at the tumor site, to be actively
targeted to cancer cells, and to be delivered across traditional biological
barriers in the body such as dense stromal tissue of the pancreas or
the blood-brain barrier that highly regulates delivery of biomolecules
to/from, our central nervous system.

Passive Tumor Accumulation

An effective cancer drug delivery should achieve high accumulation in tumor and spare the surrounding healthy tissues. The passive localization of many drugs and drug carriers due to their extravasation through leaky vasculature (named the Enhanced Permeability and Retention [EPR] effect) works very well for tumors. As tumor mass grows rapidly, a network of blood vessels needs to expand quickly to accommodate tumor cells' need for oxygen and nutrient. This abnormal and poorly regulated vessel generation (i.e., angiogenesis) results in vessel walls with large pores (40 nm to 1 um); these leaky vessels allow relatively large nanoparticles to extravasate into tumor masses. As fast growing tumor mass lacks a functioning lymphatic system, clearance of these nanoparticles is limited and further enhances the accumulation. Through the EPR effect, nanoparticles larger than 8 nm (between 8-100 nm) can passively target tumors by freely pass through large pores and achieve higher intratumoral accumulation. The majority of current nanomedicines for solid tumor treatment rely on EPR effect to ensure high drug accumulation thereby improve treatment efficacy. Without targeting cell types expressing targeting ligand of interest, this drug delivery system is called passive targeting.

Before reaching to the proximity of tumor site for EPR effect to take place, passive targeting requires drug delivery system to be long-circulating to allow sufficient level of drug to the target area. To design nano-drugs that can stay in blood longer, one can "mask" these nano-drugs by modifying the surface with water-soluble polymers such as polyethylene glycol (PEG); PEG is often used to make water-insoluble nanoparticles to be water-soluble in many preclinical research laboratories. PEG-coated liposomal doxorubicin (Doxil) is used clinically for breast cancer leveraging passive tumor accumulation. As in vivo surveillance system for macromolecules (i.e., scavenger receptors of the reticuloendothelial system, RES) reportedly showed faster uptake of negatively charged nanoparticles, nano-drugs with a neutral or positive charge are expected to have a longer plasma half-life.

Utilizing EPR effect for passive tumor targeting drug delivery is not without problems. Although EPR effect is a unique phenomenon in solid tumors, the central region of metastatic or larger tumor mass does not exhibit EPR effect, a result of an extreme hypoxic condition. For this reason, there are methods used in the clinics to artificially enhance EPR effect: slow infusion of angiotensin II to increase systolic blood pressure, topical application of NO-releasing agents to expand blood and photodynamic therapy or hyperthermia-mediated vascular permeabilization in solid tumors.

Passive accumulation through EPR effect is the most acceptable drug delivery system for solid tumor treatment. However, size or molecular weight of the nanoparticles is not the sole determinant of the EPR effect, other factors such as surface charge, biocompatibility and in vivo surveillance system for macromolecules should not be ignored in designing the nanomedicine for efficient passive tumor accumulation.

Active Tumor Targeting

EPR effect, which serves as nanoparticle "passive tumor targeting" scheme is responsible for accumulation of particles in the tumor region. However, EPR does not promote uptake of nanoparticles into cells; yet nanoparticle/drug cell internalization is required for some of the treatment modalities relying on drug activation within the cell nucleus or cytosol. Similarly, delivery of nucleic acids (DNA, siRNA, miRNA) in genetic therapies requires escape of these molecules from endosome so they can reach desired subcellular compartments. In addition, EPR is heterogenous and its strength varies among different tumors and/or patients. For these reasons, active targeting is considered an essential feature for next-generation nanoparticle therapeutics. It will enable certain modalities of therapies not achievable with EPR and improve effectiveness of treatments which can be accomplished using EPR, but with less than satisfactory effect. Active targeting of nanoparticles to tumor cells, microenvironment or vasculature, as well as directed delivery to intracellular compartments, can be attained through nanoparticle surface modification with small molecules, antibodies, affibodies, peptides or aptamers.

Passive targeting (EPR effect) is the process of nanoparticles extravasating from the circulation through the leaky vasculature to the tumor region. The drug molecules carried by nanoparticle are released in the extracellular matrix and diffuse throughout the tumor tissue. The particles carry surface ligands to facilitate active targeting of particles to receptors present on target cell or tissue. Active targeting is expected to enhance nanoparticle/drug accumulation in tumor and also promote their prospective cell uptake through receptor mediated endocytosis. The particles, which are engineered for vascular targeting, incorporate ligands that bind to endothelial cell-surface receptors. The vascular targeting is expected to provide synergistic strategy utilizing both targeting of vascular tissue and cells within the diseased tissue.

Most of the nanotechnology-based strategies which are approved for clinical use or are in advanced clinical trials rely on EPR effect. It is expected that next-generation nanotherapies will use targeting to enable and enhance intracellular uptake, intracellular trafficking, and penetration of physiological barriers which block drug access to some tumors.

Transport across Tissue Barriers

Nanoparticle or nano-drug delivery is hampered by tissue barriers before the drug can reach the tumor site. Tissue barriers for efficient transporting of nano-drugs to tumor sites include tumor stroma (e.g., biological barriers) and tumor endothelium barriers (e.g., functional barriers). Biological barriers are physical constructs or cell formation that restrict the movement of nanoparticles. Functional barriers can affect the transport of intact nanoparticles or nanomedicine into the tumor mass: elevated interstitial fluid pressure and acidic environment for examples. It is important to design nanoparticles and strategies to overcome these barriers to improve cancer treatment efficacy.

Tumor microenvironment (TME) is a dynamic system composed of abnormal vasculature, fibroblasts and immune cells, all embedded in an extracellular matrix (EMC). TME poses both biological and functional barriers to nano-drug delivery in cancer treatment. Increase cell density and abnormal vasculature elevate the interstitial fluid pressure within a tumor mass. Such pressure gradient is unfavorable for free diffusion of the nanoparticles and is often a limiting factor for the enhanced permeability and retention (EPR) effect. When tumor mass reaches 106 cells in number, metabolic strains ensue. Often, cells in the core of this proliferating cluster are distanced by 100–200 um from the source of nutrient: 200um is a limiting distance for oxygen diffusion. As a result, cancer cells in the core live at pO2 levels below 2.5–10mmHg and become hypoxic; anoxic metabolic pathway can kick in and generate lactic acid. Nanoparticles become unstable in an acidic environment and delivery of the drugs to target tumor cells will be unpredictable. EMC of the tumor provides nutrient for cancer cells and stromal cell. It is a collection of fibrous proteins and polysaccharides and expands rapidly in aggressive cancer as the result of stromal cell proliferation. The most notorious biological barrier to cancer treatment is pancreatic stroma in pancreatic ductal adenocarcinoma (PADC). Pancreatic cancer stroma has the characteristics of an abnormal and poorly functioning vasculature, altered extracellular matrix, infiltrating macrophages and proliferation of fibroblasts. Not only tumor-stroma interactions have been shown to promote pancreatic cancer cell invasion and metastasis, but TME and tumor stroma also create an unfavorable environment for drug delivery and other forms of cancer treatments.

Because EPR effect is a clinically relevant phenomenon for nano-carriers' tumor penetration, strategies have been developed to address the tumor endothelium barrier. Strategies to reduce interstitial fluid pressure to improve tumor penetration include ECM-targeting pharmacological interventions to normalize vasculature within TME; hypertonic solutions to shrink ECM cells; hyperthermia, radiofrequency (RF) or high-intensity focused ultrasound (HIFU) to enhance nano-drug transport and accumulation. These strategies can also alleviate hypoxic conditions in larger tumor mass. Although TME and tumor mass pose a harsh and acidic environment for nano-carrier stability, pH-responsive nano-carrier designs leveraging this unique feature are gaining interest in recent years. Many of the strategies described above are used to address tumor stroma barrier.

Another formidable tissue barrier for drugs and nanoparticle delivery is the blood-brain barrier (BBB). BBB is a physical barrier in the central nervous system to prevent harmful substances from entering the brain. It consists of endothelial cells which are sealed in continuous tight junction around the capillaries. Outside the layer of epithelial cell is covered by astrocytes that further contribute to the selectivity of substance passage. As BBB keeps harmful substances from the brain, it also restricts the delivery of therapeutics for brain diseases, such as brain tumors and other neurological diseases. There have been tremendous efforts in overcoming the BBB for drug delivery in general. The multi-valent feature of nanoparticles makes nano-carriers appealing in designing BBB-crossing delivering strategies. One promising nanoparticle design has transferrin receptor-targeting moiety to facilitate transportation of these nanoparticles across the BBB.

Section 28.3

Nanotechnology in Cancer

This section includes text excerpted from "Nanotechnology for Treating Cancer: Pitfalls and Bridges on the Path to Nanomedicines," National Cancer Institute (NCI), June 8, 2015.

Nanotechnology is often touted as one of the most promising drug delivery innovations in today's fight against cancer. Typically not drugs themselves, nanoparticles have the potential to deliver traditional cancer drugs to tumors with fewer side effects, or to enable nontraditional drugs (e.g., proteins or nucleic acids) to be targeted to kill cancer cells. However, since the mid-1990s only two nanoparticle cancer treatments have been approved by the U.S. Food and Drug Administration (FDA). Doxil (Janssen Biotech), a liposomal formulation of doxorubicin, was the first nanomedicine approved (1995). In 2005 the albumin-bound paclitaxel formulation Abraxane (Celgene Corp.) was approved, largely by virtue of reduced side effects in the treatment of solid tumors. The question naturally arises, why aren't there more approved nanodrugs on the market? Why is their development taking so long? Based on our experiences the lag between inception and delivery in the development of nanotechnology-based therapeutics can be ascribed to the complexity of the nanomaterials themselves. Nanomaterials are not pure entities. On the contrary, they are complex, polydisperse, and oftentimes multifunctional formulations—the term in the field is "nonbiological complex drugs" (NBCDs). Many different physical and chemical traits must be fine-tuned for each application, including nanoparticle size, charge, surface chemistry, and hydrophobicity, and this tuning process requires a suite of skills and technologies that often must be developed iteratively. "One size does not fit all" is a truism in the field of nanomedicine.

For the past ten years the Nanotechnology Characterization Lab (NCL) of the National Cancer Institute has provided comprehensive nanomaterial characterization, testing and evaluation services to nanomedicine developers around the world. The NCL has analyzed over 300 different nanoformulations and worked with nearly 100 academic, government, and commercial organizations, affording a unique opportunity to study the advantages and disadvantages of various platforms, drugs, surface coatings, targeting ligands, etc. A summary of our experience with many of the most common pitfalls encountered by nanomedicine developers was recently published.

With nanoparticle-enabled delivery of chemotherapeutics there is an opportunity to deliver more of the cytotoxic drug to the intended site, offering reduced off-target toxicities and or enhanced efficacy (because the "maximum tolerated dose" can be higher). Formulation using nanotechnology can alter biodistribution, clearance, and pharmacokinetics compared to the legacy drug. Employing what is known as the enhanced permeability and retention (EPR) effect, nanoparticles can accumulate in tumor tissues because of their leaky vasculature and compromised lymphatic drainage. To take advantage of the EPR effect, however, nanoparticles must be precisely engineered to evade the mononuclear phagocyte system (MPS). For example, nanomedicines should be small enough to avoid uptake by the liver and spleen (<250 nm), yet large enough to avoid clearance by the kidneys (>10 nm), and should remain in circulation long enough to allow for significant tumor accumulation ($t1/2 > 3$ hr). A nano-material's physicochemical properties are known to influence its biological performance. For example, a size difference as little as 2 nm has been shown to alter the route of clearance, and surface modification has been shown to alter biodistribution.

It goes without saying that the most critical step in nanomedicine evaluation is thorough and well-documented characterization of each batch of material. Without a comprehensive understanding of the formulation its biological analysis can be easily misinterpreted. Starting materials should be characterized; intermediate materials should be characterized and archived for side-by-side biological evaluation (e.g., nontargeted versus. targeted nanomaterials); and of course, the final material should be characterized. It is imperative to ascertain which parameters are the most important to measure, which ones affect biological activity, and what assay techniques are most appropriate. A short list of essential parameters to investigate includes:

1. the level of polydispersity that is acceptable to maintain the desired efficacy;

2. whether or not the surface coatings/targeting ligands are covalently attached or simply physisorbed;

3. the level of surface coverage required for optimal biological performance;

4. and the stability (temperature, pH, shelf-life, in biological matrix, etc.) of the formulation.

There are a number of excellent articles that address the importance of these and other characterization aspects.

Additional challenges arise when delivering agents such as RNA, DNA, or proteins, especially avoiding undesired immune responses. Although many nanoparticles without these agents can also elicit immunological reactions, nanoparticles containing oligos or proteins are particularly susceptible. Some commonly observed toxicities include anemia, neutropenia, thrombosis, complement activation, cytokine induction, and allergic reactions. Screening for this variety of potential adverse conditions can be a challenge, and it is often difficult to predict which assays will be most relevant for a given formulation. The NCL has more than a dozen in vitro immunological assays tailored for nanomedicine evaluation.

Sterility and endotoxin contamination are other aspects many researchers fail to address in the developmental process. Almost one-third of the materials submitted to the NCL have endotoxin levels exceeding U.S. FDA limits. Even though materials submitted to the NCL are at the preclinical stage, high levels of endotoxin can interfere with the correct interpretation of many assays. Without a proper screen for endotoxin, toxicity may be mistakenly assigned to the nanomaterial, when in fact it stems from contamination during the synthesis and/or purification process. The NCL has studied endotoxin quantification in nanomaterials extensively and has several manuscripts offering more elaboration on the trials and tribulations of this topic.

Generic versions of nanomedicines, or nano-similars, pose even more challenges. Recently the FDA approved the first "generic" nanomedicine. A generic version of Doxil (Sun Pharma) was approved for the treatment of ovarian cancer in 2013, nearly 20 years after approval of the innovator product. Researchers are now beginning to develop new and improved methods to verify the bioequivalence of these follow-on nanomedicines. However, there is an inherent challenge in defining similarity for a formulation that is naturally polydisperse, and determining whether or not these differences are meaningful. Because of the novelty of this area, the potential regulatory hurdles and additional characterization requirements for nano-similars may not yet be fully realized.

Nanomedicine research is not unrealistic or unattainable. There are many who do this work superbly. But for the novice nano-researcher, here are a few key recommendations:

- Screen for endotoxin early.

- Ensure the biocompatibility of all formulation components.

- Monitor the complete removal of potentially toxic excipients and side products from the manufacturing and purification process.

- Certify batch-to-batch consistency and define acceptance criteria.

- Assess nanoparticle stability and drug release rates in vivo or in an appropriate biological matrix.

- Don't ignore immunological assessments.

- Don't skimp on proper controls and comparisons for in vivo studies. While this may save on costs in the short term, it usually doesn't in the long term.

- It is never too early to think about the big picture and how the research product should ultimately materialize. Researchers who focus on achieving a single optimal preclinical result often lose sight of clinical and regulatory requirements and end up facing unexpected (i.e., time consuming and costly) hurdles in their development path.

A variety of NCL services are available to researchers pursuing nanomedicine translation. Researchers developing cancer nanomedicines are eligible to apply for the free NCL Assay Cascade testing services. Formulations are accepted via a quarterly application process; more information about this service, as well as acceptance and evaluation criteria can be found on the NCL's website (www.ncl.cancer. gov). Other services are also available via a Collaborative Research and Development Agreement (CRADA). These include characterization of nononcology based nanomedicines, nanotechnology reformulation services, and more. Submitting investigators must provide funding for services under the cCRADA, but NCL only charges for direct costs — there is zero profit associated with these contracts.

Chapter 29

Robotics

Chapter Contents

Section 29.1—Robots for Better Health and
        Quality of Life.. 260

Section 29.2—Robotic Cleaners... 261

Section 29.3—Image-Guided Robotic Interventions 263

Section 29.1

Robots for Better Health and Quality of Life

This section includes text excerpted from "Robots for Better Health and Quality of Life," MedlinePlus, National Institutes of Health (NIH), April 21, 2016.

"Robots are rapidly being incorporated into all aspects of our lives, from global positioning system (GPS) in cars, to speech recognition on smartphones," observes Roderic I. Pettigrew, PhD, MD, Director of the National Institute of Biomedical Imaging and Bioengineering (NIBIB), the lead institute for the National Robotics Initiative at the National Institutes of Health (NIH).

"We want to encourage leaders in the field of robotics to apply their ingenuity to improve healthcare. Such innovations have the potential to help facilitate healthy independent living."

Smart-Walker

As we age, it's harder to walk without assistance. Physical activity and quality of life decrease. To continue living at home, we often require costly modifications such as ramps or wheelchair lifts.

University of Alabama in Tuscaloosa mechanical engineer Xiangrong Shen is developing a four-legged robot to help the elderly remain active and independent—without relying on caregivers or expensive home renovations.

Says Shen, "We want to help people in their daily lives in their own homes. Our robot surrounds a person with confidence."

The new robot has two modes: power-assisted walker and smart "mule." In the first, you select the level of power to maintain a stable, steady pace. As the smart mule, the robot walks beside you while carrying "saddlebags" of groceries, for example. It uses a 3D computer vision-based system to detect your motion and surroundings. It easily bypasses obstacles that wheelchairs cannot.

Buddy: A Social Robot for Kids

Thanks to Star Wars, R2D2, and C3PO captivated Cynthia Breazeal's imagination as a child. She grew up to pioneer human-robot interactions, develop Jibo, the world's first family "companion" robot, and found and direct the Massachusetts Institute of Technology Personal Robots Group.

She and her team are working on an autonomous, long-term social robotic companion for children—an interactive "buddy"—to promote and assess a child's curiosity and intellectual growth. Not only do dedication and hard work improve one's basic abilities, Breazeal believes they also influence a child's mental health, academic achievement, and general well-being.

"Seeing-Eye" Glove for the Visually Impaired

Cang Ye is passionate about enlarging the world for the blind and visually impaired. "In the age of computers, we're still using primitive devices—the white cane—to navigate our surroundings," he says.

At his University of Arkansas laboratory, Ye and his systems engineering colleagues are creating a kind of "seeing eye" glove that combines a small, 3D camera and computerized sensors to help people detect obstacles and grasp things. A blind person could use it to walk around a chair, for instance, or open a door handle.

"It's a big challenge," Ye says. "The glove needs to be both small and powerful."

Section 29.2

Robotic Cleaners

This section includes text excerpted from "Milwaukee VA
Medical Center Zaps Germs with Robots," U.S. Department of
Veterans Affairs (VA), July 16, 2017.

The Milwaukee VA Medical Center has a new weapon against invisible critters that can spread infection, illness, or even death—a purple and silver robot about the size of a trash can that looks like R2D2 and obliterates the buggers with 67 pulses of ultraviolet light per second.

Meet Xena and Thor—two germ-zapping robots added to Milwaukee's cleaning and infection control procedures to ensure better health and safety for Veterans and employees.

VA put the machines into action this summer after holding a "Name the Robots" contest among employees. Milwaukee is the first VA hospital in this region to use the robots.

The portable devices, manufactured by Xenex, are the only mercury-free systems available and kill numerous micro-organisms in about 15 minutes.

No Unnecessary Hazardous Chemicals

This basically takes cleaning to the next level," said Jai Reneau, Environmental Management Services division manager. "We already do a good job of cleaning, but even with the best cleaning there will always be germs that can't be seen by the naked eye. We chose this system because it doesn't introduce unnecessary hazardous chemicals to the hospital, and it has a very good success rate."

Typically, after a room is manually cleaned by human hands, the robots take over. Housekeepers wheel it into position, put up orange safety cones, press a button then leave the room. The robot head rises in the air, then attacks the room with bright pulses of UV-C light. The machines are safe for humans, but you can't look directly at the light.

The light isn't the same as a tanning bed. Instead of giving bacteria a suntan, it scrambles their DNA.

"It actually exerts enough pressure to open the bacterial cell wall, scrambles the DNA and makes the bacteria inert," said Gaylyn Raduenz, a registered nurse and infection preventionist. "Then the bacteria can't reproduce and it can't infect someone."

Studies show the treatment lowers infection rates 20 to 50 percent, but Milwaukee officials won't know local results for about six months.

The robots will mostly be used in the Spinal Cord Injury Center, Community Living Center and other hospital areas where there is a higher risk of infection because of the type of care provided.

Raduenz said hospital infection rates are already lower than national benchmarks, but this takes safety a step further.

Each machine costs about $92,000 and Raduenz says it's money well spent.

"You can't put a price on the health and well-being of our Veterans," Raduenz says. "Our Veterans deserve the absolute best we can provide. That's priceless."

Section 29.3

Image-Guided Robotic Interventions

This section includes text excerpted from "Science Education—
Image-Guided Robotic Interventions," National Institute of
Biomedical Imaging and Bioengineering (NIBIB), July 2016.

What Are Image-Guided Robotic Interventions?

Image-guided robotic interventions are medical procedures that
integrate sophisticated robotic and imaging technologies, primarily to perform minimally invasive surgery. This integrated technology approach offers distinct advantages for both patients and
physicians.

Imaging: In image-guided procedures, the surgeon is guided by
images from various techniques, including magnetic resonance (MR)
and ultrasound. Images can also be obtained using tiny cameras
attached to probes that are small enough to fit into a minimal incision.
The camera allows the surgery to be performed using a much smaller
incision than in traditional surgery.

Robotics: The surgeon's hands and traditional surgical tools are
too large for small incisions. Instead, thin, finger-like robotic tools are
used to perform the surgery. As the surgeon watches the image on the
screen, she uses a tele-manipulator to transmit and direct hand and
finger movements to a robot, which can be controlled by hydraulic,
electronic, or mechanical means.

Robotic tools can also be controlled by computer. One advantage of
a computerized system is that a surgeon could potentially perform the
surgery from anywhere in the world. This type of long-distance surgery
is currently in the experimental phase. The experiments illustrate
the life-saving potential for such surgeries when a delicate operation requires a specially trained surgeon who is in a distant location.
Additionally, doctors can use image-guided robotic interventions to
more accurately target tumors when performing biopsies and radiation
treatments.

What Are the Advantages of Minimally Invasive Procedures?

Minimally invasive surgery can reduce the damage to surrounding healthy tissues, thus decreasing the need for pain medication and reducing patients' recovery time. For surgeons, image-guided interventions using robots also have the advantage of reducing fatigue during long operations, allowing the surgeon to perform the procedure while seated.

What Are Some Examples of Image-Guided Robotic Interventions and How Are They Used?

Robotic prostatectomy: Complete prostate removal is performed through a series of small incisions, compared with a single large incision of 4-5 inches in traditional surgery. The small incisions result in a shorter postoperative recovery, less scarring, and a faster return to normal activities.

Ablation techniques for early cancers: Patients with early kidney cancer can be treated with minimally invasive procedures to destroy small tumors. Cryoablation uses cold energy to destroy the tumors. Doctors use computed tomography (CT) and ultrasound imaging to position a needle-like probe within each kidney tumor. Once in position, the tip of the probe is super-cooled to encase the tumor in a ball of ice. Alternate freeze/thaw cycles kill the tumor cells. Other minimally invasive methods of destroying early kidney cancers include heating the tumor cells, and surgical removal using a robotic device. Many patients can go home the same day and are able to perform regular activities in several days.

Orthopedics: Image-guided robotic procedures are improving the precision and outcome of a number of orthopedic procedures. For example, partial knee resurfacing surgeries aim to target only the damaged sections of the knee joint. Orthopedic surgeons are combining the use of a robotic surgical arm and fiber optic cameras in such procedures, which results in patients retaining more of their normal healthy tissue. Image-guided robotic procedures also improve total knee replacements, allowing precise alignment and positioning of knee implants. The result is more natural knee function, better range of motion, and improved balance for patients.

Image-Guided Robotic Interventions to Improve Medical Care: Research and Development

Portable robot uses 3D near-infrared imaging to guide needle insertion into veins: Drawing blood and inserting intravenous (IV) lines are the most commonly performed medical procedures in hospitals and clinics. However, for many patients it can be difficult to find veins and accurately insert the needle, resulting in patient injury. Scientists are developing a portable, lightweight medical robot to help perform these procedures. The device uses 3D near-infrared imaging to identify an appropriate vein for the robot to insert the needle. The current goal is to integrate the imaging system and software into a miniaturized version of the prototype robot. The outcome will be a compact, low-cost system that will greatly improve the safety and accuracy of accessing veins.

Robot-assisted needle guidance aids removal of liver tumors: Radiofrequency ablation (RFA) is a minimally invasive treatment that kills tumors with heat and can be a life-saving option for patients who are not eligible for surgery. However, broad use of RFA has been limited because the straight paths taken by the needles that carry tumor-killing electrodes may damage lung or other sensitive organs. Also, large tumors require multiple needle insertions, which increases bleeding risk. To address the problem of tissue damage using straight needles, scientists are developing highly flexible needles that can be guided along controlled, curved paths through tissue, allowing the removal of tumors that are not accessible by a straight-line path. The technology combines needle flexibility with a 3D ultrasound guidance system that allows the doctor to correct the path of the needle to avoid unexpected obstacles as the needle advances toward the tumor. The device will ultimately increase the accuracy and reduce the damage to healthy tissue during tumor removal resulting in wider use of the technology for better patient outcomes.

Swallowable capsule identifies and biopsies abnormal tissue in the esophagus: Barrett's esophagus is a precancerous condition that requires repeated biopsies to monitor abnormal tissue. Researchers are developing a swallowable, pill-sized device to improve the management and treatment of this condition. The unsedated patient can easily swallow the pill, which is attached to a thin tether made of cable and optic fiber. The device detects microscopic areas of the esophagus that may show evidence of disease, and uses a laser to collect samples from the suspicious tissue—a technology known as laser capture micro-dissection. The physician then retrieves the device from the patient without discomfort and the collected micro-samples are examined for visual evidence of disease, as well as genetic analysis. This minimally invasive device improves patient comfort and provides a precise molecular profile of the biopsied regions, which helps the physician to better monitor and treat the disorder.

Chapter 30

Advanced Therapies

Chapter Contents

Section 30.1—Tissue Engineering and Regenerative
      Medicine... 268

Section 30.2—Cartilage Engineering.. 272

Section 30.3—Regenerative Medicine
      Biomanufacturing 274

Section 30.4—New Method Builds Bone 275

Section 30.5—Light Therapy and Brain Function.................... 277

Section 30.1

Tissue Engineering and Regenerative Medicine

This section includes text excerpted from "Tissue
Engineering and Regenerative Medicine," National Institute of
Biomedical Imaging and Bioengineering (NIBIB), June 26, 2013.
Reviewed December 2017.

What Are Tissue Engineering and Regenerative Medicine?

Tissue engineering evolved from the field of biomaterials development and refers to the practice of combining scaffolds, cells, and biologically active molecules into functional tissues. The goal of tissue engineering is to assemble functional constructs that restore, maintain, or
improve damaged tissues or whole organs. Artificial skin and cartilage
are examples of engineered tissues that have been approved by the
FDA; however, currently they have limited use in human patients.

Regenerative medicine is a broad field that includes tissue engineering but also incorporates research on self-healing – where the body
uses its own systems, sometimes with help foreign biological material
to re-create cells and rebuild tissues and organs. The terms "tissue
engineering" and "regenerative medicine" have become largely inter-
changeable, as the field hopes to focus on cures instead of treatments
for complex, often chronic, diseases.

This field continues to evolve. In addition to medical applications,
nontherapeutic applications include using tissues as biosensors to
detect biological or chemical threat agents, and tissue chips that can
be used to test the toxicity of an experimental medication.

How Do Tissue Engineering and Regenerative Medicine Work?

Cells are the building blocks of tissue, and tissues are the basic unit
of function in the body. Generally, groups of cells make and secrete
their own support structures, called extra-cellular matrix. This matrix,

or scaffold, does more than just support the cells; it also acts as a relay station for various signaling molecules. Thus, cells receive messages from many sources that become available from the local environment. Each signal can start a chain of responses that determine what happens to the cell. By understanding how individual cells respond to signals, interact with their environment, and organize into tissues and organisms, researchers have been able to manipulate these processes to mend damaged tissues or even create new ones.

The process often begins with building a scaffold from a wide set of possible sources, from proteins to plastics. Once scaffolds are created, cells with or without a "cocktail" of growth factors can be introduced. If the environment is right, a tissue develops. In some cases, the cells, scaffolds, and growth factors are all mixed together at once, allowing the tissue to "self-assemble."

Another method to create new tissue uses an existing scaffold. The cells of a donor organ are stripped and the remaining collagen scaffold is used to grow new tissue. This process has been used to bioengineer heart, liver, lung, and kidney tissue. This approach holds great promise for using scaffolding from human tissue discarded during surgery and combining it with a patient's own cells to make customized organs that would not be rejected by the immune system.

How Do Tissue Engineering and Regenerative Medicine Fit In with Current Medical Practices?

Currently, tissue engineering plays a relatively small role in patient treatment. Supplemental bladders, small arteries, skin grafts, cartilage, and even a full trachea have been implanted in patients, but the procedures are still experimental and very costly. While more complex organ tissues like heart, lung, and liver tissue have been successfully re-created in the lab, they are a long way from being fully reproducible and ready to implant into a patient. These tissues, however, can be quite useful in research, especially in drug development. Using functioning human tissue to help screen medication candidates could speed up development and provide key tools for facilitating personalized medicine while saving money and reducing the number of animals used for research.

What Are NIH-Funded Researchers Developing in the Areas of Tissue Engineering and Regenerative Medicine?

Research supported by NIBIB includes development of new scaffold materials and new tools to fabricate, image, monitor, and preserve engineered tissues. Some examples of research in this area are described below.

Controlling stem cells through their environment:

For many years, scientists have searched for ways to control how stems cells develop into other cell types, in the hopes of creating new therapies. Two NIBIB researchers have grown pluripotent cells—stem cells that have the ability to turn into any kind of cell—in different types of defined spaces and found that this confinement triggered very specific gene networks that determined the ultimate fate for the cells. Most other medical research on pluripotent stem cells has focused on modifying the combination of growth solutions in which the cells are placed. The discovery that there is a biomechanical element to controlling how stem cells transform into other cell types is an important piece of the puzzle as scientists try to harness stem cells for medical uses.

Implanting human livers in mice:

NIBIB-funded researchers have engineered human liver tissue that can be implanted in a mouse. The mouse retains its own liver as well, and therefore its normal function—but the added piece of engineered human liver can metabolize drugs in the same way humans do. This allows researchers to test susceptibility to toxicity and to demonstrate species-specific responses that typically do not show up until clinical trials. Using engineered human tissue in this way could cut down on the time and cost of producing new drugs, as well as allow for critical examinations of drug-drug interactions within a human-like system.

Engineering mature bone stem cells:

Researchers funded by NIBIB completed the first published study that has been able to take stem cells all the way from their pluripotent state to mature bone grafts that could potentially be transplanted into a patient. Previously, investigators could only differentiate the cells to a primitive version of the tissue which was not fully functional. Additionally, the study found that when the bone was implanted in immunodeficient mice there were no abnormal growths afterwards—a problem that often occurs after implanting stem cells or bone scaffolds alone.

Using lattices to help engineered tissue survive:

Currently, engineered tissues that are larger than 200 microns (about twice the width of a human hair) in any dimension cannot survive because they do not have vascular networks (veins or arteries).

Tissues need a good "plumbing system"—a way to bring nutrients to the cells and carry away the waste—and without a blood supply or similar mechanism, the cells quickly die. Ideally, scientists would like to be able to create engineered tissue with this plumbing system already built in. One NIBIB-funded researcher is working on a very simple and easily reproducible system to solve this problem: a modified ink-jet printer that lays down a lattice made of a sugar solution. This solution hardens and the engineered tissue (in a gel form) surrounds the lattice. Later, blood is added which easily dissolves the sugar lattice, leaving preformed channels to act as blood vessels.

New hope for the bum knee:

Until now, cartilage has been very difficult, if not impossible, to repair due to the fact that cartilage lacks a blood supply to promote regeneration. There has been a 50 percent long-term success rate using microfracture surgery in young adults suffering from sports injuries, and little to no success in patients with widespread cartilage degeneration such as osteoarthritis. An NIBIB-funded tissue engineer has developed a biological gel that can be injected into a cartilage defect following microfracture surgery to create an environment that facilitates regeneration. However, in order for this gel to stay in place within the knee, researchers also developed a new biological adhesive that is able to bond to both the gel as well as the damaged cartilage in the knee, keeping the newly regrown cartilage in place. The gel/adhesive combo was successful in regenerating cartilage tissue following surgery in a recent clinical trial of 15 patients, all of whom reported decreased pain at six months postsurgery. In contrast, the majority of microfracture patients, after an initial decrease in pain, returned to their original pain level within six months. This researcher worked in collaboration with another NIBIB grantee to image the patients who had undergone surgery enabling scientists to combine new, noninvasive methods to see the evolving results in real-time.

Regenerating a new kidney:

The ability to regenerate a new kidney from a patient's own cells would provide major relief for the hundreds of thousands of patients suffering from kidney disease. Experimenting on rat, pig and human kidney cells, NIDDK supported researchers broke new ground on this front by first stripping cells from a donor organ and using the remaining collagen scaffold to help guide the growth of new tissue. To regenerate viable kidney tissue, researchers seeded the kidney scaffolds with epithelial and endothelial cells. The resulting organ tissue was able to

271

clear metabolites, reabsorb nutrients, and produce urine both in vitro and in vivo in rats. This process was previously used to bioengineer heart, liver, and lung tissue. The creation of transplantable tissue to permanently replace kidney function is a leap forward in overcoming the problems of donor organ shortages and the morbidity associated with immunosuppression in organ transplants.

Section 30.2

Cartilage Engineering

This section includes text excerpted from "Engineering
Cartilage," National Institutes of Health (NIH), March 3, 2014.
Reviewed December 2017.

Researchers developed a 3-D scaffold that guides the development of stem cells into specialized cartilage-producing cells. The approach could allow for the creation of orthopedic implants to replace cartilage, bone, and other tissues.

Cartilage is the slippery tissue that covers the ends of bones in a joint. In osteoarthritis (the most common type of arthritis), cartilage breaks down and wears away. Replacing cartilage in this and other situations has been a major goal in tissue engineering.

Cartilage contains water, collagen, proteoglycans, and chondrocytes. Collagens are fibrous proteins that serve as the building blocks of skin, tendon, bone, and other connective tissues. Proteoglycans, made of proteins and sugars, form strands that interweave with collagens to form a mesh-like structure. This structure, called an extracellular matrix, allows cartilage to flex and absorb shock. Chondrocytes, cells found throughout cartilage, produce and maintain the structure.

Creating replacements for musculoskeletal tissues is challenging. Stem cells have required extensive treatment in the lab with growth factors in order to develop (or differentiate) into suitable specialized cells. These cells then need to be placed into an appropriate 3-D structure. A team led by Drs. Farshid Guilak and Charles Gersbach at Duke University set out to create an artificial scaffold that could direct stem cells within to differentiate and form extracellular matrix. Their work was supported in part by NIH's National Institute of Arthritis and Musculoskeletal and Skin Diseases (NIAMS), National Institute on Aging (NIA), and an NIH Director's New Innovator Award.

The team used human mesenchymal stem cells, which are found in adult bone marrow. These cells can differentiate into different types of musculoskeletal cells. The scientists coated a 3-D woven scaffold with a compound that can secure viruses to a surface but still allow them to transfer genes into target cells. Lentiviruses were chosen to deliver the TGF-β3 (transforming growth factor β3) gene into the cells. TGF-β3 drives stem cells to become chondrocytes. After the viruses were attached to the structure, it was seeded with human mesenchymal stem cells and incubated in culture media.

Cells within the artificial scaffold successfully differentiated into chondrocytes within 2 weeks. Without any extra prompting, the cells created a cartilage-like extracellular matrix within 4 weeks. The results appeared online on February 18, 2014, in the Proceedings of the National Academy of Sciences.

"One of the advantages of our method is getting rid of the growth factor delivery, which is expensive and unstable, and replacing it with scaffolding functionalized with the viral gene carrier," Gersbach says. "The virus-laden scaffolding could be mass-produced and just sitting in a clinic ready to go. We hope this gets us one step closer to a translatable product."

This approach could allow for implants that restore function to a joint immediately and drive development of a mature, viable tissue replacement. The technique could also be applied to other kinds of tissues using other stem cells—or even a patient's own cells. However, further refinement will be needed before it could safely be used in the clinic.

Section 30.3

Regenerative Medicine Biomanufacturing

This section includes text excerpted from "Regenerative Medicine Biomanufacturing," National Institute Standards and Technology (NIST), June 30, 2017.

Regenerative medicine and advanced therapies are demonstrating promising clinical efficacy and could change the paradigm for treating a wide range of diseases and injuries. Clinical translation of this broad class of new therapeutics requires better defined and characterized products and more robust, reliable, and cost-effective manufacturing processes.

This program is designed to assist the nascent and promising regenerative medicine industry to meet their measurement assurance and regulatory challenges. NIST contributes to this effort by:

1. developing measurement solutions,

2. serving as a neutral ground for the discussion of underpinning measurements and other manufacturing needs, and

3. leading and contributing to the development of standards.

NIST aims to improve the confidence in cell measurements needed for translation and commercialization of advanced therapies, including cell therapy, gene therapy, and tissue engineering

Description

National Institute of Standards and Technology's (NIST) laboratory programs include quantitative genomic and cell measurements, live cell imaging, tissue engineering, and quantitative flow cytometry for cells and gene-modified cells as well as measurement assurance strategies for advanced therapeutic products. Much of their laboratory programs are conducted in collaborations with industry and federal agency partners and leverage NIST expertise in measurement science to address immediate and broad industry needs. We coordinate with key stakeholders to address cell measurement challenges and development of standards.

274

Measurement Assurance—The challenges in characterization of advanced therapy products may be largely addressed with systematic approaches for assessing sources of uncertainty and improving confidence in key measurements. NIST is developing strategies to ensure measurement confidence and discusses them in terms of how they can be applied to characterization of advanced therapy products.

Standards are critical in the development and commercialization of new technologies and facilitate national and international commerce. Standards also have an important role to ensure product consistency and facilitate regulatory approval. NIST is working with key stakeholders to develop Standard Reference Materials and Documentary Standards for regenerative medicine and advanced therapy products, and is leading and contributing to various Standards Development Organizations including ISO/TC 276 and ASTM F04. In addition, NIST administers the US TAG to ISO/TC276 Biotechnology as a means to coordinate national and international standards activities for existing and emerging biotechnology sectors, including regenerative medicine and advanced therapies. In particular, WG3 Analytical Methods is developing standards to enable confident measurements of cells and nucleic acids, and WG4 Bioprocessing is developing a suite of standards aimed to improve the consistency of manufacturing processes for cellular therapeutic products.

Section 30.4

New Method Builds Bone

This section includes text excerpted from "New Method Builds Bone," National Institutes of Health (NIH), February 13, 2012. Reviewed December 2017.

Researchers have developed a way to direct the body's own stem cells to the outer bone to build new, strong bone tissue. The method, developed in mice, may lead to new treatments for osteoporosis and other bone diseases that affect millions of people.

Bones are made of a mineral and protein scaffold filled with bone cells. Bone tissues continually break down and build back up again.

When the rate of bone loss outpaces the rate of bone tissue replacement, bones weaken, eventually leading to osteoporosis. This is common in people as they age.

Osteoblasts, the cells that rebuild bone, are derived from mesenchymal stem cells. These stem cells are found in bone marrow, deep inside the bone. They transform into osteoblasts and migrate to the outer bone, where they create new bone tissue.

As we age, we lose mesenchymal stem cells, so bone tissue building slows down. A team of researchers led by Dr. Wei Yao of the University of California, Davis sought to build new bone tissue by directing mesenchymal stem cells to outer bone more quickly. Their work was funded by several NIH components, including the National Institute of Arthritis and Musculoskeletal and Skin Diseases (NIAMS), *Eunice Kennedy Shriver* National Institute of Child Health and Human Development (NICHD) and National Institute on Aging (NIA). The results appeared in the online edition of Nature Medicine on February 5, 2012.

Mesenchymal stem cells express a surface protein called β4β1 integrin as they turn into osteoblasts. This protein helps them stick to bone and tissue surfaces. The scientists reasoned that a linker binding to both the β4β1 integrins and the outer bone surface would encourage the cells to stick to the outer bone.

The researchers created a hybrid compound from 2 molecules: LLP2A, a protein-like molecule that sticks to β4β1 integrins, and alendronate, an osteoporosis drug that sticks to the outer surface of bones. They called the compound LLP2A-Ale.

After 4 weeks of treatment with LLP2A-Ale, the bones of healthy mice were stronger and had more bone tissue than those of mice treated with alendronate alone or saline. In mice with weakened bone, the compound prevented further bone loss. Because mice, like humans, lose bone as they age, the scientists also treated older mice with LLP2A-Ale. The compound increased bone tissue in the older mice and prevented age-related bone loss.

The rate of bone loss can rise steeply in women after menopause. This is because levels of estrogen, a hormone important for maintaining bone health, begin to drop. To see if LLP2A-Ale could reverse bone loss when estrogen is low, the researchers infused estrogen-deficient female mice with LLP2A-Ale or parathyroid hormone, a molecule that increases bone formation. They found that LLP2A-Ale was as effective as parathyroid hormone at increasing the rate of bone formation.

"For the first time, we may have potentially found a way to direct a person's own stem cells to the bone surface where they can regenerate bone," says coinvestigator Dr. Nancy Lane of UC Davis. "This technique could become a revolutionary new therapy for osteoporosis as well as for other conditions that require new bone formation."

More studies will be needed, however, before the compound is ready for human trials.

Section 30.5

Light Therapy and Brain Function

This section includes text excerpted from "Can Light Therapy Help the Brain?" U.S. Department of Veterans Affairs (VA), March 31, 2015.

Can Light Therapy Help the Brain?

Researchers in a study at the U.S. Department of Veterans Affairs (VA) Boston Healthcare System are testing the effects of light therapy on brain function in Veterans with Gulf War Illness. The veterans wear a helmet lined with light-emitting diodes that apply red and near-infrared light to the scalp. They also have diodes placed in their nostrils, to deliver photons to the deeper parts of the brain.

The light is painless and generates no heat. A treatment takes about 30 minutes.

The therapy, though still considered "investigational" and not covered by most health insurance plans, is already used by some alternative medicine practitioners to treat wounds and pain. The light from the diodes has been shown to boost the output of nitric oxide near where the Light-emitting diodes (LEDs) are placed, which improves blood flow in that location.

"We are applying a technology that's been around for a while," says lead investigator Dr. Margaret Naeser, "but it's always been used on the body, for wound healing and to treat muscle aches and pains, and joint problems. We're starting to use it on the brain."

Naeser is a research linguist and speech pathologist for the Boston Veterans Affairs (VA), and a research professor of neurology at Boston University School of Medicine (BUSM). She is also a licensed acupuncturist and has conducted past research on laser acupuncture to treat paralysis in stroke, and pain in carpal tunnel syndrome.

How Do the Diodes Work?

The LED therapy increases blood flow in the brain, as shown on magnetic resonance imaging (MRI) scans. It also appears to have an effect on damaged brain cells, specifically on their mitochondria. These are bean-shaped subunits within the cell that put out energy in the form of a chemical known as adenosine triphosphate (ATP). The red and near-infrared light photons penetrate through the skull and into brain cells and spur the mitochondria to produce more ATP. That can mean clearer, sharper thinking, says Naeser.

Naeser says brain damage caused by explosions, or exposure to pesticides or other neurotoxins—such as in the Gulf War—could impair the mitochondria in cells. She believes light therapy can be a valuable adjunct to standard cognitive rehabilitation, which typically involves "exercising" the brain in various ways to take advantage of brain plasticity and forge new neural networks.

"The light-emitting diodes add something beyond what's currently available with cognitive rehabilitation therapy," says Naeser. "That's a very important therapy, but patients can go only so far with it. And in fact, most of the traumatic brain injury and posttraumatic stress disorder (PTSD) cases that we've helped so far with LEDs on the head have been through cognitive rehabilitation therapy. These people still showed additional progress after the LED treatments. It's likely a combination of both methods would produce the best results."

The LED approach has its skeptics, but Naeser's group has already published some encouraging results in the peer-reviewed scientific literature.

LED Therapy with Chronic Traumatic Brain Injury (TBI)

The Journal of Neurotrauma, they reported the outcomes of LED therapy in 11 patients with chronic TBI, ranging in age from 26–62. Most of the injuries occurred in car accidents or on the athletic field. One was a battlefield injury, from an improvised explosive device (IED).

Neuropsychological testing before the therapy and at several points thereafter showed gains in areas such as executive function, verbal learning, and memory. The study volunteers also reported better sleep and fewer PTSD symptoms.

The study authors concluded that the pilot results warranted a randomized, placebo-controlled trial—the gold standard in medical research.

That's happening now, thanks to VA support. One trial, already underway, aims to enroll 160 Gulf War Veterans. Half the Veterans will get the real LED therapy for 15 sessions, while the others will get a mock version, using sham lights.

Then the groups will switch, so all the volunteers will end up getting the real therapy, although they won't know at which point they received it. After each Veteran's last real or sham treatment, he or she will undergo tests of brain function.

Naeser points out that "because this is a blinded, controlled study, neither the participant nor the assistant applying the LED helmet and the intranasal diodes is aware whether the LEDs are real or sham. So they both wear goggles that block out the red LED light." The near-infrared light is invisible to begin with.

Part Five

Rehabilitation and Assistive Technologies

Chapter 31

Rehabilitation Engineering

What Is Rehabilitation Engineering?

Rehabilitation engineering is the use of engineering principles to:

- develop technological solutions and devices to assist individuals with disabilities and

- aid the recovery of physical and cognitive functions lost because of disease or injury.

Rehabilitation engineers design and build devices and systems to meet a wide range of needs that can assist individuals with mobility, communication, hearing, vision, and cognition. These tools help people with day-to-day activities related to employment, independent living, and education.

Rehabilitation engineering may involve relatively simple observations of how individuals perform tasks, and making accommodations to eliminate further injuries and discomfort. On the other end of the spectrum, rehabilitation engineering includes sophisticated brain computer interfaces that allow a severely disabled individual to operate

This chapter contains text excerpted from the following sources: Text beginning with the heading "What Is Rehabilitation Engineering?" is excerpted from "Science Education," National Institute of Biomedical Imaging and Bioengineering (NIBIB), November 2016; Text under the heading "Telerehabilitation" is excerpted from "Polytrauma/TBI System of Care," U.S. Department of Veterans Affairs (VA), June 3, 2015.

computers and other devices simply by thinking about the task they want to perform.

Rehabilitation engineers also improve upon standard rehabilitation methods to regain functions lost due to congenital disorders, disease (such as stroke or joint replacement), or injury (such as limb loss) to restore mobility.

Role of Future Rehabilitation Engineering Research in Improving the Quality of Life for Individuals

Ongoing research in rehabilitation engineering involves the design and development of innovative technologies and techniques that can help people regain physical or cognitive functions. For example:

- **Rehabilitation robotics,** to use robots as therapy aids instead of solely as assistive devices. Smart rehabilitation robotics aid mobility training in individuals suffering from impaired movement, such as following a stroke.

- **Virtual rehabilitation,** which uses virtual reality simulation exercises for physical and cognitive rehabilitation. These tools are entertaining, motivate patients to exercise, and provide objective measures such as range of motion. The exercises can be performed at home by a patient and monitored by a therapist over the Internet (known as tele-rehabilitation), which offers convenience as well as reduced costs.

- **Physical prosthetics,** such as smarter artificial legs with powered ankles, exoskeletons, dextrous upper limbs and hands. This is an area where researchers continue to make advances in design and function to better mimic natural limb movement and user intent.

- **Advanced kinematics,** to analyze human motion, muscle electrophysiology and brain activity to more accurately monitor human functions and prevent secondary injuries.

- **Sensory prosthetics,** such as retinal and cochlear implants to restore some lost function to provide navigation and communication, increasing independence and integration into the community.

- **Brain computer interfaces,** to enable severely impaired individuals to communicate and access information. These technologies use the brain's electrical impulses to allow individuals to move a computer cursor or a robotic arm that can reach and grab items, or send text messages.

- **Modulation of organ function,** as interventions for urinary and fecal incontinence and sexual disorders. Recent developments in neuromodulation of the peripheral nervous system offer the promise to treat organ function in the case of a spinal cord injury.

- **Secondary disorder treatment,** such as pain management.

Telerehabilitation

Telerehabilitation care involves the use of electronic information and telecommunication technologies when patients and providers are separated by geographic distances. Telerehabilitation technologies may include video teleconferencing to link a speech pathologist located at one of the Polytrauma System of Care locations with a Veteran patient at the local VA community-based outpatient clinic, or using home telehealth technologies to connect with Veterans at home to monitor their functional status and equipment needs. The advantages of doing this are:

1. it expedites access to care,

2. it improves clinical communication and transitions between locations of care, and

3. it eliminates unnecessary travel for Veterans and their families.

Early experience with telerehabilitation has shown that it can provide continuity and coordination of care across a continuum to help patients in their transition back to their local communities. Before leaving Department of Defense medical facilities or the Polytrauma Rehabilitation Centers, Veterans and their families have the opportunity to meet clinicians at the next location of care via video teleconferencing. This builds confidence in the continuum of services and promotes ongoing relationships with treatment teams across locations of care.

Telerehabilitation reduces the need for Veterans and their families to travel to receive specialized rehabilitation care. Over the past five years, telereahabilitation services have increased exponentially, with over 20 times more Veterans with polytrauma and TBI receiving rehabilitation care using video teleconferencing in 2013 than in 2008.

Increasingly, video teleconferencing is available between medical facilities and Veterans' homes. By connecting with Veterans in their homes, clinicians are able to observe how Veterans participate in activities of daily living, what assistive devices may be indicated, and how the home environment may be modified to facilitate greater independence. Home video teleconferencing is useful option for providing rehabilitation care for Veterans who have a difficulties traveling outside their homes.

Chapter 32

Rehabilitation Medicine: Research Activities and Scientific Advances

Through its intramural and extramural organizational units, the *Eunice Kennedy Shriver* National Institute of Child Health and Human Development (NICHD) supports and conducts a broad range of research projects that fall under the rehabilitation medicine umbrella, as well as research on conditions that cause disabilities.

Institute Activities and Advances

Several NICHD organizational units support and conduct research related to rehabilitation medicine. Some of this research aims to establish an evidence base for the development of best practices; other activities aim to improve health outcomes related to specific diseases and conditions that cause disability, such as traumatic brain injury (TBI) and stroke.

The Institute's National Center for Medical Rehabilitation Research (NCMRR) fosters the development of scientific knowledge to enhance the health, productivity, independence, and quality of life of people

This chapter includes text excerpted from "Rehabilitation Medicine: Research Activities and Scientific Advances," *Eunice Kennedy Shriver* National Institute of Child Health and Human Development (NICHD), September 2, 2015.

with physical disabilities through basic and clinical research. The NCMRR also serves as the coordinating body for rehabilitation research across the NIH and seeks collaborative opportunities with other NIH Institutes.

The NCMRR supports the development and application of devices to improve the human-environment interface and to restore or enhance an individual's capacity to function in his or her environment. This type of applied research and rehabilitation technology includes, but is not limited to, prosthetics, wheelchairs, biomechanical modeling, and other devices that aim to enhance mobility, communication, cognition, and environmental control.

The center supports some of these activities through the Small Business Innovative Research (SBIR) and Small Business Technology Transfer (STTR) programs. For example, NCMRR recently awarded funding to IntelliWheels, Inc. to develop ultra-lightweight, multi-geared wheels for manual wheelchairs to give users increased mobility and independence. Another NICHD-funded SBIR grant involves development and testing of an instrumented glove for rehabilitation of individuals who have lost hand function from stroke. The glove requires the user to practice gripping movements by playing a computer game.

Through its research programs, the NCMRR addresses specific issues in rehabilitation medicine:

- The Behavioral Sciences and Rehabilitation Technologies (BSRT) Program supports research related to development or redevelopment of emotional, cognitive, and physical processes and characteristics. This work includes interventions to encourage behavioral development in children with disabilities, as well as research on behavioral plasticity. The rehabilitative technology portion of the BSRT Program supports research that applies bioengineering principles to developing assistive technology to help people with disabilities perform daily tasks and activities.

- Projects within the Biological Sciences and Career Development (BSCD) Program support basic research on substrate responses to injury and on strategies to promote regeneration, plasticity, adaptation, and recovery. This research includes studies on topics ranging from activity-mediated processes, such as treadmill training and constrained-use therapy, to genomic influences on outcomes and recovery. This program also includes research on secondary conditions, such as pain, depression, and cardiovascular dysfunction.

- Projects within the Traumatic Brain Injury (TBI) and Stroke Rehabilitation (TSR) Program involve studying how to improve recovery of abilities that can be affected by TBI and stroke, including movement, mobility, and language, as well as mental health problems. Other ongoing areas of research include studies of combinations of pharmacological, surgical, and physical therapies to improve outcomes; the effect of compensatory training for unimpaired extremities; and measuring caregiver burden at different times following a stroke.

- Scientists supported by the Spinal Cord and Musculoskeletal Disorders and Assistive Devices (SMAD) Program conduct research to develop rehabilitation technology for individuals with spinal cord injury (SCI) and musculoskeletal disorders such as cerebral palsy, muscular dystrophy, multiple sclerosis, arthritis, osteoporosis, and systemic lupus erythematosus.

A few advances by NCMRR-funded scientists are described below. Additional advances are available in the right column of this page.

- NCMRR-funded scientists are currently working on major breakthroughs in walking technologies for lower-limb amputees. For example, at the University of Alabama, Tuscaloosa, a muscle-actuated robotic below-knee prosthesis is being developed that will give amputees a powered ankle joint capable of better meeting the demands of human locomotion than the passive ankle joints found in current prostheses. Scientists at Vanderbilt University are developing paired, coordinated robotic ankle and knee prostheses for bilateral transfemoral amputees. This will restore awareness and stability between the prostheses to enhance patients' ability to walk. At the University of Texas, scientists are studying the mechanics of falling in lower-limb amputees and designing rehabilitative interventions to prevent falls.

- Scientists supported in part by the NICHD, the National Institute of Biomedical Imaging and Bioengineering (NIBIB), the National Science Foundation, and the Defense Advanced Research Projects Agency developed and implanted a wireless sensor into the brains of pigs and monkeys that recorded and transmitted information about brain activity for more than a year. The sensor could be used to study the brain's muscle and movement control mechanisms in animals that are able to interact more naturally with their environments. It could also

289

eventually be used in severely neurologically impaired patients for wireless control of prosthetics that move with the power of thought, as well as in controlling motorized wheelchairs or other assistive technologies.

- Experts previously believed that recovery from TBI could occur only within a year after sustaining the injury. However, new findings from University of Texas at Dallas researchers indicate that a type of brain training called "gist-reasoning training" can improve cognitive performance months and even years after injury. Adolescents who experienced TBI at least six months prior to study enrollment completed eight 45-minute training sessions over the course of a month. The gist-reasoning training involved reading texts and creating summaries and recalling important facts. Compared to a control group, the gist training group displayed significant improvement in several cognitive functions. The results suggest that this kind of cognitive training can be effective at improving brain functioning at 6 months and beyond the injury.

- Researchers supported in part by NICHD reported on results from on ongoing clinical trial of a brain-computer interface called BrainGate that allows paralyzed individuals to use their thoughts to control a robotic arm that makes reach-and-grasp movements. The published report documented the ability of a paralyzed study participant to reach for and sip from a drink with no assistance. The article reported on several other tasks that the participants were able to complete. While the device requires additional testing before it can be widely used in paralyzed patients, it could eventually represent a way to restore some level of everyday function in these individuals.

In addition to NCMRR, the several other NICHD components also address rehabilitation medicine research, including (but not limited to):

In the Division of External Research (DER), the Intellectual and Developmental Disabilities Branch (IDDB) sponsors research and research training intended to prevent and ameliorate a variety of intellectual and developmental disabilities. These efforts include support of national research networks and programs that include some rehabilitation medicine-related work: Autism Centers of Excellence (ACE) Program, the *Eunice Kennedy Shriver* Intellectual & Developmental Disabilities Research Centers (EKS-IDDRCs), the Fragile X Syndrome

Research Center (FXSRC) Program, and the Paul D. Wellstone Muscular Dystrophy Cooperative Research Centers (MDCRCs).

The DER Pediatric Trauma and Critical Illness Branch supports research that addresses the prevention, treatment, management, and outcomes of physical and psychological trauma and the surgical, medical, psychosocial, and systems interventions needed to improve outcomes for critically ill and injured children across the developmental trajectory. The Branch also focuses on the continuum of psychosocial, behavioral, biological, and physiological influences that affect child health outcomes in trauma, injury, and acute care.

In the Division of Intramural Research (DIR), the Section on Nervous System Development and Plasticity conducts research on the development of the nervous system and nervous system plasticity during fetal and early postnatal life. Studies include investigations of mechanisms of synaptic plasticity, neuron-glia signaling, development of neural precursor cells, and implications for learning and memory.

The DIR Program on Pediatric Imaging and Tissue Sciences develops and evaluates noninvasive imaging methods for assessing normal development, screening, diagnosis, and prognosis of diseases, disorders, and disabilities in pediatric populations. Studies include both basic and applied explorations of the science of tissues, physics and imaging. The Program's Section on Tissue Biophysics and Biomimetics invents, develops, and implements novel quantitative in vivo methods for imaging tissues and organs. For example, an ongoing study uses multimodal magnetic resonance imaging to evaluate cerebral reorganization caused by various rehabilitation approaches in children with cerebral palsy and TBI. Another line of investigation examines plasticity changes after rehabilitation in military personnel affected by TBI.

Other Activities and Advances

- Medical Rehabilitation Research Infrastructure Network (MRRIN). MRRIN, funded through the NCMRR, the National Institute of Neurological Disorders and Stroke and the NIBIB, is a centralized medical rehabilitation research infrastructure that provides investigators with access to expertise, courses, workshops, technologies, core services, research training, pilot project funding, and collaborative, multidisciplinary opportunities. The Network currently consists of seven medical center sites across the country.

291

- Blue Ribbon Panel on Rehabilitation Research. The NICHD convened a panel comprising 13 non-NIH scientific experts who were tasked with reviewing medical rehabilitation research within NCMRR and across NIH to identify promising research opportunities. The NICHD, along with the National Institute of Neurological Disorders and Stroke (NINDS) and the National Institute on Deafness and Other Communication Disorders (NIDCD), administers grants funded by the Foundation for the National Institutes of Health (FNIH) and the National Football League intended to answer some of the fundamental questions about TBI. These cooperative awards will allow teams of scientists to correlate brain scans with changes in brain tissue, possibly making it possible to diagnose chronic effects of TBI in living individuals.

- The NICHD has also teamed up with NINDS to fund an eight-center, randomized clinical trial for the study of arm rehabilitation following stroke. Called ICARE, the trial compared an experimental upper-extremity rehabilitation protocol with usual care.

- NIH Clinical Center. At the Clinical Center, rehabilitation medicine professionals collaborate with NICHD and other NIH IC investigators in support of biomedical rehabilitation research. They initiate research in rehabilitation sciences by providing innovative rehabilitation services and developing, investigating and applying measurements and treatments of impairments, disabilities and handicaps pertaining to human function. The team also provides consultations, clinical assessments, and treatments for patients.

- NIH Pain Consortium. The consortium is an initiative consisting of representative members of most of the NIH ICs with programs related to pain, including the NICHD. The Consortium was designed to promote increased pain research across the NIH.

- From 2002–2012, NCMRR supported the TBI Clinical Trials Network. This network comprised eight level-1 trauma centers throughout the United States and designed and executed a clinical trial of citicoline (2,000 mg daily for 90 days) versus. placebo to treat complicated mild, moderate, and severe TBI. The Citicoline Brain Injury treatment Trial (COBRIT) was a phase III, double-blind, randomized clinical trial which ran from

2007 through 2011. The main outcome measures were functional and cognitive status, assessed at 90 days after injury using a core test battery developed by the Network. Rates of favorable outcome did not significantly differ between the treatment and placebo groups at the post-injury times evaluated. The data from the COBRIT trial are available to requesting investigators through the Federal Interagency Traumatic Brain Injury Research Informatics System (FITBIR).

Chapter 33

Vision and Hearing Loss

Chapter Contents

Section 33.1—Low Vision and Blindness
        Rehabilitation 296

Section 33.2—Artificial Retina 299

Section 33.3—Cochlear Implants: Different Kind of
        Hearing 302

Section 33.1

Low Vision and Blindness Rehabilitation

This section includes text excerpted from "Vision
Research Needs, Gaps, and Opportunities," National Eye
Institute (NEI), August 2012. Reviewed December 2017.

Rehabilitation Highlights of Recent Progress

Assistive Technology

Because most content on the Internet is displayed visually, several new applications are geared to interpret this content for visually impaired users such as dynamic pin displays for online Braille and tactile graphics. Recent advances in computing power and image-processing have revolutionized applications for the visually impaired. Screen-magnifying and screen-reading software are widely deployed so that computers and smartphones are now accessible to low-vision and blind users, without the need for costly third-party software accessories. The latest generation of smartphones has stimulated development of innovative products to aid the visually impaired. These include flexible image magnifiers, mobile optical character recognition, bar code readers, and indoor wayfinding aids. In the past five years, research and development of global positioning system based navigation aids for visually impaired people has refined commercially available products.

Behavioral and Neuroscience Basic Research

When we move around our environment, in our mind's eye, we construct a picture of the world around us. This picture, or cognitive map, is attributed to a neural network thought to be located in the medial temporal brain area. The parietal area of the brain is closely tied to accrual of perceptual information. The interaction between the parietal and temporal regions may explain how ongoing perceptual input leads to the formation of cognitive maps and has implications for understanding how visually impaired individuals learn different strategies for orienting and navigating.

Following pathological insult to retina or brain, perceptual training techniques have been examined using videogames. Behavioral studies have demonstrated that extensive practice can improve visual sensitivity. Infants with congenital cataracts or other treatable eye conditions experience visual deprivation during a period of robust visual development. Studies of these children are finding that once vision is restored, substantial functional and organizational changes in the visual cortex occur; whether the same holds true later in life is an actively debated topic. This neuroplasticity can now be studied non-invasively with functional magnetic resonance imaging. These findings regarding plasticity hold promise for informing vision rehabilitation efforts. Different areas of the brain respond to different types of perceptual stimuli (vision, touch, sound). Perception depends on integrating this multisensory information. Research shows that normally sighted, as well as visually impaired individuals recruit the visual cortex when interpreting tactile or auditory information. The functional roles of such cross-modal activations are not well understood, but are hot topics of current research and may provide the neural basis for sensory substitution, where perceptual processing for one sensory modality is largely replaced for another.

Implications of Vision Loss

With an increased understanding of the interdependence of physical and mental health, vision loss has been shown to be an independent predictor of depression. Depression (both major depressive disorders and subthreshold depression) affects roughly one-third of older adults with vision loss, which is similar to rates found among medically ill populations and those with other chronic conditions. In the visually impaired, depression further exacerbates functional disability in everyday activities. Thus, visual impairment has been found to have widespread negative effects on quality of life, and psychological and social well-being.

Quality of Life

Quality-of-life issues are gaining increased attention in vision impairment and rehabilitation research. With the development of standardized metrics (e.g., NEI Visual Functioning Questionnaire), quality-of-life measurements complement objective measures of visual function. Furthermore, there is a growing recognition that quality of life is a multidimensional concept that includes financial status, employment, physical and mental health, social relationships, and recreation and leisure time activities.

Activities of Daily Living

Research on activities of daily living includes reading, mobility, and orientation in lab settings and real-world environments. Recent research has focused on the complicated visual environment encountered in the real world to appreciate how normally sighted and visually impaired individuals process a visually rich.

New Mobile Assistive Technologies

For visually impaired individuals, smartphone apps are emerging as important tools for everyday functioning and independence. NEI-funded researchers are developing apps to assist individuals to maneuver around obstacles, read, and recognize faces and objects. For example, researchers are developing products that will allow the visually impaired to use smartphone cameras for identifying packaged food content and prices at the grocery store by scanning the barcodes on the package labels. Another app scans money to determine bill denominations, which provides confidence to the user for transactions at the cash register. Several assistive devices also are under development for the home or the workplace. For example, researchers are developing an app that immediately converts an image of the clock on a microwave oven or the temperature setting on a thermostat into an audio report on the phone's speaker. Indoor wayfinding systems use scannable signs or other locators so that the visually impaired can navigate unfamiliar locations. For outdoor navigation, researchers are developing apps to capture images of intersections and analyze them to identify crosswalks, curbs, and the status of "Walk/Don't Walk" signs in real-time. Others are creating services that provide subscribers with on-demand assistance, where a caller describes a situation or snaps a picture of an item, and an offsite assistant immediately calls back and describes the scene or item to the subscriber. The latest mobile technologies have opened up seemingly unlimited possibilities for assisting the visually impaired, and NEI remains committed to supporting the development of these and other cutting edge technologies.

Section 33.2

Artificial Retina

This section includes text excerpted from "Overview of
the Artificial Retina Project," U.S. Department of
Energy (DOE), July 10, 2017.

The DOE Artificial Retina Project was a multi-institutional collaborative effort to develop and implant a device containing an array of microelectrodes into the eyes of people blinded by retinal disease. The ultimate goal was to design a device to help restore limited vision that enables reading, unaided mobility, and facial recognition.

The device is intended to bypass the damaged eye structure of those with retinitis pigmentosa and macular degeneration. These diseases destroy the light-sensing cells (photoreceptors, or rods and cones) in the retina, a multilayered membrane located at the back of the eye.

How the Artificial Retina Works

Normal vision begins when light enters and moves through the eye to strike specialized photoreceptor (light-receiving) cells in the retina called rods and cones. These cells convert light signals to electric impulses that are sent to the optic nerve and the brain. Retinal diseases like age-related macular degeneration and retinitis pigmentosa destroy vision by annihilating these cells.

With the artificial retina device, a miniature camera mounted in eyeglasses captures images and wirelessly sends the information to a microprocessor (worn on a belt) that converts the data to an electronic signal and transmits it to a receiver on the eye. The receiver sends the signals through a tiny, thin cable to the microelectrode array, stimulating it to emit pulses. The artificial retina device thus bypasses defunct photoreceptor cells and transmits electrical signals directly to the retina's remaining viable cells. The pulses travel to the optic nerve and, ultimately, to the brain, which perceives patterns of light and dark spots corresponding to the electrodes stimulated. Patients learn to interpret these visual patterns.

Technological Challenges in Engineering a Retinal Implant

Researchers face numerous challenges in developing retinal prosthetic devices that are effective, safe, and durable enough to last for the lifetime of the individual.

The retinal device bypasses the eye's lost light-gathering function of the rods and cones with a video camera. The information captured by the camera is used to electrically stimulate the part of the retina not destroyed by disease. Stimulation is done with a thin, flexible metal electrode array that has been patterned on soft plastic material similar to that of a contact lens.

The device must be biocompatible with delicate eye tissue, yet tough enough to withstand the corrosive effect of the salty environment. It should remain stably tacked to the retinal macula and not overly compress or pull at the tissue--the resilience of which can be compared to that of a wet Kleenex®. The apparatus also needs to be powered at a high enough level to stimulate the electrodes, yet not generate enough heat to damage the remaining functional retinal cells.

Moreover, just as the resolution of graphic images on a computer screen improves with greater pixel density, researchers assume that increased electrode densities will translate into higher-resolution images for patients. However, the area of the retina targeted for electrical stimulation is less than 5 mm by 5 mm. Consequently, as the number of electrodes increases, their size and spacing must decrease.

Furthermore, image processing needs to be performed in real time so there is no delay in interpreting an object in view. Development of effective surgical approaches is also critically important to ensure a successful implant (see sidebar, Ensuring Surgical Reproducibility, below).

In other words, engineering a retinal prosthesis is somewhat analogous to constructing a miniature iPod® on a foldable contact lens that works in seawater.

Ensuring Surgical Reproducibility

Designing a robust, biocompatible retinal prosthesis is one thing. However, another challenge lies in developing easily replicable surgical techniques to place the implant in just the right spot on the retinal macula and keep it there.

Many of the maneuvers surgeons perform during implantation of the Argus™ II are standard techniques any experienced retinal surgeon has used numerous times, says Mark Humayun, a vitreoretinal surgeon and associate director of research at the University of Southern California's Doheny Eye Institute. Introducing the electrode array into the eye and tacking it to the retina are new tasks requiring novel, advanced approaches not within a retinal surgeon's normal arsenal.

Consequently, "We tried to tailor the approach to processes mimicking those that surgeons already follow," says Humayun, who pioneered the implantation procedure. Another key to achieving surgical reproducibility is using easy-to-handle materials whose look and feel are like those with which surgeons already are comfortable. For example, the telemetry coil is mounted on a scleral buckle, which surgeons place around the eye for retinal detachments.

"We've really reduced this technique more to science than art so that it can be more easily reproduced," Humayun says.

Although still a complex procedure, "It's a surgery that's doable, and I think it's very reasonable that this will become a much more widely used technique," says Lyndon da Cruz, a vitreoretinal surgeon at Moorfields Eye Hospital in London who is participating in the Argus™ II clinical trials. "We feel we're part of something that's genuinely new, innovative, and cutting edge," he adds.

Promising Advances

Three devices of increasing resolution are now in testing or development. Several pioneering technological advances in fabrication and packaging by DOE national laboratories have helped make the third-generation device a reality. For example, the significantly higher electrode density required new lithographic and etching techniques to pattern platinum films on soft polymer materials. Additionally, new stacking techniques were needed to layer metals and polymers on top of each other to achieve a narrower prosthesis in the section that delivers electrical charges to the electrodes. Other advances by DOE national laboratories include softening the rim of the array that is in contact with delicate retinal neurons and improving techniques to ensure none of the electrodes short-circuit.

Because the device's advanced electronics operate in the eye's saltwater environment, DOE's national laboratories have spearheaded critical innovations in packaging. These innovations include higher interconnect densities of the individual contacts and attachment to the electronic chip while still preserving a leak-tight electrical connection. A novel, dual-sided integrated circuit also has been developed

301

for stacking components and interconnecting them. Research also is under way on various bioadhesives that could be used to attach the microelectrode array to the retinal surface.

Section 33.3

Cochlear Implants: Different Kind of Hearing

This section includes text excerpted from "Cochlear Implants: A Different Kind of 'Hearing," U.S. Food and Drug Administration (FDA), February 10, 2017.

Your elderly uncle is hard of hearing and has a difficult time under-standing conversation—so much so that he's feeling frustrated and left out. His hearing aids aren't helping much.

Your 1-year-old daughter was diagnosed with severe hearing loss in both ears, and you're worried about her ability to learn and understand speech. How will she learn to communicate?

For both of these cases, a cochlear implant may be an option.

What are cochlear implants? Who uses them and why? And how does the U.S. Food and Drug Administration (FDA) play a role? The cochlea is the part of the inner ear that contains the endings of the nerve which carries sound to the brain. A cochlear implant is a small, electronic device that when surgically placed under the skin, stimu-lates the nerve endings in the cochlea to provide a sense of sound to a person who is profoundly deaf or severely hard of hearing.

"A severe to profound hearing loss in both ears prevents a person from understanding speech and communicating in everyday conver-sations. Cochlear implants can increase hearing and communication abilities for people who don't receive enough benefit from traditional hearing aids," says Srinivas Nandkumar, Ph.D., chief of the Ear, Nose and Throat (ENT) Devices Branch at FDA.

How Does It Work?

A cochlear implant consists of an external part that sits behind the ear and an internal part that is surgically placed under the skin.

Usually, a magnet holds the external system in place next to the implanted internal system. The FDA has approved cochlear implants for use by individuals aged one year and older.

Here's how it works:

- A surgeon places the cochlear implant under the skin next to the ear.

- The cochlear implant receives sound from the outside environment, processes it, and sends small electric currents near the auditory nerve.

- These electric currents activate the nerve, which then sends a signal to the brain.

- The brain learns to recognize this signal and the wearer experiences this as "hearing."

"A cochlear implant is quite different from a typical hearing aid, which simply amplifies sound," says Nandkumar. "Using one is not just a matter of turning up the volume; the nerves are being electrically stimulated to send signals and the brain translates and does the rest of the work." Moreover, cochlear implant wearers need to undergo intensive speech therapy to understand how to process what they are hearing.

Cochlear implants don't restore normal hearing, says Nandkumar. But depending on the individual, they can help the wearer recognize words and better understand speech, including when using a telephone.

Does Age Matter?

According to the National Institute on Deafness and other Communication Disorders (NIDCD) at the National Institutes of Health (NIH), for young children who are deaf or severely hard-of-hearing, using a cochlear implant while they are young exposes them to sounds during an optimal period to develop speech and language skills. Several research studies have shown that when these children receive a cochlear implant at a relatively young age (for example, at 18 months) followed by intensive therapy, they tend to hear and speak better than those who receive implants at an older age.

But adults and older children who have acquired severe to profound hearing loss after they have acquired speech can also do very well with an implant, partly because they are postlingual (that is,

303

already have learned to speak a language). "At that point, a person has to get used to the fact that what he hears sounds differently and more 'machine-like' than it did when he had more hearing," Nandkumar says. "Whereas someone who was profoundly deaf at birth will adapt at a very early age to a cochlear implant and the way in which it processes sound."

Conversely, people who are deaf since birth and have not gotten implants until they are a bit older (for example, 8 years of age) may not derive as much benefit from cochlear implants.

FDA Regulation of Cochlear Implants

Before manufacturers can bring a new cochlear implant to market, they must submit studies and data to FDA scientists, who will review the information for safety and effectiveness. Cochlear implants are designated as Class III devices, meaning they receive the highest level of regulatory scrutiny. This is because they are surgically implanted near the brain, which increases health risk. Other risks, while minimal, include injury to the facial nerve, meningitis, perilymph fluid leak (fluid from the inner ear leaks through the hole created to place the implant), and dizziness or vertigo.

The Future of Cochlear Implants

Scientists continue to look for ways to improve cochlear implants and how they function once implanted. For example:

Companies are developing more sophisticated strategies that help to minimize background noise and increase the noise-to-sound ratio, helping the user to better focus and understand speech.

Hearing science researchers also are looking at the potential benefits of pairing a cochlear implant in one ear with either another cochlear implant or a hearing aid in the other ear.

"A cochlear implant won't restore hearing the way that eyeglasses can fully restore vision," Nandkumar says. "But companies are developing increasingly sophisticated processing strategies that can reduce background noise and increase the signal-to-noise ratio, in an effort to improve the quality of speech the wearer hears."

Chapter 34

Robotics in Rehabilitation

Chapter Contents

Section 34.1—Cybernetics 306

Section 34.2—Prosthetic Engineering 310

Section 34.3—New Robotic Wheelchair 314

Section 34.1

Cybernetics

This section includes text excerpted from "Cybernetics"
U.S. Department of Energy's National Nuclear Security
Administration (NNSA), September 18, 2013.
Reviewed December 2017.

Cybernetics includes the development of mechanical, physical, biological, and cognitive systems that enable the development of advanced man-machine interface technologies. U.S. Department of Energy's National Nuclear Security Administration's (NNSA) work in this area has led to the development of dynamic prosthetics technology, implantable sensors with neural interfaces, and modular integrated microsystems.

Dynamic Socket

Challenge

A prosthetic socket is the interface between an amputee's residual limb and a prosthetic limb. Unlike the tissues under the foot, the soft tissues of the residual limb aren't well adapted to tolerate weight-bearing loads. Prosthetists are tasked with creating a comfortable, custom interface for the amputee that appropriately distributes pressures across the socket surface. Some pressure must be applied everywhere to avoid blistering but local high-pressure points should be avoided, with special care taken to limit pressure on load-intolerant regions, such as bony areas. Exacerbating these challenges is the fact that the volume and shape of the residual limb change over time. The limb often shrinks over the course of the day as interstitial fluid is pumped out while the amputee walks. Longer-term changes due to weight gain/loss and muscle atrophy are also common.

Need

Current approaches to residual limb volume management are crude and inconvenient. Most commonly, amputees will remove the socket and don socks on the residual limb to accommodate lost volume. This approach results in a global volume adjustment, which does not accurately reflect the nonuniform nature of the limb shape change. A more intelligent and convenient approach is needed to meet the needs of active amputees, who are more likely to lose limb volume quickly.

Technical Challenges

A practical solution to limb volume management must be simple for both the amputee and prosthetist to use. It should require little or no special fitting, donning/doffing procedures or maintenance. The size and weight of the system should also not dominate the prosthetic device.

Solution

A dynamic prosthetic socket system that monitors and adjusts to limb volume changes is being developed. The Dynamic Socket consists of an elastomeric liner (similar in geometry and material properties to what most amputees currently wear) with embedded sensing elements and fluidic bladders and channels. The sensors monitor the socket fit continuously and compare to a baseline established by the prosthetist. As the fit deviates from the baseline, incompressible fluid (liquid) is moved into or out of bladders to reach the desired fit.

Features / Benefits

- Can chronically monitor socket fit
- Intelligent volume adjustments based on sensor readings
- Both global and local adjustments
- Uses ubiquitous socket fitting procedure, requiring minimal extra procedures

Applications

The Dynamic Socket is targeted primarily to lower-limb amputees who experience large volume fluctuations. Active amputees, such as injured soldiers, are of primary interest as the high activity levels often result in larger volume loss throughout the day. These amputees also require a higher-performance fit. The technology is also applicable to vascular disease amputees who lack sensitivity on the residual limb and have unique tissue-health concerns.

Neural Control of Prosthetics

Researchers in High Consequence, Automation, and Robotics are working on ways to improve amputees' control over prosthetics with direct help from their own nervous systems.

Neural interfaces operate where the nervous system and an artificial device intersect. Interfaces can monitor nerve signals or provide inputs that let amputees control prosthetic devices by direct neural signals, the same way they would control parts of their own bodies.

Challenge

Interfaces must be:

- structured so nerve fibers can grow through,

- mechanically compatible so they don't harm the nervous system or surrounding tissues,

- biocompatible to integrate with tissue and promote nerve fiber growth,

- conductive to allow electrode sites to connect with external circuitry, and the electrical properties must be tuned to transmit neural signals.

Need

The Amputee Coalition estimates 2 million people in the United States are living with limb loss. The Congressional Research Service reports more than 1,600 amputations involving U.S. troops between 2001 and 2010, more than 1,400 of those associated with the fighting in Iraq and Afghanistan. Most were major limb amputations.

Solution

Robotics approached the problem from a technical point of view, looking at improving implantable and wearable neural interface electronics.

Sandia's research focused on biomaterials and peripheral nerves at the interface site. The idea was to match material properties to nerve fibers with flexible, conductive materials that are biocompatible so they can integrate with nerve bundles.

Features / Benefits

Improved prosthetics with flexible nerve-to-nerve or nerve-to-muscle interfaces let amputees control prosthetic devices by direct neural signals, the same way they would control parts of their own bodies.

Applications

This proof-of-concept work is being used to obtain third-party funding so researchers can bring the technology to wounded warriors, amputees, and victims of peripheral nerve injury.

Pressure Measurement Sensors

Challenge

Tactile (touch) sensing has many engineering and medical applications. Robotic and prosthetic hands can use tactile sensing to manipulate objects or provide feedback to the user. Sensors can also measure the interface pressure and shear loads on human soft tissues (e.g., skin) in a prosthetic device, exoskeleton, or shoe.

Need

While several commercially available tactile sensors exist, most are limited in some way in relation to the applications described above. Most notably, a tactile sensor that can measure both normal and shear pressures is not commercially available. Shear measurement is especially important for robotic manipulation and human interface load measurement.

Technical Challenge

Designing a tactile sensor presents many unique challenges. Almost all force or pressure sensors actually measure displacement or strain and the challenge is to create a mechanical transducer that reliably converts loads to strain. This is particularly difficult in multiple directions, which is required when both pressure and shear are desired.

Solution

Multiple (patent pending) tactile sensors that offer unique performance have been developed. A bubble pressure sensor that consists of a fluid pressure sensor encapsulated in a fluid-filled bubble has been designed. This sensor has performed better than other tactile sensors we've tested in many areas, such as hysteresis and drift. A three-axis optical sensor that can measure both normal and shear (in two directions) has also been developed.

Features/Benefits

- Bubble pressure sensor has less drift and other inaccuracies than many commercial sensors

- Optical sensor can sense multi-axis loads and has a thin profile

- Optical sensor uses inexpensive integrated circuit components

Applications

Both the bubble pressure sensor and the optical sensor have been integrated into a prosthetic socket liner for socket/limb interface load measurement. The optical sensor has been integrated into a robotic hand and a shoe sole. The insole can be used to monitor local pressure and shear loads and has been effective at measuring the ground reaction force for mobile biomechanics applications.

Section 34.2

Prosthetic Engineering

This section includes text excerpted from "Prosthetic Engineering—Overview," U.S. Department of Veterans Affairs (VA), March 30, 2017.

The aim of U.S. Department of Veterans Affairs (VA) Center for Limb Loss and MoBility is to improve prosthetic prescription by investigating the efficacy of prosthetic components used in current clinical practice and by developing novel approaches to improve the current standard of care. Their amputee-centric research encompasses improving patient mobility and comfort and preventing injury. Support for this research (2000 to present) includes funding from the U.S.

Department of Veterans Affairs Rehabilitation Research and Development Service (RR&D) and the National Institutes of Health (NIH).

Mobility Research

Disturbance Response in Amputee Gait

Errors in foot placement while avoiding obstacles and maneuvering in the household and community environments may lead to falls and injuries. This research aims to develop an ankle that can invert and evert and thereby control the center of pressure under the prosthetic foot; enhancing balance and stability of lower limb amputees.

Foot-Ankle Stiffness

Many ambulatory lower limb amputees exhibit fatigue, asymmetrical gait, and the inability to walk at varying speeds. A rapid prototyping approach is being used to fabricate feet of varying stiffness for exploring the effects of foot stiffness on amputee gait.

Turning Gait

Turning corners and maneuvering around obstacles are essential abilities for successful community and household ambulation. The aim of this research is to test the efficacy of a compliant torque adapter in the pylons of transtibial amputees.

Energy Storage and Release

Many ambulatory lower limb amputees exhibit fatigue, asymmetrical gait, and the inability to walk at varying speeds. VA Center for Limb Loss and MoBility developing and testing several approaches aimed at providing the propulsive forces necessary to alleviate these problems.

Stochastic Resonance

Stochastic resonance (sub-threshold vibration) may enhance peripheral sensation sufficiently to result in improved postural stability and locomotor function. This research explores application of this phenomenon to the residual limb and intact plantar surface of diabetic lower limb amputees.

Research in Robotics and Biomechanics

Dr. Aubin's research spans robotics and biomechanics with applications in health and mobility. He motivates his research by engaging with patients and stakeholders to understand shortcomings in the areas of rehabilitation, prosthetics, orthotics, and physical therapy. Dr. Aubin strives to address these unmet patient and caregiver needs by establishing multidisciplinary research teams that leverage state of the art technologies in robotics, neuroscience, and computational intelligence. Dr. Aubin's research goal is to develop and utilizes novel sensors, algorithms, assistive powered devices, and robotic tools that can augment human performance and/or improve mobility and function for those affected by disease, age or trauma.

Smart Cane System

People with pain or arthritis in their knee often walk with a cane to reduce knee pain and to improve or maintain their mobility. Increased pressure on the knee joint likely causes knee arthritis and reducing the pressure on the knee joint may slow the progression of arthritis. Walking with a cane reduces the pressure inside the knee joint, but only if the cane supports 10 percent to 20 percent of a person's weight. Many people may not be using their cane in the best way they can because they don't know how much force (percent of their body weight) they are putting on the cane when they walk. In this study, VA Center for Limb Loss and MoBility is looking at how using a computerized cane that beeps or vibrates (like a cell phone) when a certain amount of force is applied to it might help people learn to more effectively use a cane. They are also examining how walking with a cane changes the pressure in the knee joint. They hypothesize that giving the user biofeedback, a sound or vibration signal from the cane, will help them apply the optimal amount of force on the cane. Their secondary hypothesis is that increased cane loading will result in a decrease in knee joint pressure.

Sensory Feedback for Prosthetic Limbs

It has long been recognized that restoring movement function after amputation is a priority. We are now entering an era in which restoration of sensation may be possible as well through the use of smart sensorized prosthetic devices and haptic feedback. VA Center for Limb Loss and MoBility is working on understanding how feedback of forces and events on the foot—for example the placement of the prosthetic foot as the user is walking down stairs—can lead to improved function.

Injury Prevention Research

Vacuum Suspension Systems

Many amputees live with an ill-fitting socket and can experience limb pistoning within the socket, which in turn may result in skin irritation, tissue breakdown, discomfort, and a reduction in activity. The aims of this research are to characterize the response of the lower residual limb to a vacuum suspension system and to measure changes in limb volume with a structured light scanning system.

Socket Systems and Tissue O_2

Limb health and wound healing capacity is closely related to the amount of oxygen present in limb tissues. Using their fiber-optic video-oximetry imaging system, they aim to discover if prosthetic prescription can influence residual limb tissue oxygenation during both rest and gait.

Distributed Sensing

The goal of the proposed project is to develop enabling sensing technology based on a flexible array and to build a prototype of a prosthetic liner with distributed, unimodal field sensing capability. The specific aims include:

1. The design of the flexible sensing array for measurement of moisture, temperature, pressure, and shear stress;

2. Integration of this array into a prosthetic liner/socket; and

3. Testing of device performance.

Torsional Prosthesis

This research seeks to develop a prosthetic limb whose torsional characteristics can adapted depending activity. Their goal is to reduce torsional stresses and the incidence of residual limb injuries.

Patient Comfort Research

Thermal Comfort

Lower limb amputations often experience discomfort related in part to higher skin temperatures within their prosthetic socket. Their research has found prosthetic liners and sockets are excellent

313

insulators that can retain heat. Activity can cause a dramatic increase in skin temperature within the prosthesis requiring substantially long periods of inactivity to restore resting state temperatures. Their current work involves developing active cooling systems and embedded sensor networks to monitor skin temperature.

Evaporative Cooling and Perspiration Removal

Amputees often complain about uncomfortably warm residual limb skin temperatures and the accumulation of perspiration within their prosthesis. This research will discover if a novel evaporative cooling system can provide ameliorate these problems.

Section 34.3

New Robotic Wheelchair

This section contains text excerpted from the following sources: Text under the heading "MeBot: Futuristic Robotic Wheelchair" is excerpted from "MeBot: Robotic Wheelchair Wows Judges in Scotland," U.S. Department of Veterans Affairs (VA), February 13, 2017; Text under the heading "MeBot's Features" is excerpted from "New Robotic Wheelchair in the Works at Pittsburgh Lab," U.S. Department of Veterans Affairs (VA), February 3, 2016.

MeBot: Futuristic Robotic Wheelchair

A robotic wheelchair created by a team led by Dr. Rory Cooper from the Human Engineering Research Laboratory (HERL) in Pittsburgh earned international recognition by winning "Best New Concept" in the Blackwood Design Awards.

"It caught the attention of the judges," a Blackwood dispatch said, "in part because it was very clear that it was designed by wheelchair users, for wheelchair users and with very full inclusion from the outset."

The Mobility Enhancement Robotic Wheelchair, or "MeBot," was born when the Marine Wounded Warrior Regiment challenged Cooper to design a wheelchair that not only moves smoothly from inside to outside over steps and curbs, but also handles trails during their staff rides at Gettysburg National Military Park.

MeBot's automatic seat, height and inclination adjustments prevent slips and falls on rough terrain and steps, ensuring a smoother, safer ride. The seat adjustment feature also gives users better access to objects in high places, and in social situations, allows them to rise to standing level during conversations.

MeBot's Features

It has six wheels, an onboard computer and software, and an array of high-tech sensors and actuators. It's designed to smoothly navigate over gravely or muddy roads, uneven slopes, wet grass, and other difficult terrain.

Highly Functional Indoors and Outdoors

The model is still in development. So far it's been tested only at HERL, using equipment such as a 180-pound test dummy and a large elevated mechanical platform that tilts and lurches in all sorts of directions. It's not quite the mechanical bull at Gilley's in Dallas, but it's robust enough to simulate a fairly rugged outdoor excursion.

The device still has to go through rigorous user testing, both in the lab and in the field. Even if all goes well in further tests, the MEBot probably won't be ready commercially for another five years or so, says Cooper.

But he is enthusiastic about what the device could mean for Veterans and others who depend on wheelchairs to get around. He says it would give them unprecedented freedom and independence, as a daily mobility device both in the great outdoors and inside homes, shops, and offices.

"MEBot can go up or down curbs or steps, and maintain a level seat—forward, backwards, and left and right—over uneven terrain," says Cooper. "It has traction control, antiskid braking, and all the features of an electric powered wheelchair with powered seat functions—tilt, recline, leg-rest, elevation. It's highly functional indoors and outdoors, in both ADA (Americans with Disabilities Act) and non-ADA environments."

The self-levelling feature is crucial because it keeps the chair from dangerously spilling its driver onto the ground when traversing rough, sloping, or otherwise uneven surfaces, including ramps and curb-cuts.

315

Wheels Pivot up and down, Backwards and Forwards

The inner workings of this feature, like just about every other aspect of the chair, are complex but elegant. Various sensors detect the positions of the seat, the wheels, and the electric and pneumatic actuator motors that control them. Algorithms programmed into the MEBot instantaneously analyze the sensor input and determine the desired position of the actuators in order to keep the seat level.

A key feature of the MEBot is its six wheels—two compact but muscular drive wheels on either side, along with smaller front and rear casters on either side. Each wheel can pivot up or down, independent of the others, and the drive wheels can also adjust backwards or forwards.

Picture someone trying to maneuver the chair along the side of a hill, on a slight angle: The wheels on one side of the chair could be a full 20 degrees lower than their counterparts on the opposite side, to help keep the seat level. Cooper uses the term "float" to describe how the seat—and the user on top of it—maintain their center of gravity amid pitching, rolling, and yawing.

Curbs? No problem. The onboard curb-climbing app kicks in automatically when it senses a curb or step. It leverages the up-and-down motion of all six wheels, and the forward motion of the drive wheels, to mount the curb while keeping the chair and its user stable. Cooper says MEBot is designed to handle curbs up to 8 inches high.

MEBot should also allow users to avoid getting stuck on snow or ice. The unit is surprisingly agile for its 365 pounds: It can balance on its two drive wheels, like a segway. Also, the drive wheels can be repositioned to help regain traction. Plus, the traction-control app senses when a wheel or two have lost their grip on the ground and adjusts other components to maintain the desired course.

Chapter 35

Electrical Signals and Stimulations

Chapter Contents

Section 35.1—Electrical Signals to Restore
　　　　　Functioning.. 318

Section 35.2—BrainGate 322

Section 35.3—Noninvasive Spinal Cord Stimulation
　　　　　for Paralysis.. 326

Section 35.1

Electrical Signals to Restore Functioning

This section includes text excerpted from "Spinal
Stimulation Helps Four Patients with Paraplegia Regain Voluntary
Movement," National Institutes of Health (NIH), April 8, 2014.
Reviewed December 2017.

Four people with paraplegia are able to voluntarily move previously paralyzed muscles as a result of a novel therapy that involves electrical stimulation of the spinal cord, according to a study funded in part by the National Institutes of Health and the Christopher and Dana Reeve Foundation. The participants, each of whom had been paralyzed for more than two years, were able to voluntarily flex their toes, ankles, and knees while the stimulator was active, and the movements were enhanced over time when combined with physical rehabilitation. Researchers involved in the study say the therapy has the potential to change the prognosis of people with paralysis even years after injury.

"When we first learned that a patient had regained voluntary control as a result of spinal stimulation, we were cautiously optimistic," said Roderic Pettigrew, Ph.D., M.D., director of the National Institute of Biomedical Imaging and Bioengineering (NIBIB) at National Institutes of Health (NIH), which provided support for the study. "Now that spinal stimulation has been successful in 4 out of 4 patients, there is evidence to suggest that a large cohort of individuals, previously with little realistic hope of any meaningful recovery from spinal cord injury, may benefit from this intervention."

One of the most impressive and unexpected findings of the study is that two of the patients who benefited from the spinal stimulation had complete motor and sensory paralysis. In these patients, the pathway that sends information about sensation from the legs to the brain is disrupted, in addition to the pathway that sends information from the brain to the legs in order to control movement. The researchers were surprised by the outcome; they had assumed that at least some of the sensory pathway needed to be intact for the therapy to be effective.

The study is the continuation of a groundbreaking pilot trial initiated in 2009 to determine whether spinal stimulation, in conjunction with daily training on a treadmill, could help patients with paralysis regain some ability to move. In that trial, Rob Summers, a young man paralyzed below his chest, had a 16-electrode array implanted on his spinal cord. He then underwent daily training in which he was suspended in a harness over a treadmill while a team of researchers supported his legs, helping him to either stand or walk. At the same time, the array delivered electrical pulses to his spinal cord just below his injury.

According to the researchers, the goal of the stimulation was to increase the sensitivity of local circuits within the spinal cord that carry out basic motor functions without input from the brain—such as the knee jerk that occurs after stepping on a tack, or even more complex patterned movements like stepping. While not strong enough to directly induce muscle activation by itself, the researchers believed the stimulation could lead to movement when combined with sensory input from stepping on a treadmill.

With his stimulator active, Summers was able to gradually bear his own weight and could eventually stand without assistance from physical therapists for up to four minutes. Surprisingly, seven months into the trial, Summers also discovered that he had regained some voluntary control of his legs. The researchers were amazed by this latter outcome, as intentional movement requires information to travel from the brain down to the lower spinal cord, a path that had been rendered nonfunctional by his injury. Other impairments caused by Summers' injury also began to improve over time, in the absence of stimulation, such as blood pressure control, body temperature regulation, bladder control, and sexual function.

Now, in this follow-up study, Claudia Angeli, Ph.D., assistant professor at the University of Louisville's Kentucky Spinal Cord Injury Research Center and her research colleagues report that three additional patients with paralysis have recovered voluntary muscle control following electrical stimulation of the spine. Their report, which also includes results from new tests conducted on Summers, was published in the April 8 online issue of Brain.

The three patients in the new study include two with complete motor and sensory paralysis, and one, similar to Summers, with complete motor paralysis but some ability to experience sensation below his injury. Within just a few days of the start of stimulation, all three patients regained some voluntary control of previously paralyzed muscles.

The first person they implanted after Summers was unable to move or experience any sensation below his injury and was initially meant to be their baseline patient. "What was astounding about him was that not only was there voluntary movement, but we saw it in the first week of stimulation. We then saw it in the next two patients as well," said Susan Harkema, Ph.D., the director of rehabilitation research at the Kentucky Spinal Cord Injury Research Center at the University of Louisville, and a researcher in the study.

The researchers point to the speed at which each subject recovered voluntary movement as evidence that there may be dormant connections that exist in patients with complete motor paralysis. "Rather than there being a complete separation of the upper and lower regions relative to the injury, it's possible that there is some contact, but that these connections are not functional," said V. Reggie Edgerton, Ph.D., a UCLA distinguished professor of integrative biology and physiology, and the researcher responsible for developing the novel approach to rehabilitation. "The spinal stimulation could be reawakening these connections."

An important aspect of the new study involved assessing the ability of each patient to modulate his movements in response to auditory and visual cues. "We hoped to determine if they could voluntarily move in the presence of stimulation, and also how controlled they could be about their movements," said Angeli.

All participants, including Summers, were able to synchronize leg, ankle, and toe movements in unison with the rise and fall of a wave displayed on a computer screen, and three out of the four were able to change the force at which they flexed their leg, depending on the intensity of three different auditory cues.

"The fact that the brain is able to take advantage of the few connections that may be remaining, and then process this complicated visual, auditory, and perceptual information, is pretty amazing. It tells us that the information from the brain is getting to the right place in the spinal cord, so that the person can control, with fairly impressive accuracy, the nature of the movement," said Edgerton.

The same tests were also administered following several months of spinal stimulation applied in conjunction with locomotor training. During this time, patients also carried out home-based training, which consisted of hour-long stimulation while practicing intentional movements lying down. At the end of the training, some subjects were able to execute voluntary movements with greater force and with reduced stimulation, while others experienced enhanced movement accuracy. Harkema says it's unclear whether the improvement was a result of the training or due to the cumulative effects of stimulation over time. They plan to test this distinction in their next study.

"With this study the investigators show that their findings about a motor complete patient regaining movement, reported three years ago in The Lancet, were not an anomaly," said Susan Howley, executive vice president for research at the Christopher and Dana Reeve Foundation, Short Hills, N.J., which provides patient advocacy and funding for spinal cord injury research. "The implications of this study for the entire field are quite profound and we can now envision a day where epidural stimulation might be part of a cocktail of therapies used to treat paralysis."

With support from NIBIB, Edgerton, along with collaborators Joel Burdick and Y.C. Tai, professors of mechanical and electrical engineering and bioengineering at Caltech, are also working to develop a new high-density, 27-electrode array in rats to determine if it can provide finer, more robust control of locomotion.

"The technology we used in these four individuals was initially designed for the suppression of back pain, and our animal experiments have told us that we can do much better," said Edgerton. "For a given type of movement, we want to be able to select exactly where and how to stimulate the spinal cord. We just don't have that flexibility in the current technology."

Edgerton is also working with various collaborators on NIBIB-funded projects to explore whether epidural stimulation can be used to help patients with paralysis of the upper limbs. They are also developing a technology that can deliver spinal stimulation through the skin (transcutaneously), which would bypass the need for surgical implantation.

Though there is much work to be done, Harkema believes the results from this newest study already provide enough evidence to challenge currently held beliefs about the prognosis of patients with severe spinal cord injuries.

"Right now, the clinical perspective for individuals with complete motor paralysis is that there is nothing we can do," said Harkema. "I think we need to rethink that. In our study, we demonstrated potential beyond any expectation. We need to relook at what the perceived potential is for this group of individuals."

"This is a wake-up call for how we see motor complete spinal cord injury," said Edgerton. "We don't have to necessarily rely on regrowth of nerves in order to regain function. The fact that we've observed this in all four patients suggests that this is actually a common phenomenon in those with complete paralysis."

This work was supported by the National Institute of Biomedical Imaging and Bioengineering and the National Institute of General Medical Sciences at NIH under the award numbers EB007615 and GM103507, the Christopher and Dana Reeve Foundation, the Kessler Foundation, the Leona M. and Harry B. Helmsley Charitable Trust, University of Louisville Foundation, and Jewish Hospital and St. Mary's Foundation, Frazier Rehab Institute and University Hospital.

Section 35.2

BrainGate

This section contains text excerpted from the following sources:
Text in this section begins with excerpts from "Office of Research and Development," U.S. Department of Veterans Affairs (VA), June 6, 2017; Text under the heading "NIH-Funded Study Shows Progress in Brain-Computer Interface Technology" is excerpted from "Paralyzed Individuals Use Thought-Controlled Robotic Arm to Reach and Grasp," National Institutes of Health (NIH), May 16, 2012. Reviewed December 2017.

U.S. Department of Veterans Affairs (VA) has played a major role in supporting the development of BrainGate. The system, spearheaded by researchers at the Providence, Rhode Island, VA Medical Center and Brown University, relies on microelectrodes implanted in the brain to pick up neural signals.

The electrodes are placed in a part of the brain that controls voluntary movement. They send signals to an external decoder that translates them into commands for electronic or robotic devices.

The research team developing BrainGate hopes to create a technology that will restore movement, control, and independence to people with paralysis or limb loss from conditions including ALS, brainstem stroke, and spinal cord injury.

BrainGate studies—A study, described above in the "neural prosthesis studies" subtopic of this page, found that the system continued to control a computer cursor accurately through brain activity more than 1,000 days after it was initially implanted.

In 2015, the BrainGate team reported the system could allow point-and-click communication by someone with incomplete locked-in syndrome, which can be caused by a spinal cord injury. In locked-in syndrome, patients are fully conscious but unable to move any muscles except for those that control eye movement.

They can see, hear, smell, taste, and even feel, but may be unable to speak or vocalize at all. Those with incomplete locked-in syndrome can make small movements of the head, fingers, and toes.

Another 2015 BrainGate study found that volunteers using the system were able to acquire "targets" on a computer screen, such as letters on a keyboard, more than twice as quickly as in previous studies, thanks to advances in the system.

The BrainGate team is now studying whether the system can be effective as a means of natural, intuitive control of prosthetic limbs, or as a way to help patients move their own paralyzed limbs. The latter work is being carried out in partnership with the Cleveland Functional Electrical Stimulation (FES) Center.

NIH-Funded Study Shows Progress in Brain-Computer Interface Technology

In an ongoing clinical trial, a paralyzed woman was able to reach for and sip from a drink on her own—for the first time in nearly 15 years—by using her thoughts to direct a robotic arm. The trial, funded in part by the National Institutes of Health, is evaluating the safety and feasibility of an investigational device called the BrainGate neural interface system. This is a type of brain-computer interface (BCI) intended to put robotics and other assistive technology under the brain's control.

A report published in Nature describes how two individuals—both paralyzed by stroke —learned to use the BrainGate system to make reach-and-grasp movements with a robotic arm, as part of the Brain-Gate2 clinical trial. The report highlights the potential for long-term use and durability of the BrainGate system, part of which is implanted in the brain to capture the signals underlying intentional movement. It also describes the most complex functions to date that anyone has been able to perform using a BCI.

For the woman, it was the first time since her stroke that she was able to sip a drink without help from a caregiver.

"The smile on her face was a remarkable thing to see. For all of us involved, we were encouraged that the research is making the kind of progress that we had all hoped," said the trial's lead investigator, Leigh Hochberg, M.D., Ph.D., who is an associate professor of engineering at

Brown University in Providence, R.I., and a critical care neurologist at Massachusetts General Hospital (MGH)/Harvard Medical School in Boston.

"Years after the onset of paralysis, we found that it was still possible to record brain signals that carry multi-dimensional information about movement and that those signals could be used to move an external device," Dr. Hochberg said.

He noted that the technology is years away from practical use and that the trial participants used the BrainGate system under controlled conditions in their homes with a technician present to calibrate it.

The BrainGate neural interface system consists of a sensor to monitor brain signals and computer software and hardware that turns these signals into digital commands for external devices. The sensor is a baby aspirin-sized square of silicon containing 100 hair-thin electrodes, which can record the activity of small groups of brain cells. It is implanted into the motor cortex, a part of the brain that directs movement.

"This technology was made possible by decades of investment and research into how the brain controls movement. It's been thrilling to see the technology evolve from studies of basic neurophysiology and move into clinical trials, where it is showing significant promise for people with brain injuries and disorders," said Story Landis, Ph.D., director of NIH's National Institute of Neurological Disorders and Stroke (NINDS). The institute funds BCI research in hopes of restoring function and improving quality of life for people coping with limb amputations or paralysis from spinal cord injury, stroke or neuromuscular disorders.

NIH has supported basic and applied research in this area for more than 30 years. The analysis from the BrainGate2 trial focused on two participants—a 58-year-old woman and a 66-year-old man. Both individuals are unable to speak or move their limbs because of brainstem strokes they had years ago—the woman's in 1996 and the man's in 2006. In the trial, both participants learned to perform complex tasks with a robotic arm by imagining the movements of their own arms and hands.

In one task, several foam targets were mounted on levers on a tabletop and programmed to pop up one at a time, at different positions and heights. The participants had less than 30 seconds to grasp each target using the DEKA Arm System (Generation 2), which is designed to work as a prosthetic limb for people with arm amputations. One participant was able to grasp the targets 62 percent of the time, and the other had a 46 percent success rate.

In some sessions, the woman controlled a DLR Light-Weight Robot III arm, which is heavier than the DEKA arm and designed to be used as an external assistive device. She used this arm prior to the DEKA arm in the foam target task, and had a success rate of 21 percent. In other sessions with the DLR arm, her task was to reach for a bottled drink, bring it to her mouth and sip from a straw. She was able to complete four out of six attempts.

This is not the first glimmer of hope from human BCI research. Participants in the BrainGate trial and other studies have also used BCI technology to perform point-and-click actions with a computer cursor, a level of control that has been used for communication.

"This is another big jump forward to control the movements of a robotic arm in three-dimensional space. We're getting closer to restoring some level of everyday function to people with limb paralysis," said John Donoghue, Ph.D., who leads the development of BrainGate technology and is the director of the Institute for Brain Science at Brown University.

Dr. Donoghue said the woman's ability to use the BrainGate was especially encouraging because her stroke occurred nearly 15 years ago and her sensor was implanted more than five years ago. Some researchers have wondered whether neurons in the motor cortex might die or stop generating meaningful signals after years of disuse. Researchers in the field have also worried that years after implantation, the sensor might break down and become less effective at enabling complex motor functions.

Roderic Pettigrew, M.D., Ph.D., director of NIH's National Institute of Biomedical Imaging and Bioengineering (NIBIB), which supports the research, indicated that the technology is promising, but at present is still undergoing development and evaluation. "The researchers have begun the long, difficult process of testing and refining the system with feedback from patients, and they've found that it is possible for a person to mentally control a robotic limb in three-dimensional space. This represents a remarkable advance," he said.

As the trial continues, the BrainGate research team needs to test the technology in more individuals, they said. They envision a system that would be stable for decades, wireless and fully automated. For now, the sensor—and therefore the user—must be connected via cables to the rest of the system. Prior to each session with the robotic arms, a technician had to perform a calibration procedure that lasted 31 minutes on average. Improvements are also needed to enhance the precision and speed of control. In the foam target task, for example, a successful reach-and-grasp motion typically took almost 10 seconds.

The ultimate goal for helping people with paralysis is to reconnect the brain directly to paralyzed limbs rather than robotic ones, the researchers said. In the future, the BrainGate system might be used to control a functional electrical stimulation (FES) device, which delivers electrical stimulation to paralyzed muscles. Such technology has shown promise in monkeys. The *Eunice Kennedy Shriver* National Institute for Child Health and Human Development (NICHD) has long supported the clinical trial research for BrainGate, with the goal of enabling mental control of an FES system for limb movement. In previous reports from the BrainGate2 trial, a participant was able to use the BrainGate system to direct the movements of a virtual, computer-animated arm designed to simulate FES control of a real arm.

Section 35.3

Noninvasive Spinal Cord Stimulation for Paralysis

The section includes text excerpted from "Noninvasive Spinal Cord Stimulation for Paralysis," National Institutes of Health (NIH), July 30, 2015.

Spinal Stimulation Helps Four Patients with Paraplegia

Five men with complete motor paralysis were able to voluntarily generate step-like movements thanks to a new strategy that noninvasively delivers electrical stimulation to their spinal cords, according to a study funded in part by the National Institutes of Health (NIH). The strategy, called transcutaneous stimulation, delivers electrical current to the spinal cord by way of electrodes strategically placed on the skin of the lower back. This expands to nine the number of completely paralyzed individuals who have achieved voluntary movement while receiving spinal stimulation, though this is the first time the stimulation was delivered noninvasively. Previously it was delivered via an electrical stimulation device surgically implanted on the spinal cord.

In the study, the men's movements occurred while their legs were suspended in braces that hung from the ceiling, allowing them to move freely without resistance from gravity. Movement in this environment is not comparable to walking; nevertheless, the results signal significant progress towards the eventual goal of developing a therapy for a wide range of individuals with spinal cord injury.

"These encouraging results provide continued evidence that spinal cord injury may no longer mean a life long sentence of paralysis and support the need for more research," said Roderic Pettigrew, Ph.D., M.D., director of the National Institute of Biomedical Imaging and Bioengineering at NIH. "The potential to offer a life-changing therapy to patients without requiring surgery would be a major advance; it could greatly expand the number of individuals who might benefit from spinal stimulation. It's a wonderful example of the power that comes from combining advances in basic biological research with technological innovation."

The study was conducted by a team of researchers at the University of California, Los Angeles; University of California, San Francisco; and the Pavlov Institute, St. Petersburg, Russia. The team was led by V. Reggie Edgerton, Ph.D., a distinguished professor of integrative biology and physiology at UCLA and Yury Gerasimenko, Ph.D., director of the laboratory of movement physiology at Pavlov Institute and a researcher in UCLA's Department of Integrative Biology and Physiology. They reported their results in the Journal of Neurotrauma.

In a little older study, Edgerton—along with Susan Harkema, Ph.D., and Claudia Angeli, Ph.D., from the University of Louisville, Kentucky—reported that four men with complete motor paralysis were able to generate some voluntary movements while receiving electrical stimulation to their spinal cords. The stimulation came from a device called an epidural stimulator that was surgically implanted on the surface of the men's spinal cords. On the heels of that success, Edgerton and colleagues began developing a strategy for delivering stimulation to the spinal cord noninvasively, believing it could greatly expand the number of paralyzed individuals who could potentially benefit from spinal stimulation.

"There are a lot of individuals with spinal cord injury that have already gone through many surgeries and some of them might not be up to or capable of going through another," said Edgerton. "The other potentially high impact is that this intervention could be close to one-tenth the cost of an implanted stimulator."

327

During this study, five men—each paralyzed for more than two years—underwent a series of 45-minute sessions, once a week, for approximately 18 weeks, to determine the effects of noninvasive electrical stimulation on their ability to move their legs.

In addition to stimulation, the men received several minutes of conditioning each session, during which their legs were moved manually for them in a step-like pattern. The goal of the conditioning was to assess whether physical training combined with electrical stimulation could enhance efforts to move voluntarily. For the final four weeks of the study, the men were given the pharmacological drug buspirone, which mimics the action of serotonin and has been shown to induce locomotion in mice with spinal cord injuries. While receiving the stimulation, the men were instructed at different points to either try to move their legs or to remain passive.

At the initiation of the study, the men's legs only moved when the stimulation was strong enough to generate involuntary step-like movements. However, when the men attempted to move their legs further while receiving stimulation, their range of movement significantly increased. After just four weeks of receiving stimulation and physical training, the men were able to double their range of motion when voluntarily moving their legs while receiving stimulation. The researchers suggest that this change was due to the ability of electrical stimulation to reawaken dormant connections that may exist between the brain and the spinal cord of patients with complete motor paralysis.

Surprisingly, by the end of the study, and following the addition of buspirone, the men were able to move their legs with no stimulation at all and their range of movement was—on average—the same as when they were moving while receiving stimulation.

"It's as if we've reawakened some networks so that once the individuals learned how to use those networks, they become less dependent and even independent of the stimulation," said Edgerton.

The researchers also made extensive recordings of electrical signals generated in the calf muscle and the muscle directly below the calf while the men attempted to flex their feet during stimulation. Over time, these signals increased with the same amount of stimulation, further supporting the hypothesis of re-established communication between the brain and spinal cord.

Edgerton has already initiated another study to see whether these same men can be trained with noninvasive spinal stimulation to fully bear their weight, a feat that the four men with surgically implanted stimulators have already achieved. In addition, he is interested in determining whether, similar to epidural stimulation, noninvasive stimulation can help individuals regain some autonomic functions lost due to paralysis such as the ability to sweat, regulate blood pressure, and control bladder, bowel, and sexual function.

The hope is that further research can help determine whether non-invasive stimulation can restore function that will truly impact patient lives.

Edgerton also wants to test noninvasive stimulation on individuals who have partial paralysis. "We have focused on individuals with complete paralysis throughout this whole process because we knew that was going to be the toughest patient population to see changes in. We've always thought, and we have every reason to believe, that those individuals with partial injuries have even more room for improvement," said Edgerton.

Though a noninvasive stimulation could offer advantages over a surgically implanted device, Edgerton says both need to continue to be developed. For example, a noninvasive stimulator might be useful in determining whether a patient will be receptive to neuromodulation, which could then help determine whether undergoing surgery to implant a stimulator is warranted. Alternatively, Edgerton speculates it may be possible early after an injury for noninvasive stimulation to help patients achieve a certain level of motor control that then allows them to continue to improve with physical rehabilitation and avoid surgery altogether.

"All patients are going to need something slightly different, and maybe noninvasive stimulation is going to be best in some cases and epidural stimulation in others," said Edgerton. "What we need to do is maximize the clinical tool box that we have so that the physician and the patient can select a therapy that is best for them."

The three patients in the study include two with complete motor and sensory paralysis, and one, similar to Summers, with complete motor paralysis but some ability to experience sensation below his injury. Within just a few days of the start of stimulation, all three patients regained some voluntary control of previously paralyzed muscles.

The first person they implanted after Summers was unable to move or experience any sensation below his injury and was initially meant to be their baseline patient. "What was astounding about him was that not only was there voluntary movement, but we saw it in the first week of stimulation. We then saw it in the next two patients as well," said Susan Harkema, Ph.D., the director of rehabilitation research at the Kentucky Spinal Cord Injury Research Center at the University of Louisville, and a researcher in the study.

The researchers point to the speed at which each subject recovered voluntary movement as evidence that there may be dormant connections that exist in patients with complete motor paralysis. "Rather than there being a complete separation of the upper and lower regions relative to the injury, it's possible that there is some contact, but that these connections are not functional," said V. Reggie Edgerton, Ph.D., a UCLA distinguished professor of integrative biology and physiology, and the researcher responsible for developing the novel approach to rehabilitation. "The spinal stimulation could be reawakening these connections."

An important aspect of the study involved assessing the ability of each patient to modulate his movements in response to auditory and visual cues. "We hoped to determine if they could voluntarily move in the presence of stimulation, and also how controlled they could be about their movements," said Angeli.

All participants, including Summers, were able to synchronize leg, ankle, and toe movements in unison with the rise and fall of a wave displayed on a computer screen, and three out of the four were able to change the force at which they flexed their leg, depending on the intensity of three different auditory cues.

"The fact that the brain is able to take advantage of the few connections that may be remaining, and then process this complicated visual, auditory, and perceptual information, is pretty amazing. It tells us that the information from the brain is getting to the right place in the spinal cord, so that the person can control, with fairly impressive accuracy, the nature of the movement," said Edgerton.

The same tests were also administered following several months of spinal stimulation applied in conjunction with locomotor training. During this time, patients also carried out home-based training, which consisted of hour-long stimulation while practicing intentional movements lying down. At the end of the training, some subjects were able to execute voluntary movements with greater force and with reduced stimulation, while others experienced enhanced movement accuracy. Harkema says it's unclear whether the improvement was a result of the training or due to the cumulative effects of stimulation over time. They plan to test this distinction in their next study.

"With this study the investigators show that their findings about a motor complete patient regaining movement, reported three years ago in The Lancet, were not an anomaly," said Susan Howley, executive vice president for research at the Christopher & Dana Reeve

Foundation, Short Hills, N.J., which provides patient advocacy and funding for spinal cord injury research. "The implications of this study for the entire field are quite profound and we can now envision a day where epidural stimulation might be part of a cocktail of therapies used to treat paralysis."

Chapter 36

Physical Therapists of the Future

Rehabilitation robots are mechanical devices that provide physical therapy assessment and training to patients whose muscles have been weakened by cerebral palsy, traumatic brain injury (TBI), or other neurological disorders. The machines can even be operated remotely. For example, a clinician in an office could control a robot that is providing therapy to a patient at home.

"We are coming to a Renaissance in robotics," said Leighton Chan, chief of the Clinical Center (CC) Rehabilitation Medicine Department. They "can play a huge role" in physical therapy. Guided by computers, these first-of-their-kind rehabilitation robots can help patients by assessing muscle-related tasks or training weakened muscles to regain their strength. Hyung-Soon Park, a staff scientist in the CC's Functional and Applied Biomechanics Section (FABS), leads the design and development of the robots. FABS chief Diane Damiano works with patients and develops clinical questions that robotics technology can address.

Usually a patient who needs physical therapy must come to a clinical facility. But Park is developing a tele-rehabilitation system that can remotely assess a patient's condition and provide treatment. Patients could be helped without ever having to leave home.

This chapter includes text excerpted from "Robotic Arms—Physical Therapists of the Future?" Intramural Research Program (IRP), National Institute of Health (NIH), June 30, 2011. Reviewed December 2017.

Park's lab developed two robotic mechanisms that work together to rehabilitate the elbow joint. The first, which resembles a human arm, is a haptic mannequin device (HMD) that relies on the sense of touch. It is attached to a computer in the clinician's office. The second is a mechanical arm brace, called a wearable stretching device (WSD). The patient wears the WSD and can be at home or in some other location but must be near a computer that is connected to the Internet.

Patients who suffer from involuntary muscle spasms caused by neurological impairments are one group that could benefit from this robotic tele-rehabilitation system. Normally a clinician has to have physical contact with a patient to feel the muscles, diagnose problems, and provide physical therapy. But with the HMD-WSD set up, the clinician moves the HMD mechanical arm; a signal travels via the Internet to the patient; the WSD arm brace that the patient is wearing mimics the movement and stretches the muscles. The WSD records muscle resistance and relays the information back to the HMD so it moves and feels just like the patient's arm. The two devices talk to each other, sharing information instantaneously as if the patient and the clinician are sitting in the same room.

Clinical trials with the HMD-WSD system are expected to begin in the near future. After the system has been perfected, Park hopes to develop devices that focus on the knee, ankle, wrist, and shoulder. Whether patients are being clinically managed or participating in clinical trials, "you could test people remotely all over the country and monitor them at home," said Damiano.

The robotic arm can also be used as a tool to standardize medical assessments and to train clinicians who want to improve their physical therapy skills. It is programmed using patient data and can provide realistic, consistent movements, including imitating spasticity (muscle stiffness) and contracture (a permanent shortening of the muscle).

Park and Damiano are also developing other robotic devices. Their robotic leg may help to eliminate crouch gait in children with cerebral palsy. Crouch gait causes a child's knees to flex and turn inward, makes walking difficult and exhausting, and often leads to the permanent use of a walking aid. The robotic device could improve leg strength and help children with cerebral palsy to stand more upright.

The researchers have also developed a self-paced treadmill that is helping patients who have suffered a TBI relearn how to walk. The machine allows patients to choose their speed via sensors that are attached to the body and linked to a computer program developed by FABS. The treadmill faces a large screen onto which a virtual world is projected. Patients walk through the mock terrain, turn corners, and even navigate crowded hallways, actions that can be difficult for someone who has suffered a TBI.

"If your brain is engaged, the response to training [is] greater," said Damiano. The system also "gives you practice in a more real-world setting."

Rehabilitation Chair

With microgravity in space, astronauts were found to be losing 1 percent of bone mass per month due to lack of weight-bearing physical activity. This led to the discovery of VibeTech One, a reha-bilitation chair. This chair uses a biomimetic approach to therapy, meaning it uses human-made means to mimic something that happens naturally.

(Source: "Space Grant Research Launches Rehabilitation Chair," National Aeronautics and Space Administration (NASA).)

Chapter 37

Assistive Devices

Chapter Contents

Section 37.1—Rehabilitative and Assistive
                  Technology: Overview 338

Section 37.2—Assistive Devices for Communication 343

Section 37.3—Hearing Aids.. 346

Section 37.4—Mobility Aids 348

Section 37.1

Rehabilitative and Assistive Technology: Overview

This section includes text excerpted from "Rehabilitative and Assistive Technology: Condition Information," *Eunice Kennedy Shriver* National Institute of Child Health and Human Development (NICHD), December 5, 2012. Reviewed December 2017.

What Is Rehabilitative and Assistive Technology?

Rehabilitative and assistive technology refers to tools, equipment, or products that can help a person with a disability to function successfully at school, home, work, and in the community. Assistive technology can be as simple as a magnifying glass or as complex as a computerized communication system. An assistive device can be as large as an automated wheelchair lift for a van or as small as a handheld hook to assist with buttoning a shirt.

The term "rehabilitative technology" is sometimes used to refer to aids used to help people recover their functioning after injury or illness. But the term often is used interchangeably with the term "assistive technology."

Rehabilitative engineering involves the application of engineering and scientific principles to study how people with disabilities function in society. It includes studying barriers to optimal function and designing solutions so that people with disabilities can interact successfully in their environments.

How Many People Use Assistive Devices?

The Centers for Disease Control and Prevention (CDC) estimated that:

- One in five Americans—about 53 million people—has a disability of some kind.

- 33 million Americans have a disability that makes it difficult for them to carry out daily activities; some have challenges with everyday activities, such as attending school or going to work, and may need help with their daily care.

- 2.2 million people in the United States depend on a wheelchair for day-to-day tasks and mobility.

- 6.5 million people use a cane, a walker, or crutches to assist with their mobility.

What Are Some Types of Assistive Devices and How Are They Used?

Some examples of assistive technologies are:

- People with physical disabilities that affect movement can use mobility aids, such as wheelchairs, scooters, walkers, canes, crutches, prosthetic devices, and orthotic devices, to enhance their mobility.

- Hearing aids can improve hearing ability in persons with hearing problems.

- Cognitive assistance, including computer or electrical assistive devices, can help people function following brain injury.

- Computer software and hardware, such as voice recognition programs, screen readers, and screen enlargement applications, help people with mobility and sensory impairments use computer technology.

- In the classroom and elsewhere, assistive devices, such as automatic page-turners, book holders, and adapted pencil grips, allow learners with disabilities to participate in educational activities.

- Closed captioning allows people with hearing impairments to enjoy movies and television programs.

- Barriers in community buildings, businesses, and workplaces can be removed or modified to improve accessibility. Such modifications include ramps, automatic door openers, grab bars, and wider doorways.

- Lightweight, high-performance wheelchairs have been designed for organized sports, such as basketball, tennis, and racing.

- Adaptive switches make it possible for a child with limited motor skills to play with toys and games.

- Many types of devices help people with disabilities perform such tasks as cooking, dressing, and grooming. Kitchen implements are available with large, cushioned grips to help people with weakness or arthritis in their hands. Medication dispensers with alarms can help people remember to take their medicine on time. People who use wheelchairs for mobility can use extendable reaching devices to reach items on shelves.

What Are Some Types of Rehabilitative Technologies?

Rehabilitative technologies are any technologies that help people recover function after injury or illness. Just a few examples include the following:

- **Robotics.** Specialized robots help people regain function in arms or legs after a stroke.

- **Virtual reality.** People who are recovering from injury can retrain themselves to perform motions within a virtual environment.

- **Musculoskeletal modeling and simulations.** These computer simulations of the human body can pinpoint the underlying mechanical problems in a person with a movement-related disability. This can help design better assistive aids or physical therapies.

- **Transcranial magnetic stimulation (TMS).** TMS sends magnetic impulses through the skull to stimulate the brain. This system can help people who have had a stroke recover movement and brain function.

- **Transcranial direct current stimulation (tDCS).** In tDCS, a mild electrical current travel through the skull and stimulates the brain of patients recovering from stroke. This can help recover movement.

- **Motion analysis.** Motion analysis captures video of human motion with specialized computer software that analyses the motion in detail. The technology gives healthcare providers a detailed picture of a person's specific movement challenges to be used as a guide for proper therapy.

For What Conditions Are Assistive Devices Used?

Some disabilities are quite visible, and others are "hidden." Most disabilities can be grouped into four major categories:

- **Cognitive disability**: intellectual and learning disabilities/disorder, distractibility, reading disorders, inability to remember or focus on large amounts of information

- **Hearing disability**: hearing loss or impaired hearing

- **Physical disability**: paralysis, difficulties with walking or other movement, inability to use a computer mouse, slow response time, limited fine or gross motor control

- **Visual disability**: blindness, low vision, color blindness

Mental illness, including anxiety disorders, mood disorders, eating disorders, and psychosis, for example, is also a disability.

Hidden disabilities can include some people with visual impairments and those with dexterity difficulties, such as repetitive strain injury. People who are hard of hearing or have mental health difficulties also may be included in this category.

Some people have disabling medical conditions that may be regarded as hidden disabilities—for example, epilepsy; diabetes; sickle cell conditions; human immunodeficiency virus (HIV)/acquired immunodeficiency syndrome (AIDS); cystic fibrosis; cancer; and heart, liver or kidney problems. The conditions may be short term or long term, stable or progressive, constant or unpredictable and fluctuating, controlled by medication or another treatment, or untreatable. Many people with hidden disabilities can benefit from assistive technologies for certain activities or during certain stages of their diseases or conditions.

People who have spinal cord injuries, traumatic brain injury (TBI), cerebral palsy, muscular dystrophy, spina bifida, osteogenesis imperfecta, multiple sclerosis, demyelinating diseases, myelopathy, progressive muscular atrophy, amputations, or paralysis often benefit from complex rehabilitative technology. This means that the assistive devices these people use are individually configured to help each person with his or her own unique disability.

How Does Rehabilitative and Assistive Technology Benefit People with Disabilities?

Deciding which type of rehabilitative or assistive technology would be most helpful for a person with a disability is usually made by the disabled person and his or her family and caregivers, along with a team of professionals and consultants. The team is trained to match particular assistive technologies to specific needs to help the person function more independently. The team may include family doctors, regular and special education teachers, speech-language pathologists, rehabilitation engineers, occupational therapists, and other specialists, including representatives from companies that manufacture assistive technology.

Assistive technology enables students with disabilities to compensate for the impairments they experience. This specialized technology promotes independence and decreases the need for other educational support.

Appropriate assistive technology helps people with disabilities overcome or compensate, at least in part, for their limitations. Rehabilitative technology can help restore function in people who have developed a disability due to disease, injury, or aging. Rehabilitative and assistive technology can enable individuals to:

- Care for themselves and their families

- Work

- Learn in schools and other educational institutions

- Access information through computers and reading

- Enjoy music, sports, travel, and the arts

- Participate fully in community life

Assistive technology also benefits employers, teachers, family members, and everyone who interacts with users of the technology. Increasing opportunities for participation benefits everyone.

As assistive technologies are becoming more commonplace, people without disabilities are benefiting from them. For example, people who are poor readers or for whom English is a second language are taking advantage of screen readers. The aging population is making use of screen enlargers and magnifiers.

ReWalk

ReWalk is a walking assistance system that helps individuals with spinal cord injuries (SCI) to stand upright, walk, and turn. Based on an Israeli technology, the wearable robotic exoskeleton system powers the hip and the knee motions for paraplegics to stand, walk, and climb stairs.

(Source: "ReWalk 'Exoskeleton'," U.S. Department of Veterans Affairs (VA).)

Section 37.2

Assistive Devices for Communication

This section includes text excerpted from "Assistive Devices for People with Hearing, Voice, Speech, or Language Disorders," National Institute on Deafness and Other Communication Disorders (NIDCD), March 6, 2017.

What Types of Augmentative and Alternative Communication (AAC) Devices Are Available for Communicating Face-to-Face?

The simplest augmentative and alternative communication (AAC) device is a picture board or touch screen that uses pictures or symbols of typical items and activities that make up a person's daily life. For example, a person might touch the image of a glass to ask for a drink. Many picture boards can be customized and expanded based on a person's age, education, occupation, and interests.

Keyboards, touch screens, and sometimes a person's limited speech may be used to communicate desired words. Some devices employ a text display. The display panel typically faces outward so that two people can exchange information while facing each other. Spelling and word prediction software can make it faster and easier to enter information.

Speech-generating devices go one step further by translating words or pictures into speech. Some models allow users to choose from several different voices, such as male or female, child or adult, and even some regional accents. Some devices employ a vocabulary of prerecorded words while others have an unlimited vocabulary, synthesizing speech as words are typed in. Software programs that convert personal computers into speaking devices are also available.

What Augmentative and Alternative Communication Devices Are Available for Communicating by Telephone?

For many years, people with hearing loss have used text telephone or telecommunications devices, called TTY or TDD machines, to communicate by phone. This same technology also benefits people with speech difficulties. A TTY machine consists of a typewriter keyboard that displays typed conversations onto a readout panel or printed on paper. Callers will either type messages to each other over the system or, if a call recipient does not have a TTY machine, use the national toll-free telecommunications relay service at 711 to communicate. Through the relay service, a communications assistant serves as a bridge between two callers, reading typed messages aloud to the person with hearing while transcribing what's spoken into type for the person with hearing loss.

With today's new electronic communication devices, however, TTY machines have almost become a thing of the past. People can place phone calls through the telecommunications relay service using almost any device with a keypad, including a laptop, personal digital assistant, and cell phone. Text messaging has also become a popular method of communication, skipping the relay service altogether.

Another system uses voice recognition software and an extensive library of video clips depicting American Sign Language to translate a signer's words into text or computer-generated speech in real time. It is also able to translate spoken words back into sign language or text.

Finally, for people with mild to moderate hearing loss, captioned telephones allow you to carry on a spoken conversation, while providing a transcript of the other person's words on a readout panel or computer screen as back-up.

What Types of Alerting Devices Are Available?

Alerting or alarm devices use sound, light, vibrations, or a combination of these techniques to let someone know when a particular event is occurring. Clocks and wake-up alarm systems allow a person to choose to wake up to flashing lights, horns, or a gentle shaking.

Visual alert signalers monitor a variety of household devices and other sounds, such as doorbells and telephones. When the phone rings, the visual alert signaler will be activated and will vibrate or flash a light to let people know. In addition, remote receivers placed around the house can alert a person from any room. Portable vibrating pagers can let parents and caretakers know when a baby is crying. Some baby monitoring devices analyze a baby's cry and light up a picture to indicate if the baby sounds hungry, bored, or sleepy.

What Research Is Being Conducted on Assistive Technology?

The National Institute on Deafness and Other Communication Disorders (NIDCD) funds research into several areas of assistive technology, such as those described below.

Improved Devices for People with Hearing Loss

Eunice Kennedy Shriver National Institute of Child Health and Human Development (NICHD)-funded researchers are developing devices that help people with varying degrees of hearing loss communicate with others. One team has developed a portable device in which two or more users type messages to each other that can be displayed simultaneously in real time. Another team is designing an ALD that amplifies and enhances speech for a group of individuals who are conversing in a noisy environment.

Improved Devices for Nonspeaking People

- **More natural synthesized speech.** NIDCD-sponsored scientists are also developing a personalized text-to-speech synthesis system that synthesizes speech that is more intelligible and natural sounding to be incorporated in speech-generating devices. Individuals who are at risk of losing their speaking ability can prerecord their own speech, which is then converted into their personal synthetic voice.

- **Brain–computer interface research.** A relatively new and exciting area of study is called brain-computer interface research. NIDCD-funded scientists are studying how neural signals in a person's brain can be translated by a computer to help someone communicate. For example, people with amyotrophic lateral sclerosis (ALS, or Lou Gehrig disease) or brainstem stroke lose their ability to move their arms, legs, or body. They can also become locked-in, where they are not able to express words, even though they are able to think and reason normally. By implanting electrodes on the brain's motor cortex, some researchers are studying how a person who is locked-in can control communication software and type out words simply by imagining the movement of his or her hand. Other researchers are attempting to develop a prosthetic device that will be able to translate a person's thoughts into synthesized words and

345

sentences. Another group is developing a wireless device that monitors brain activity that is triggered by visual stimulation. In this way, people who are locked-in can call for help during an emergency by staring at a designated spot on the device.

Section 37.3

Hearing Aids

This section includes text excerpted from "Hearing Aids—Other Products and Devices to Improve Hearing," U.S. Food and Drug Administration (FDA), December 7, 2016.

Assistive listening devices (ALDs) or assistive listening systems include a large variety of devices designed to help you hear sounds in everyday activities. ALDs are available in some public places such as auditoriums, movie theaters, houses of worship, and meeting rooms. They may be used by both normal hearing and hearing impaired people to improve listening in these settings.

ALDs can be used to overcome the negative effects of distance, poor room acoustics, and background noise. To achieve this purpose, many ALDs consist of a microphone near the source of the sound and a receiver near the listener. The listener can usually adjust the volume of the receiver as needed. Careful microphone placement allows the level of the speaker's voice to stay constant regardless of the distance between the speaker and the audience. The speaker's voice is also heard clearly over room noises such as chairs moving, fan motors running, and people talking.

ALDs can be used with or without hearing aids.

Cochlear Implants

A cochlear implant is an implanted electronic device that can produce useful hearing sensation by electrically stimulating nerves inside the inner ear. Cochlear implants currently consist of two main components:

- external component, comprised of an externally worn micro-phone, sound processor and transmitter system,

- internal component, comprised of an implanted receiver and electrode system, which contains the electronic circuits that receive signals from the external system and send electrical signals to the inner ear.

Cochlear implants are different from hearing aids in some aspects:

Table 37.1. Difference between Cochlear Implants and Hearing Aids

Hearing Aids	Cochlear Implants
Hearing aids are indicated for individuals with all degrees of hearing loss (from mild to profound).	Cochlear implants are indicated only for individuals with severe-profound hearing loss.
Most hearing aids are not implanted (although some bone-conduction hearing aids have an implanted component).	Cochlear implants are composed of both internal (implanted) and external components. A surgical procedure is needed to place the internal components.
In hearing aids, sound is amplified and conveyed through both the outer and middle ear and finally to the sensory receptor cells (hair cells) in the inner ear. The hair cells convert the sound energy into neural signals that are picked up by the auditory nerve.	Cochlear implants bypass the outer and middle ears, and the damaged hair cells and replace their functions by converting sound energy into electrical energy that directly stimulates the auditory nerve.

Implantable Middle Ear Hearing Devices

Implantable Middle Ear Hearing Devices (IMEHD) help increase the transmission of sound to the inner ear. IMEHDs are small implantable devices that are typically attached to one of the tiny bones in the middle ear. When they receive sound waves, IMEHDs vibrate and directly move the middle ear bones. This creates sound vibrations in the inner ear, which helps you to detect the sound. This device is generally used for people with sensorineural hearing loss.

Bone-Anchored Hearing Aids

A bone-anchored hearing aid (BAHA), like a cochlear implant, has both implanted and external components. The implanted component is a small post that is surgically attached to the skull bone behind your ear. The external component is a speech processor which converts sound into vibrations; it connects to the implanted post and transmits sound vibrations directly to the inner ear through the skull, bypassing the middle ear. BAHAs are for people with middle ear problems (usually a mixed hearing loss) or who have no hearing in one ear.

Personal Sound Amplification Products

Personal Sound Amplification Products (PSAPs), or sound amplifiers, increase environmental sounds for nonhearing impaired consumers. Examples of situations when these products would be used include hunting (listening for prey), bird watching, listening to a lecture with a distant speaker, and listening to soft sounds that would be difficult for normal hearing individuals to hear (e.g., distant conversations, performances). PSAPs are not intended to be used as hearing aids to compensate for hearing impairment.

Section 37.4

Mobility Aids

This section includes text excerpted from "Wheelchairs, Mobility Aids, and Other Power-Driven Mobility Devices," ADA.gov, U.S. Department of Justice (DOJ), January 31, 2014. Reviewed December 2017.

People with mobility, circulatory, respiratory, or neurological disabilities use many kinds of devices for mobility. Some use walkers, canes, crutches, or braces. Some use manual or power wheelchairs or electric scooters. In addition, advances in technology have given rise to new devices, such as Segways®, that some people with disabilities use as mobility devices, including many veterans injured while serving in the military. And more advanced devices will inevitably be invented, providing more mobility options for people with disabilities.

This section is designed to help title II entities (state and local governments) and title III entities (businesses and nonprofit organizations that serve the public) (together, "covered entities") understand how the new rules for mobility devices apply to them. These rules went into effect on March 15, 2011.

- Covered entities must allow people with disabilities who use manual or power wheelchairs or scooters, and manually-powered mobility aids such as walkers, crutches, and canes, into all areas where members of the public are allowed to go.

- Covered entities must also allow people with disabilities who use other types of power-driven mobility devices into their facilities, unless a particular type of device cannot be accommodated because of legitimate safety requirements. Where legitimate safety requirements bar accommodation for a particular type of device, the covered entity must provide the service it offers in alternate ways if possible.

- The rules set out five specific factors to consider in deciding whether or not a particular type of device can be accommodated.

Wheelchairs

Most people are familiar with the manual and power wheelchairs and electric scooters used by people with mobility disabilities. The term "wheelchair" is defined in the new rules as "a manually-operated or power-driven device designed primarily for use by an individual with a mobility disability for the main purpose of indoor or of both indoor and outdoor locomotion."

Other Power-Driven Mobility Devices

In recent years, some people with mobility disabilities have begun using less traditional mobility devices such as golf cars or Segways®. These devices are called "other power-driven mobility device" (OPDMD) in the rule. OPDMD is defined in the new rules as "any mobility device powered by batteries, fuel, or other engines—that is used by individuals with mobility disabilities for the purpose of locomotion, including golf cars, electronic personal assistance mobility devices... such as the Segway® PT, or any mobility device designed to operate in areas without defined pedestrian routes, but that is not a wheelchair." When an OPDMD is being used by a person with a mobility disability, different rules apply under the Americans with Disabilities Act (ADA) than when it is being used by a person without a disability.

Choice of Device

People with disabilities have the right to choose whatever mobility device best suits their needs. For example, someone may choose to use a manual wheelchair rather than a power wheelchair because it enables her to maintain her upper body strength. Similarly, someone who is able to stand may choose to use a Segway® rather than a manual wheelchair because of the health benefits gained by standing. A facility may be required to allow a type of device that is generally prohibited when being used by someone without a disability when it is being used by a person who needs it because of a mobility disability. For example, if golf cars are generally prohibited in a park, the park may be required to allow a golf car when it is being used because of a person's mobility disability, unless there is a legitimate safety reason that it cannot be accommodated.

Requirements Regarding Mobility Devices and Aids

Under the new rules, covered entities must allow people with disabilities who use wheelchairs (including manual wheelchairs, power wheelchairs, and electric scooters) and manually-powered mobility aids such as walkers, crutches, canes, braces, and other similar devices into all areas of a facility where members of the public are allowed to go.

In addition, covered entities must allow people with disabilities who use any OPDMD to enter the premises unless a particular type of device cannot be accommodated because of legitimate safety requirements. Such safety requirements must be based on actual risks, not on speculation or stereotypes about a particular type of device or how it might be operated by people with disabilities using them.

- For some facilities—such as a hospital, a shopping mall, a large home improvement store with wide aisles, a public park, or an outdoor amusement park—covered entities will likely determine that certain classes of OPDMDs being used by people with disabilities can be accommodated. These entities must allow people with disabilities using these types of OPDMDs into all areas where members of the public are allowed to go.

- In some cases, even in facilities such as those described above, an OPDMD can be accommodated in some areas of a facility, but not in others because of legitimate safety concerns. For example, a cruise ship may decide that people with disabilities using Segways® can generally be accommodated, except in constricted areas, such as passageways to cabins that are very narrow and have low ceilings.

- For other facilities—such as a small convenience store, or a small town manager's office—covered entities may determine that certain classes of OPDMDs cannot be accommodated. In that case, they are still required to serve a person with a disability using one of these devices in an alternate manner if possible, such as providing curbside service or meeting the person at an alternate location.

Covered entities are encouraged to develop written policies specifying which kinds of OPDMDs will be permitted and where and when they will be permitted, based on the following assessment factors.

Assessment Factors

In deciding whether a particular type of OPDMD can be accommodated in a particular facility, the following factors must be considered:

- the type, size, weight, dimensions, and speed of the device;

- the facility's volume of pedestrian traffic (which may vary at different times of the day, week, month, or year);

- the facility's design and operational characteristics (e.g., whether its business is conducted indoors or outdoors, its square footage, the density and placement of furniture and other stationary devices, and the availability of storage for the OPDMD if needed and requested by the user);

- whether legitimate safety requirements (such as limiting speed to the pace of pedestrian traffic or prohibiting use on escalators) can be established to permit the safe operation of the OPDMD in the specific facility; and

- whether the use of the OPDMD creates a substantial risk of serious harm to the immediate environment or natural or cultural resources, or poses a conflict with Federal land management laws and regulations.

It is important to understand that these assessment factors relate to an entire class of device type, not to how a person with a disability might operate the device. All types of devices powered by fuel or combustion engines, for example, may be excluded from indoor settings for health or environmental reasons, but may be deemed acceptable in some outdoor settings. Also, for safety reasons, larger electric devices such as golf cars may be excluded from narrow or crowded settings where there is no valid reason to exclude smaller electric devices like Segways®.

Based on these assessment factors, the Department of Justice expects that devices such as Segways® can be accommodated in most circumstances. The Department also expects that, in most circumstances, people with disabilities using ATVs and other combustion engine-driven devices may be prohibited indoors and in outdoor areas with heavy pedestrian traffic.

Policies on the Use of OPDMDs

In deciding whether a type of OPDMD can be accommodated, covered entities must consider all assessment factors and, where appropriate, should develop and publicize rules for people with disabilities using these devices. Such rules may include:

- requiring the user to operate the device at the speed of pedestrian traffic;

- identifying specific locations, terms, or circumstances (if any) where the devices cannot be accommodated;

- setting out instructions for going through security screening machines if the device contains technology that could be harmed by the machine; and

- specifying whether or not storage is available for the device when it is not being used.

Credible Assurance

An entity that determines it can accommodate one or more types of OPDMDs in its facility is allowed to ask the person using the device to provide credible assurance that the device is used because of a disability. If the person presents a valid, State-issued disability parking placard or card or a State-issued proof of disability, that must be accepted as credible assurance on its face. If the person does not have this documentation, but states verbally that the OPDMD is being used because of a mobility disability, that also must be accepted as credible assurance, unless the person is observed doing something that contradicts the assurance. For example, if a person is observed running and jumping, that may be evidence that contradicts the person's assertion of a mobility disability. However, it is very important for covered entities and their staff to understand that the fact that a person with a disability is able to walk for a short distance does not necessarily contradict a verbal assurance—many people with mobility disabilities can walk, but need their mobility device for longer distances or uneven terrain. This is particularly true for people who lack stamina, have poor balance, or use mobility devices because of respiratory, cardiac, or neurological disabilities. A covered entity cannot ask people about their disabilities.

Chapter 38

Space Technologies in the Rehabilitation of Movement Disorders

More than 50 years have passed since the first human spaceflight. As the duration of the flights has increased considerably, and the amount of in-orbit activities has become greater, the need to maintain healthy bones and muscles in space has become more critical. Bones and muscles rely on performing daily activities in the presence of Earth's gravity to stay healthy. In space, traditional Earth-based methods to maintain bones and muscles, such as physical exercise, are challenging due to constraints that include such factors as crew time and vehicle size.

To meet these challenges, specialists from the Institute of Biomedical Problems in Russia and their commercial partner, Zvezda, developed the Penguin suit to provide loading along the length of the body (axial loading) in a way that compensates for the lack of daily loading that the body usually experiences under the Earth's gravity. The first testing of the suit in space was performed in 1971 aboard the Salyut-1 station. Now the Penguin suit is actively used on the International Space Station as a regular component of the Russian countermeasure system of health maintenance.

This chapter includes text excerpted from "Space Technologies in the Rehabilitation of Movement Disorders," National Aeronautics and Space Administration (NASA), August 4, 2017.

Since the early 1990s, Professor Inessa Kozlovskaya and her team at the Institute of Biomedical Problems in Russia have implemented the use of this axial loading suit in clinical rehabilitation practice. The clinical version of the Penguin suit, the Adeli, was developed at the Institute of Pediatrics Russian Academy of Science under the leadership of Professor Ksenia Semyonova and is used for the comprehensive treatment of cerebral palsy in children. The treatment method is focused on restoring functional links of the body through a corrective flow of sensory information to the muscles, thereby improving the health of the tissues being loaded. This results in the correction of walking patterns and stabilization of balance in a relatively short period of time, including for those children with cerebral palsy who have deep motor disturbances. The Adeli suit was licensed in 1992 and has been continuously developed since. These methods have become one of the most popular and widely used in Russian medical clinics for rehabilitation of children with infantile cerebral paralysis.

New methods were also developed for patients undergoing motor rehabilitation after stroke and brain trauma. Paralytic and paretic alterations of motor functions that are the most frequent after-effects of these diseases typically lead to significant limitations in motor and social activity of these patients, decrease their functional abilities and obstruct their rehabilitation. Given all of the complexities and importance of the rehabilitation of these patients, another clinical modification of the Penguin suit was developed called the "Regent suit." The complex effect of the Regent suit on the body is based on an increase of the axial loading on skeletal structures and an increase in resistive loads on muscles during movement, which results in an increase of sensory information to the nervous system that is important for counteracting the development of pathological posture and for normalization of vertical stance and walking control. The Regent suit is effectively used at the early stage of rehabilitation for patients having movement disorders after cerebrovascular accident and cranium-brain traumas.

The clinical studies of the efficacy of the Regent suit in the rehabilitation of motor disorders in patients with limited lesions of the central nervous system were performed in acute and chronic studies with the participation of hundreds of stroke and brain trauma patients in the hospital No 83 Federal Medical-Biological Agency of Russia under leadership of professor Sergey Shvarkov, and in the Center of Speech Pathology and Neurorehabilitation under leadership of professor Vicktor Shklovsky. The efficacy of the suit in patients with post-stroke hemiparesis was assessed at the Scientific Center of Neurology under leadership of professor Ludmila Chernikova. These studies have shown that use of the suit results in a significant decrease in paresis and spasticity in the lower leg muscle groups, as well as an improvement of sensitivity in distal parts of lower limbs, and an overall improvement of locomotor functions. The positive effect on high mental functions was noticed at the same time; namely, an improvement of speech characteristics, an increase of active vocabulary, and an improvement in the patient's ability to recognize objects.

The use of the Regent suit is a complex, drug-free approach to the treatment of motor disorders. The method is closely related to the natural function of walking, activates all of the muscles involved in posture and spatial orientation, and is very safe. It allows for shorter treatment time, can be used both under hospital and outpatient conditions, and allows for a wide range of adjustments that allow individualized rehabilitation programs based on uniqueness of the neurological deficit and functional abilities of each patient. Today the Regent suit is applied in 43 medical institutions in Russia and abroad, and the results related to using both the Adeli and Regent suits are based on numerous observations and clinical studies.

Part Six

Health Information Technology

Chapter 39

Understanding Health Information Technology

Chapter Contents

Section 39.1—Basics of Health Information Technology
.... 362

Section 39.2—Benefits of Health IT.. 364

Section 39.3—Consumer Health IT Applications 366

Section 39.4—Trends in Use 368

Section 39.1

Basics of Health Information Technology

This section contains text excerpted from the following sources:
Text under the heading "What Is Health Information Technology?"
is excerpted from "Health Information Technology," Substance
Abuse and Mental Health Services Administration (SAMHSA),
September 15, 2017; Text beginning with the heading "What
Does Health Information Technology Comprise of?" is excerpted
from "Basics of Health IT," HealthIT.gov, Office of the National
Coordinator for Health Information Technology (ONC),
January 15, 2013. Reviewed December 2017.

What Is Health Information Technology?

Health information technology, or health IT, involves the secure
exchange of health information using computer systems.

Health IT makes it faster and easier for patients, families, providers, and health insurers to securely share information. Health IT helps
behavioral health professionals manage patient records, while giving
patients and families more control over their care.

What Does Health Information Technology Comprise of?

Health information technology includes:

Electronic health records (EHRs). Your doctor keeps records of
your health information, such as your history of diseases and which
medications you're taking. Up until now, most doctors stored these in
paper files. EHRs (sometimes called "electronic medical records") are
electronic systems that store your health information.

EHRs allow doctors to more easily keep track of your health information and may enable them to access your information when you
have a problem even if their office is closed. EHRs also make it easier
for your doctor to share information with specialists and others so
that everyone who needs your information has it available when they
need it.

Some EHRs may also allow you to log in to a web portal to view your own health record, lab results, and treatment plan, and to email your doctor.

Personal health records (PHRs). A PHR is a lot like an EHR, except that you control what kind of information goes into it.

You can use a PHR to keep track of information from your doctor visits, but the PHR can also reflect your life outside the doctor's office and your health priorities, such as tracking your food intake, exercise, and blood pressure. Sometimes, your PHR can link with your doctor's EHR.

E-prescribing. A paper prescription can get lost or misread. E-prescribing allows your doctor to communicate directly with your pharmacy. This means you can go to the pharmacy to pick up medicine without having to bring the paper prescription.

Other Types of Health Information Technology: e-Health Tools

There are other "e-Health tools" that you can use on your own, if you wish, that may be considered a part of the broader health IT world. These include:

Personal health tools. These are tools that help you check your health, get feedback, and keep track of your progress to better manage your health. Examples include smartphone "apps" that can help you set and monitor fitness goals and cell phone text reminders to take your medicine on time.

Online communities. Online communities can help people connect with one another to try to maximize good health (such as during pregnancy) or to respond to concerns about poor health.

Through online communities you can share information with—and emotionally support—others facing similar concerns about a particular disease or disability.

These e-health tools are designed to place you at the center of your care—helping to put the "I" in health IT.

Section 39.2

Benefits of Health IT

This section includes text excerpted from "Benefits of
Health IT," HealthIT.gov, Office of the National Coordinator for
Health Information Technology (ONC), February 4,
2013. Reviewed December 2017.

Information Technology in Healthcare: The Next Consumer Revolution

Over the past 20 years, our nation has undergone a major transformation due to information technology (IT). Today, we have at our fingertips access to a variety of information and services to help us manage our relationships with the organizations that are part of our lives: banks, utilities, Government offices—even entertainment companies.

Until now, relatively few Americans have had the opportunity to use this kind of technology to enhance some of the most important relationships: those related to your health. Relationships with your doctors, your pharmacy, your hospital, and other organizations that make up your circle of care are now about to benefit from the next transformation in information technology: health IT.

For patients and consumers, this transformation will enhance both relationships with providers and providers' relationships with each other. This change will place you at the center of your care—in effect, helping to put the "I" in health IT.

Although it will take years for healthcare to realize all these improvements and fully address any pitfalls, the first changes in this transformation are already underway. At the same time, numerous technology tools are becoming available to improve health for you, your family, and your community.

Most consumers will first encounter the benefits of health IT through an electronic health record, or EHR, at their doctor's office or at a hospital.

Benefits of Health IT for You and Your Family

On a basic level, an Electronic Health Record (EHR) provides a digitized version of the "paper chart" you often see doctors, nurses, and others using. But when an EHR is connected to all of your healthcare providers (and often, to you as a patient), it can offer so much more:

- **EHRs reduce your paperwork.** The clipboard and new patient questionnaire may remain a feature of your doctor's office for some time to come. But as more information gets added to your EHR, your doctor and hospital will have more of that data available as soon as you arrive. This means fewer and shorter forms for you to complete, reducing the healthcare "hassle factor."

- **EHRs get your information accurately into the hands of people who need it.** Even if you have relatively simple healthcare needs, coordinating information among care providers can be a daunting task, and one that can lead to medical mistakes if done incorrectly. When all of your providers can share your health information via EHRs, each of them has access to more accurate and up-to-date information about your care. That enables your providers to make the best possible decisions, particularly in a crisis.

- **EHRs help your doctors coordinate your care and protect your safety.** Suppose you see three specialists in addition to your primary care physician. Each of them may prescribe different drugs, and sometimes, these drugs may interact in harmful ways. EHRs can warn your care providers if they try to prescribe a drug that could cause that kind of interaction. An EHR may also alert one of your doctors if another doctor has already prescribed a drug that did not work out for you, saving you from the risks and costs of taking ineffective medication.

- **EHRs reduce unnecessary tests and procedures.** Have you ever had to repeat medical tests ordered by one doctor because the results weren't readily available to another doctor? Those tests may have been uncomfortable and inconvenient or have posed some risk, and they also cost money. Repeating tests— whether a $20 blood test or a $2,000 magnetic resonance imaging (MRI)—results in higher costs to you in the form of bigger bills and increased insurance premiums. With EHRs, all of your care providers can have access to all your test results and records at once, reducing the potential for unnecessary repeat tests.

- **EHRs give you direct access to your health records.** In the United States, you already have a Federally guaranteed right to see your health records, identify wrong and missing information, and make additions or corrections as needed. Some healthcare providers with EHR systems give their patients direct access to their health information online in ways that help preserve privacy and security. This access enables you to keep better track of your care, and in some cases, answer your questions immediately rather than waiting hours or days for a returned phone call. This access may also allow you to communicate directly and securely with your healthcare provider.

Section 39.3

Consumer Health IT Applications

This section includes text excerpted from "Consumer Health IT Applications," Agency for Healthcare Research and Quality (AHRQ), U.S. Department of Health and Human Services (HHS), May 30, 2013. Reviewed December 2017.

As patients become more responsible for managing an increasing volume of health information, including their medical history, lab results, and medications, new consumer health information technology (health IT) applications are being developed that allow patients to manage, share, and control their health information electronically and to assume a more active role in the management of their health.

While the term "consumer health IT applications" is not yet well-defined, in general, it refers to a wide range of hardware, software, and web-based applications that allows patients to participate in their own healthcare via electronic means. The American Medical Informatics Association (AMIA) has developed a working definition for the field of consumer health informatics stating that it is "a subspecialty of medical informatics which studies from a patient/consumer perspective the use of electronic information and communication to improve medical outcomes and the healthcare decision-making process." In addition, as defined by Eysenbach, the study of consumer health informatics includes analyzing consumers' information needs, studying and implementing methods of making information accessible to consumers, and modeling and integrating consumers' preferences into medical information systems.

New consumer health IT applications are being developed to be used on a variety of different platforms, including via the web, messaging systems, PDAs, and cell phones, and their use can benefit both patients and providers. These applications have various purposes including assisting with self-management through reminders and educational prompts, delivering real-time data on a patient's health condition to both patients and providers, facilitating web-based support groups, and compiling and storing personal health information in an easily accessible format. One example of the potential benefits of these kinds of applications is illustrated by the use of messaging capabilities available in certain consumer health IT applications that enable timely communication between patients and their providers. Moreover, consumer health IT applications that allow gathering and integrating data from various healthcare sources can serve as a comprehensive resource for patients and their providers. In addition to convenience, consumer health IT applications also can be important in emergency situations to provide critical health information to medical staff.

As described by Jimison et al., consumer health IT applications differ to the degree with which they integrate information about the patient in the application itself and the degree to which they provide patient-specific recommendations back to the user. Some examples of the range of applications are listed below.

Self-Management Systems. This includes systems that are highly varied and include different combinations of functionality utilizing multiple platforms. The most effective systems provide a timely response to information about the current or evolving status of the user. Some of them allow for monitoring and transmission of information, such as blood pressure or blood glucose. Depending on system design, feedback to a patient regarding his/her health status can be received from the system directly or from the provider who receives information from the system.

Electronic Personal Health Records and Patient Portals. Electronic personal health records (PHRs) are defined as "an electronic record of health-related information on an individual that conforms to nationally recognized interoperability standards and that can be drawn from multiple sources while being managed, shared, and controlled by the individual." An electronic PHR can exist as a stand-alone application that allows information to be exported to or imported from other sources or applications or as a "tethered" application that is linked to a specific healthcare organization's information system. Tethered PHRs, also referred to as patient portals, typically allow patients to view, but not modify, data from the provider's electronic health record (EHR). Relevant information that is often retained in a PHR include personal identifiers, contact information, health provider information, problem list, medication history, allergies, immunizations, lab and test results, and other relevant medical history. Some applications also allow patients to communicate electronically with their providers.

Peer Interaction Systems. Peer interaction can take the form of stand alone applications or can sometimes be a part of multicomponent applications. These applications can increase the perceived peer support and improve personal and social outcomes. Through online forums, discussion groups, and other peer communication features, patients can interact electronically with others who have similar conditions.

Section 39.4

Trends in Use

This section includes text excerpted from "Trends in Consumer Access and Use of Electronic Health Information," HealthIT.gov, Office of the National Coordinator for Health Information Technology (ONC), October 30, 2015.

The ability of individuals to easily and securely access and use their health information electronically serves as one of the cornerstones of nationwide efforts to increase patient and family engagement, and advance person-centered health. With access to their electronic health information, individuals can serve as intermediaries of information exchange among providers and use innovative applications to better manage their health. Over the past few years, a number of policy changes have been put in place to increase individuals' access to their personal electronic health information. HIPAA was modified to clarify that if an individual's health information is available electronically, individuals have a right to obtain that information electronically. In Stage 2 Meaningful Use, CMS requires eligible providers and hospitals participating in the Medicare and Medicaid EHR Incentive Program to use certified EHR technology with the capability for patients to electronically view, download, and transmit (VDT) their health information electronically. From 2011 to 2014, participation in the Blue Button Initiative, a public-private partnership to increase consumer access and use of their health data grew from 30 organizations to more than 650. This brief provides national estimates of consumers' access and use of their electronic health information based upon nationally representative surveys conducted from 2012–2014.

Individuals' electronic access to their medical records increased significantly in 2014.

- In 2014, nearly 4 in 10 Americans were offered electronic access to their medical record.

- The proportion of Americans offered online access to their medical records rose by more than a third between 2013 and 2014.

In 2014, over half of individuals who were offered access viewed their record at least once within the last year.

- About one-third of individuals accessed their medical record one to two times in 2014 whereas about one-fifth of individuals accessed their online record once or twice in 2013.

- In both 2013 and 2014, about one in ten individuals accessed their online medical record more than 6 times over a one-year period.

Almost all individuals report having access to laboratory results within their online medical record.

- Among individuals using online medical records, more than 90 percent report having laboratory test results in their record.

- Among individuals who have used an online medical record, almost 8 in 10 report having a list of health and medical problems in their online medical record.

- Approximately three-quarters of individuals report having access to a current list of medications within their online medical record.

369

Summary

Over the past several years there have been a number of initiatives, policies, and regulations designed to increase individuals' electronic access to their health information that are connected to the broader goals of increasing patient engagement and improving health. Since 2012, individuals' electronic access to their medical record has increased significantly, from 28 percent of individuals being offered online access to their medical record in 2013 to 38 percent in 2014.

This increase in individuals' electronic access to their medical record may reflect significant growth in office-based physicians' and hospitals' VDT capabilities. As of 2014, almost half of office-based physicians and over 6-in-10 hospitals possessed these VDT capabilities. This represents significant increases from 2013, before the start of Stage 2 of Meaningful Use. Although there has been some concern expressed that individuals' receipt of multiple online medical records or portals may dampen individuals' usage, these results show that few individuals endorsed this as a reason for not accessing their online medical record.

Furthermore, these results indicate that over half of individuals are taking advantage of their online medical record and most individuals who use their online medical record value the information.

Individuals are using online medical records to better manage their health and healthcare needs. Monitoring health was consistently the most common use of online medical records. Individuals who reported accessing their online record, reported high rates of access to information that enabled monitoring, such as their list of medications, medical or health problems, and laboratory test results. In both 2013 and 2014, at least 8 in 10 individuals who had accessed their online medical record considered the information provided as very or somewhat useful, and in 2014, less than 5 percent of individuals did not consider it useful. Although gaps in health information exchange remain persistent, these findings show that individuals are engaging in activities to help address these gaps. In 2014, over one-third of individuals who visited a healthcare provider in the last year experienced at least one gap in information exchange among their healthcare providers or between themselves and their healthcare provider. The most frequent gaps in information exchange related to healthcare providers not sharing medical records and test results. Individuals are beginning to use their online medical record to address potential gaps in interoperability among providers by directly sharing information with other healthcare providers or making requests of healthcare providers to send information to another provider on their behalf. Among individuals who did access their online medical record, 11 percent shared their electronic health information with a healthcare provider and 12 percent transmitted their health information to a PHR or app. Additionally, among individuals whose provider had an EHR, almost one in five individuals requested their healthcare provider electronically transmit their health information to another healthcare provider. There is a significant opportunity for consumer outreach to increase individuals' awareness regarding electronic access and use of online medical records. Individuals' who were aware of their right to a copy of their electronic medical record had significantly higher rates of being offered online access compared to those who were unware or incorrectly believed they didn't have this right. A lack of need remains the most frequently cited reason for not accessing an online medical record. Illustrating the value of using an online medical record to manage one's health and address information gaps among providers could increase usage among those individuals who cited a lack of need as a reason for not accessing an online medical record.

Chapter 40

Integrating Technology and Healthcare

Chapter Contents

Section 40.1—Health Information Technology
    Integration.. 374

Section 40.2—Information and Communication
    Technology.. 375

Section 40.3—E-Health 377

Section 40.1

Health Information Technology Integration

This section includes text excerpted from "Prevention and Chronic
Care—Improving Primary Care Practice—Health Information
Technology Integration," Agency for Healthcare Research and
Quality (AHRQ), U.S. Department of Health and Human Services
(HHS), May 1, 2012. Reviewed December 2017.

The integration of health information technology (IT) into primary
care includes a variety of electronic methods that are used to manage
information about people's health and healthcare, for both individual
patients and groups of patients. The use of health IT can improve the
quality of care, even as it makes healthcare more cost effective.

Health IT makes it possible for healthcare providers to better manage patient care through the secure use and sharing of health information. By developing secure and private electronic health records for
most Americans and making health information available electronically when and where it is needed, health IT can improve the quality
of care, even as it makes healthcare more cost effective.

With the help of health IT, healthcare providers will have:

- Accurate and complete information about a patient's health.
  That way, providers can give the best possible care, whether
  during a routine visit or a medical emergency.

- The ability to better coordinate the care given. This is especially
  important if a patient has a serious medical condition.

- A way to securely share information with patients and their
  family caregivers over the Internet, for patients who opt for this
  convenience. This means patients and their families can more
  fully take part in decisions about their healthcare.

- Information to help diagnose health problems sooner, reduce
  medical errors, and provide safer care at lower costs.

Section 40.2

Information and Communication Technology

This section includes text excerpted from "Health Communication and Health Information Technology," Office of Disease Prevention and Health Promotion (ODPHP), U.S. Department of Health and Human Services (HHS), October 7, 2017.

Why Are Health Communication and Health Information Technology Important?

Effective use of communication and technology by healthcare and public health professionals can bring about an age of patient- and public-centered health information and services. By strategically combining health IT tools and effective health communication processes, there is the potential to:

- Improve healthcare quality and safety

- Increase the efficiency of healthcare and public health service delivery

- Improve the public health information infrastructure

- Support care in the community and at home

- Facilitate clinical and consumer decision-making

- Build health skills and knowledge

Understanding Health Communication and Health Information Technology

All people have some ability to manage their health and the health of those they care for. However, with the increasing complexity of health information and healthcare settings, most people need additional information, skills, and supportive relationships to meet their health needs.

Disparities in access to health information, services, and technology can result in lower usage rates of preventive services, less knowledge of chronic disease management, higher rates of hospitalization, and poorer reported health status.

Both public and private institutions are increasingly using the Internet and other technologies to streamline the delivery of health information and services. This results in an even greater need for health professionals to develop additional skills in the understanding and use of consumer health information.

The increase in online health information and services challenges users with limited literacy skills or limited experience using the Internet. For many of these users, the Internet is stressful and overwhelming—even inaccessible. Much of this stress can be reduced through the application of evidence-based best practices in user-centered design.

In addition, despite increased access to technology, other forms of communication are essential to ensuring that everyone, including nonweb users, is able to obtain, process, and understand health information to make good health decisions. These include printed materials, media campaigns, community outreach, and interpersonal communication.

Emerging Issues in Health Communication and Health Information Technology

During the coming decade, the speed, scope, and scale of adoption of health IT will only increase. Social media and emerging technologies promise to blur the line between expert and peer health information. Monitoring and assessing the impact of these new media, including mobile health, on public health will be challenging.

Equally challenging will be helping health professionals and the public adapt to the changes in healthcare quality and efficiency due to the creative use of health communication and health IT. Continual feedback, productive interactions, and access to evidence on the effectiveness of treatments and interventions will likely transform the traditional patient-provider relationship. It will also change the way people receive, process, and evaluate health information. Capturing the scope and impact of these changes—and the role of health communication and health IT in facilitating them—will require multidisciplinary models and data systems.

Such systems will be critical to expanding the collection of data to better understand the effects of health communication and health IT on population health outcomes, healthcare quality, and health disparities.

Section 40.3

E-Health

This section includes text excerpted from "eHealth Tools You Can Use," HealthIT.gov, Office of the National Coordinator for Health Information Technology (ONC), March 3, 2014. Reviewed December 2017.

How Can I Use Health IT and eHealth Tools to Manage My Health?

Nearly everything you do to affect your health and the health of your loved ones happens outside of the doctor's office. Patients and family caregivers today have access to more resources and tools than ever before to enhance personal health and become more involved with their healthcare.

But finding high-quality tools among the thousands of apps, websites, and devices that meet your needs can be hard. On just one of the leading smartphone platforms, users can download any of 14,000 apps related to health and medicine.

How Do I Know If I Can Trust the Information I Find Online? How Do I Know If an eHealth Tool Is Right for Me or for My Family?

With thousands of webpages, online services, and apps related to health, it can be hard to find high-quality, trusted, relevant resources to meet your needs and the needs of your family.

In some cases, you can get trustworthy recommendations from doctors and nurses, from other experts, or from consumer organizations. But when doing your own research, it's in your best interest to look at resources carefully, particularly before making a purchase or making a decision about a health condition.

Here are some questions to consider while you decide whether or not a given tool or resource is right for you.

Is It Up-to-Date?

Generally, webpages will indicate when they were last updated, and apps will indicate when the latest version was released. But even without exact information, you can often make educated guesses about whether or not a resource is up-to-date by looking at the material. For example, if an article about a health condition mentions research from the last five years, it's probably more up-to-date than an article that only mentions research from twenty years ago. But keep in mind that not everything needs to be updated frequently. For example, the science of basic care of cuts and bruises doesn't change much from year to year, or even decade to decade.

Whose Name Is on It and Who Provides It?

Some resources are sponsored or sold by private companies. Others are sold or provided free-of-charge by government offices, nonprofit organizations, or educational institutions. One type of sponsorship is not necessarily better than another. But keep in mind that the sponsor of a resource may have an interest or agenda different from your own.

Is the Information Accurate?

While medicine is based on science, some health information on the web and provided through apps may be biased. Consider sources carefully, particularly when they guide you towards specific treatment options or towards a specific product.

For Apps and Devices, Do They Work as Advertised?

More than ever before, people have access to a mix of product reviews written by professionals and by individuals like themselves. Try to find unbiased sources of reviews and read them carefully to learn more about whether or not a product performs as promised, and whether or not it will address the specific needs you have. Also, look for endorsements by professional organizations like medical associations, or certifications by government agencies like the U.S. Food and Drug Administration (FDA).

Are the Tools or Resources Easily Usable?

On a website, is it easy to search for the information you need? In an app, is it easy for you to understand how it works and how to use it? If you have a disability, does the resource include accessibility features or work with assistive software?

Does It Work with Other Tools and Resources?

For example, does a device give you choices about what to do with the data it collects, or are you limited to seeing it on the device itself, or just the product's website? Does a website that tracks information for you offer ways to connect that information to other resources either automatically or through options to export your information?

Is It Secure? Does It Protect Your Privacy?

Any resource that collects personal health information about you or your family can expose you to potential risks. When evaluating such tools, look for privacy and security policies that protect your data and ensure that no one can access your information without your explicit permission. (The Office of the National Coordinator for Health IT (ONC) offers a model privacy policy for companies offering personal health records.)

Chapter 41

Digital Health Records

Chapter Contents

Section 41.1—Blue Button 382

Section 41.2—Personal Health Record (PHR)........................... 389

Section 41.3—Benefits of Electronic Health
             Records (EHRs) 391

Section 41.4—E-Prescription... 397

Section 41.1

Blue Button

This section includes text excerpted from "Your Health Records—
About Blue Button," HealthIT.gov, Office of the National Coordinator
for Health Information Technology (ONC), September 21, 2016.

The Blue Button symbol signifies that a site has functionality for customers to go online and download health records. You can use your health data to improve your health, and to have more control over your personal health information and your family's healthcare.

- Do you want to feel more in control of your health and your personal health information? Do you have a health issue?

- Are you caring for an elderly parent?

- Are you changing doctors?

- Do you need to find the results of a medical test or a complete and current list of your medications?

Blue Button may be able to help. Look for the Blue Button symbol and take action using your personal health information.

Your Health Records

Health information about you may be stored in many places, such as doctors' offices, hospitals, drug stores, and health insurance companies. The Blue Button symbol signifies that an organization has a way for you to access your health records electronically so you can:

- Share them with your doctor or trusted family members or caregivers

- Check to make sure the information, such as your medication list, is accurate and complete

- Keep track of when your child had his/her last vaccination

- Have your medical history available in case of emergency, when traveling, seeking a second opinion, or switching health insurance companies

- Plug your health information into apps and tools that help you set and reach personalized health goals.

You have a legal right to receive your personal health information. Look for the Blue Button symbol, and ask your healthcare providers or health insurance company if they offer you the ability to view online, download, and share your health records.

Your Rights

As Americans, we each have the legal right to access our own health records held by doctors, hospitals, and others who provide healthcare services for us. And we have the option of getting our records on paper or electronically, depending on how they are stored. You can exercise your rights by downloading your health records through an online portal, or by asking how to get a copy of your health records. Some doctors or hospitals may not be familiar with your rights to access your information about your own health.

What Kind of Information Is Available to You?

It depends on whether you are getting information from your healthcare provider (doctor, hospital, nursing home, etc.), your health insurance company, or another source such as a drug store or a lab since each has different kinds of information. In general, you may expect to be able to electronically access important information such as:

- Current medications you are taking

- Any allergies you may have

- Medical treatment information from your doctor or hospital visits

- Your lab test results

- Your health insurance claims information (financial information, clinical information, and more)

Until recently, many health records were stored in paper files, so it wasn't very easy for you to access or use this information. But all that is changing as more doctors and hospitals adopt electronic health records (EHRs) and other health information technologies, including mobile health apps.

Medicare beneficiaries can view and download their Medicare claims data in a more timely and user-friendly format than ever before. And that information now covers three years of your health history, including claims information on services covered under Medicare Parts A and B, and a list of medications that were purchased under Part D. Look for the Blue Button symbol on the MyMedicare website.

Veterans can find the Blue Button symbol on the MyHealtheVet website, and download demographic information (age, gender, ethnicity, and more); emergency contacts; a list of their prescription medications, clinical notes; and wellness reminders.

Users visiting the Blue Button Connector will be able to see a complete list of organizations offering their members the ability to view and download their health records securely online.

You may want to check back often as more and more organizations join the Blue Button movement. Online health records are not yet available to everyone, but access is rapidly growing, and if you ask for access you can help grow it faster.

Blue Button Movement

"Blue Button" is not only an image displayed on patient portals and other secure websites that lets you know you can get your health information electronically, but it is also becoming a symbol of a movement toward an improved healthcare system in which patients and healthcare providers use information technology to work together and improve health.

Blue Button originated at the Veteran's Administration as a symbol on its patient portal that beneficiaries could click to securely download their own health record electronically. Since then the Blue Button has spread beyond VA to other government agencies and the private sector. Responsibility for encouraging broader use of Blue Button and enhancing its technical standards website Disclaimers was transferred to the Office of the National Coordinator for Health Information Technology (ONC), part of the U.S. Department of Health and Human Services (HHS), in 2012.

Now, via the Blue Button Pledge Program, more than 450 organizations are making personal health data available to Americans via their healthcare providers, health insurance companies, labs, and drug stores; building tools to make health information actionable for patients; and/or spreading the word about why all this matters.

As America's healthcare system rapidly goes digital, these organizations are starting to give patients and consumers access to their health records electronically through the "Blue Button" *mechanism* which allows consumers to take action—download your own health information and use it!

Blue Button has also become a rallying cry for achieving the potential of patients and their families to engage via better health information and tools Blue Button and is becoming a *movement*.

Benefits of Blue Button

Blue Button allows you to be in control of your healthcare and your family's healthcare.

Having secure, electronic access to view and download your health records online means you can:

- Share your information with people you trust, like your family doctor, specialists, and caregivers

- Check your information to make sure it is correct and complete

- Keep track of important health information like medications, vaccination records, and test results

- Have your medical history available if you are changing doctors or visiting a specialist

- Find specific information about your health and healthcare when you need it, like in an emergency situation or when you are traveling out of town away from your usual healthcare providers

You can also plug your health information into mobile apps and other health tools. This can help you to stay in control of your health and your family's health. It's your health record and it's about you so you should have it readily accessible when you need it!

Why Is This Important?

The ability to electronically access and use your health records is critically important. Having this information available can:

- Prevent someone from giving you the wrong medication

- Avoid duplicate tests and procedures which can save you time, money, and even risks to your safety

- Avoid costly delays in treatment by having important information at your fingertips

- Make sure everyone caring for you or your family is on the same page

How to Begin Downloading and Using Your Health Records

Get started by finding out if your doctor, hospital, drug store, lab, or health insurance company offers Blue Button. Although Blue Button is in its early stages, it is expanding rapidly.

Go to the Blue Button Connector

Today, millions of Americans have access to their health records through their healthcare providers or health insurance company, along with Medicare beneficiaries, veterans, and uniformed service members.

In 2014, The Office of the National Coordinator for Health Information Technology (ONC) did an early launch of the online Blue Button Connector tool to help consumers find out which healthcare providers offer electronic access to their health records, what to do with them, and useful tools to help meet their health needs and lifestyle. Various Blue Button-capable products and tools will be featured to help patients better navigate online resources tailored to help them manage their health needs. ONC continues to improve and populate the site and will rely on your to help.

Ask Your Healthcare Providers

More and more healthcare providers are giving patients easy-to-use tools to securely access, reliably download, and easily share their own health records. If you do not see your healthcare providers listed on the Blue Button Connector, ask them if they offer a way for you to view and download your health records online so you have this information available when you need it.

Check Your Data

One of the first things you should do with copies of your medical record is check it for accuracy. Doctors and other healthcare providers rely on your medical records in order to make correct diagnoses, identify potential problems. Health insurers rely on information in your medical history to approve medicines and procedures and process payments.

It's important to make sure your information is accurate and complete. You should carefully review all the information in your records, which may include:

Your personal information

- Is the information that identifies you correct?
- Is your contact information and your emergency contact information up to date?

Your diagnoses

- Is the record of your health conditions correct and up-to-date?
- Is anything missing or mistaken?
- Has anything changed?

Your medications

- Is the list of medications you take complete and are the dosages accurate?
- Are there any medications on the list that you no longer take?

Your tests

- Are any test results missing?
- Do your doctor's notes reflect the test results accurately?

Your care team

- Is the list of doctors and other providers you see accurate and up-to-date?

Your advanced directives

- Do you have documentation of your preferences regarding extraordinary measures and end-of-life care?
- Are they up to date?

Errors

You have the right to go back to the healthcare provider and request amendments and corrections.

Step 1: Make a list of all items that require a correction, focusing on errors in your personal information, test results, diagnoses, procedures, medications, and anything else that might have an impact on your care or insurance in the future.

Note that some minor errors may not require correction, and use your best judgment.

Step 2: Contact the provider's office and ask if they have a form to use when requesting corrections. If they do, follow the instruction on that form. If they do not, you will need to summarize your request in a letter.

Step 3: Document the errors. Include copies of the parts of the record with errors and note any needed corrections. In some cases, you may need to provide additional explanations.

Step 4: Return your request to your provider's office, noting when you dropped it off or when you sent it. If you send your request through the U.S. Mail via a shipping company, you may want to use a service that provides proof of receipt.

The provider must respond within 60 days, although they may take an additional 30 days if they provide you with an explanation.

If your provider refuses to make some or all of the corrections, they must provide you with an explanation. If you still disagree with their explanation, you have the right to submit a letter of disagreement, which by law the provider must insert into your record.

Section 41.2

Personal Health Record (PHR)

This section includes text excerpted from "Personal Health
Records and the HIPAA Privacy Rule," U.S. Department of
Health and Human Services (HHS), December 16, 2008.
Reviewed December 2017.

A personal health record (PHR) is an emerging health information
technology that individuals can use to engage in their own healthcare
to improve the quality and efficiency of that care. In this rapidly developing market, there are several types of PHRs available to individuals
with varying functionalities. Some PHRs are offered by healthcare
providers and health plans covered by the Health Insurance Portability and Accountability Act of 1996 (HIPAA) Privacy Rule, known
as HIPAA-covered entities. The HIPAA Privacy Rule applies to these
PHRs and protects the privacy of the information in them. Alternatively, some PHRs are not offered by HIPAA-covered entities, and,
in these cases, it is the privacy policies of the PHR vendor as well as
any other applicable laws, which will govern how information in the
PHR is protected.

What Is a Personal Health Record (PHR)?

There is currently no universal definition of a PHR, although several relatively similar definitions exist within the industry. In general,
a PHR is an electronic record of an individual's health information
by which the individual controls access to the information and may
have the ability to manage, track, and participate in his or her own
healthcare. A PHR should not be confused with an electronic health
record (EHR). An EHR is held and maintained by a healthcare provider
and may contain all the information that once existed in a patient's
paper medical record, but in electronic form. PHRs universally focus
on providing individuals with the ability to manage their health information and to control, to varying extents, who can access that health
information. A PHR has the potential to provide individuals with a
way to create a longitudinal health history and may include common

information such as medical diagnoses, medications, and test results. Most PHRs also provide individuals with the capability to control who can access the health information in the PHR, and because PHRs are electronic and generally accessible over the Internet, individuals have the flexibility to view their health information at any time and from any computer at any location. The accessibility of health information in a PHR may facilitate appropriate and improved treatment for conditions or emergencies that occur away from an individual's usual healthcare provider. Additionally, the ability to access one's own health information in a PHR may assist individuals in identifying potential errors or mistakes in their information.

Depending on the type of PHR, individuals also may be able to input family histories and emergency contact information, to track and chart their own health information and the health information of their children or others whose care they manage, to schedule and receive reminders about upcoming appointments or procedures, to research medical conditions, to renew prescriptions, and to communicate directly with their healthcare providers through secure messaging systems. The PHR also may function as a way for both individuals and healthcare providers to streamline the administrative processes involved in transferring patient records or for coordinating patient care.

Types of PHRs

The PHR market continues to evolve at a rapid pace, with new types of PHRs continually emerging. For the purposes of this document, however, the universe of PHRs can be broken down into two categories: those subject to the Privacy Rule and those that fall outside of its scope. PHRs that are subject to the Privacy Rule are those that a covered healthcare provider or health plan offers. Examples of PHRs that fall outside the scope of the Privacy Rule are those offered by an employer (separate from the employer's group health plan) or those made available directly to an individual by a PHR vendor that is not a HIPAA-covered entity. Some standalone software packages or portable devices also may be available for use by individuals as PHRs. However, while third parties may provide individuals with information to upload into these tools, since they are solely in the custody of the individual and are not offered by or connected to a third party, they will not be addressed in this document.

Section 41.3

Benefits of Electronic Health Records (EHRs)

This section includes text excerpted from "For Providers and
Professionals—Benefits of Electronic Health Records (EHRs),"
HealthIT.gov, Office of the National Coordinator for Health
Information Technology (ONC), July 30, 2015.

Our world has been radically transformed by digital technology—
smart phones, tablets, and web-enabled devices have transformed
our daily lives and the way we communicate. Medicine is an informa-
tion-rich enterprise. A greater and more seamless flow of information
within a digital healthcare infrastructure, created by electronic health
records (EHRs), encompasses and leverages digital progress and can
transform the way care is delivered and compensated. With EHRs,
information is available whenever and wherever it is needed.

The Health Information Technology for Economic and Clinical
Health (HITECH) Act, a component of the American Recovery and
Reinvestment Act of 2009, represents the Nation's first substantial
commitment of Federal resources to support the widespread adoption of EHRs. As of August 2012, 54 percent of the Medicare- and
Medicaid-eligible professionals had registered for the meaningful use
incentive program.

Healthcare Quality and Convenience

Electronic health records (EHRs) can improve healthcare quality.
EHRs can also make healthcare more convenient for providers and
patients.

Snapshot of Improved Healthcare Quality and Convenience for Providers

- Quick access to patient records from inpatient and remote locations for more coordinated, efficient care

- Enhanced decision support, clinical alerts, reminders, and medical information

- Performance-improving tools, real-time quality reporting
- Legible, complete documentation that facilitates accurate coding and billing
- Interfaces with labs, registries, and other EHRs
- Safer, more reliable prescribing

Snapshot of Improved Healthcare Quality and Convenience for Patients

- Reduced need to fill out the same forms at each office visit
- Reliable point-of-care information and reminders notifying providers of important health interventions
- Convenience of e-prescriptions electronically sent to pharmacy
- Patient portals with online interaction for providers
- Electronic referrals allowing easier access to follow-up care with specialists

EHRs Improve Information Availability

With EHRs, patients' health information is available in one place, when and where it is needed. Providers have access to the information they need, at the time they need it to make a decision.

EHRs Can Be the Foundation for Quality Improvements

Reliable access to complete patient health information is essential for safe and effective care. EHRs place accurate and complete information about patients' health and medical history at the fingertips of providers. With EHRs, providers can give the best possible care, at the point of care. This can lead to a better patient experience and, most importantly, better patient outcomes.

Practices also report that they utilize extracted reports on patient and disease registries to track patient care as well as facilitate quality improvement discussions during clinical meetings.

EHRs Support Provider Decision Making

EHRs can help providers make efficient, effective decisions about patient care, through:

- Improved aggregation, analysis, and communication of patient information

- Clinical alerts and reminders

- Support for diagnostic and therapeutic decisions

- Built-in safeguards against potential adverse events

How EHRs Foster Patient Participation

Electronic health records (EHRs) can help providers:

- **Ensure high-quality care.** With EHRs, providers can give patients full and accurate information about all of their medical evaluations. Providers can also offer follow-up information after an office visit or a hospital stay, such as self-care instructions, reminders for other follow-up care, and links to web resources.

- **Create an avenue for communication with their patients.** With EHRs, providers can manage appointment schedules electronically and exchange e-mail with their patients. Quick and easy communication between patients and providers may help providers identify symptoms earlier. And it can position providers to be more proactive by reaching out to patients.

Improved Diagnostics and Patient Outcomes

When healthcare providers have access to complete and accurate information, patients receive better medical care. Electronic health records (EHRs) can improve the ability to diagnose diseases and reduce—even prevent—medical errors, improving patient outcomes.

A national survey of doctors who are ready for meaningful use offers important evidence:

- 94 percent of providers report that their EHR makes records readily available at point of care.

- 88 percent report that their EHR produces clinical benefits for the practice.

- 75 percent of providers report that their EHR allows them to deliver better patient care.

EHRs Can Aid in Diagnosis

With EHRs, providers can have reliable access to a patient's complete health information. This comprehensive picture can help providers diagnose patients' problems sooner.

EHRs Can Reduce Errors, Improve Patient Safety, and Support Better Patient Outcomes

How? EHRs don't just contain or transmit information; they "compute" it. That means that EHRs manipulate the information in ways that make a difference for patients. For example:

- A qualified EHR not only keeps a record of a patient's medications or allergies, it also automatically checks for problems whenever a new medication is prescribed and alerts the clinician to potential conflicts.

- Information gathered by a primary care provider and recorded in an EHR tells a clinician in the emergency department about a patient's life-threatening allergy, and emergency staff can adjust care appropriately, even if the patient is unconscious.

- EHRs can expose potential safety problems when they occur, helping providers avoid more serious consequences for patients and leading to better patient outcomes.

- EHRs can help providers quickly and systematically identify and correct operational problems. In a paper-based setting, identifying such problems is much more difficult, and correcting them can take years.

Risk Management and Liability Prevention: Study Findings

EHRs may improve risk management by:

- Providing clinical alerts and reminders

- Improving aggregation, analysis, and communication of patient information

- Making it easier to consider all aspects of a patient's condition

- Supporting diagnostic and therapeutic decision making

- Gathering all relevant information (lab results, etc.) in one place

- Support for therapeutic decisions

- Enabling evidence-based decisions at point of care

- Preventing adverse events

- Providing built-in safeguards against prescribing treatments that would result in adverse events

- Enhancing research and monitoring for improvements in clinical quality

- Certified EHRs may help providers prevent liability actions by:

- Demonstrating adherence to the best evidence-based practices

- Producing complete, legible records readily available for the defense (reconstructing what actually happened during the point of care)

- Disclosing evidence that suggests informed consent

EHRs Can Improve Public Health Outcomes

EHRs can also have beneficial effects on the health of groups of patients.

Providers who have electronic health information about the entire population of patients they serve can look more meaningfully at the needs of patients who:

- Suffer from a specific condition

- Are eligible for specific preventive measures

- Are currently taking specific medications

This EHR function helps providers identify and work with patients to manage specific risk factors or combinations of risk factors to improve patient outcomes.

For example, providers might wish to identify:

- How many patients with hypertension have their blood pressure under control

- How many patients with diabetes have their blood sugar measurements in the target range and have had appropriate screening tests

This EHR function also can detect patterns of potentially related adverse events and enable at-risk patients to be notified quickly.

Medical Practice Efficiencies and Cost Savings

Many healthcare providers have found that electronic health records (EHRs) help improve medical practice management by increasing practice efficiencies and cost savings.

A national survey of doctors who are ready for meaningful use offers important evidence:

- 79 percent of providers report that with an EHR, their practice functions more efficiently

- 82 percent report that sending prescriptions electronically (e-prescribing) saves time

- 68 percent of providers see their EHR as an asset with recruiting physicians

- 75 percent receive lab results faster

- 70 percent report enhances in data confidentiality

Based on the size of a health system and the scope of their implementation, benefits for large hospitals can range from $37 million to $59 million over a five-year period in addition to incentive payments.

Electronic Health Records Create More Efficient Practices

EHR-enabled medical practices report:

- Improved medical practice management through integrated scheduling systems that link appointments directly to progress notes, automate coding, and managed claims

- Time savings with easier centralized chart management, condition-specific queries, and other shortcuts

- Enhanced communication with other clinicians, labs, and health plans through:

- Easy access to patient information from anywhere

- Tracking electronic messages to staff, other clinicians, hospitals, labs, etc.

- Automated formulary checks by health plans

- Order and receipt of lab tests and diagnostic images

- Links to public health systems such as registries and communicable disease databases

Electronic Health Records Reduce Paperwork

EHRs can reduce the amount of time providers spend doing paperwork.

Administrative tasks, such as filling out forms and processing billing requests, represent a significant percentage of healthcare costs. EHRs can increase practice efficiencies by streamlining these tasks, significantly decreasing costs.

In addition, EHRs can deliver more information in additional directions. EHRs can be programmed for easy or even automatic delivery of information that needs to be shared with public health agencies or for the purpose of quality measurement.

Electronic Health Records Reduce Duplication of Testing

Because EHRs contain all of a patient's health information in one place, it is less likely that providers will have to spend time ordering—and reviewing the results of—unnecessary or duplicate tests and medical procedures. Less utilization means fewer costs.

Section 41.4

E-Prescription

This section includes text excerpted from "A Prescription for e-Prescribers: Getting the Most Out of Electronic Prescribing," HealthIT.gov, Office of the National Coordinator for Health Information Technology (ONC), February 13, 2015.

Ninety percent of pharmacies in the United States are enabled to accept electronic prescriptions (e-prescriptions). Seventy percent of physicians are e-prescribing using an electronic health record (EHR), and each state has an e-prescribing rate of 41 percent or above. If you are using ONC certified health IT, then you are one of the many providers nationwide with EHR technology enabled to prescribe electronically.

This section highlights some key questions to consider and potential changes you or your practice can make to better manage medication use through the e-prescribing process. Some of these changes can result in decreased pharmacy call backs to the practice, increased patient satisfaction, and improved e-prescribing productivity. Recommendations to create unambiguous prescriptions with standardized information enables effective clinical decision support and enhanced patient safety. While stand-alone e-prescribing systems are available, many of the optimal features and functions described in this guide are only possible through an e-prescribing application integrated with an electronic health record.

Think about your current e-prescribing process as you read through this guide and identify areas you can improve. What issues do you typically face? What is your e-prescribing system capable of doing? Select through each of the steps in the e-prescribing process to learn more about what you should expect from your e-prescribing system, and what you can do to improve the prescriptions you send electronically.

Process for Creating and Managing a Prescription Electronically

Identify Patient

Providers or staff gather patient information, review stored data using sources within the electronic health record (EHR) and select the correct patient.

Review Current Patient Data

Providers or staff review patient medications using historical information from EHR sources and patient/caregiver interview

Select Drug

Providers select the drug to be prescribed from a menu in the EHR.

Enter Parameters

Provider enters directions for use and provides all required information to be transmitted to the pharmacy.

Review Alerts and Advisories

Provider reviews warnings such as duplicate therapy or drug-drug interactions, and other messages, as well as formulary status and drug benefits.

Select Pharmacy; Print or Send Rx

Provider selects pharmacy from patient's stored preferences and reviews the final prescription before sending.

Pharmacy Review and Process

Provider reviews e-prescribing expectations with patients, has staff dedicated to monitoring e-prescription logs, and electronically manages renewal requests.

Part Seven

Medical Technology—Legal and Ethical Concerns

Chapter 42

Health Information Privacy Law and Policy

The Health Insurance Portability and Accountability Act (HIPAA) Privacy Rule is a federal privacy law that sets a baseline of protection for certain individually identifiable health information ("health information").

The Privacy Rule generally permits, but does not require, covered healthcare providers to give patients the choice as to whether their health information may be disclosed to others for certain key purposes. These key purposes include treatment, payment, and healthcare operations.

Are There Privacy Laws That Require Patient Consent?

Yes. There are some federal and state privacy laws (e.g., 42 Code of Federal Regulations (CFR) Part 2, Title X of the Public Health Service Act) that require healthcare providers to obtain patients' written

This chapter contains text excerpted from the following sources: Text in this chapter begins with excerpts from "Patient Consent for eHIE—Health Information Privacy Law and Policy," HealthIT.gov, Office of the National Coordinator for Health Information Technology (ONC), October 31, 2014. Reviewed December 2017; Text beginning with the heading "Does an Individual Have a Right under HIPAA to Access Their Health Information in Human Readable Form?" is excerpted from "Individual Privacy and HIPAA," U.S. Department of Health and Human Services (HHS), January 27, 2017.

consent before they disclose their health information to other people and organizations, even for treatment. Many of these privacy laws protect information that is related to health conditions considered "sensitive" by most people.

How Does HIPAA Affect These Other Privacy Laws?

HIPAA created a baseline of privacy protection. It overrides (or "preempts") other privacy laws that are less protective. But HIPAA leaves in effect other laws that are more privacy-protective. Under this legal framework, healthcare providers and other implementers must continue to follow other applicable federal and state laws that require obtaining patients' consent before disclosing their health information.

Does an Individual Have a Right under HIPAA to Access Their Health Information in Human Readable Form?

In general, a covered entity must provide an individual with access to protected health information (PHI) about the individual in a designated record set in the form and format requested by the individual, if it is readily producible in such form and format. In cases where the PHI is not readily producible in the requested form and format, the covered entity must provide the PHI in a readable alternative form and format as agreed to by the covered entity and the individual. Thus, individuals have a right under HIPAA to access PHI about themselves in human readable form.

Under the HIPAA Privacy Rule, Do Individuals Have the Right to an Electronic Copy of Their PHI?

Yes, in most cases. If the PHI is maintained by a covered entity electronically, an individual has a right to receive an electronic copy of the information upon request (assuming the covered entity does not have a ground for denial under 45 CFR 164.524(a)(2) or (a)(3)). The covered entity must provide the individual with access to the PHI in the electronic form and format requested by the individual, if it is readily producible in that form and format, or if not, in a readable alternative electronic format as agreed to by the individual and covered entity. Where an individual requests access to PHI that is maintained electronically by a covered entity, the covered entity may provide the individual with a paper copy of the PHI to satisfy the request only in cases where the individual declines to accept any of the electronic formats readily producible by the covered entity.

Under HIPAA, When Can a Family Member of an Individual Access the Individual's PHI from a Healthcare Provider or Health Plan?

The HIPAA Privacy Rule provides individuals with the right to access their medical and other health records from their healthcare providers and health plans, upon request. The Privacy Rule generally also gives the right to access the individual's health records to a personal representative of the individual. Under the Rule, an individual's personal representative is someone authorized under State or other applicable law to act on behalf of the individual in making healthcare related decisions. With respect to deceased individuals, the individual's personal representative is an executor, administrator, or other person who has authority under State or other law to act on behalf of the deceased individual or the individual's estate. Thus, whether a family member or other person is a personal representative of the individual, and therefore has a right to access the individual's PHI under the Privacy Rule, generally depends on whether that person has authority under State law to act on behalf of the individual.

Chapter 43

Health Information Technology Legislation and Regulations

The Office of the National Coordinator for Health Information Technology's (ONC) work on health information technology (IT) is authorized by the Health Information Technology for Economic and Clinical Health (HITECH) Act.

The HITECH Act established ONC in law and provides the U.S. Department of Health and Human Services (HHS) with the authority to establish programs to improve healthcare quality, safety, and efficiency through the promotion of health IT, including electronic health records (EHRs) and private and secure electronic health information exchange.

Other legislation related to ONC's work includes Health Insurance Portability and Accountability Act (HIPAA) the Affordable Care Act (ACA), and the FDA Safety and Innovation Act.

HITECH Act

The Health Information Technology for Economic and Clinical Health (HITECH) Act of 2009 provides HHS with the authority

---

This chapter includes text excerpted from "Health IT Legislation and Regulations," HealthIT.gov, Office of the National Coordinator for Health Information Technology (ONC), May 12, 2016.

to establish programs to improve healthcare quality, safety, and efficiency through the promotion of health IT, including electronic health records and private and secure electronic health information exchange.

FDASIA

Section 618 of the Food and Drug Administration Safety and Innovation Act (FDASIA) of 2012 directed the Secretary of Health and Human Services, acting through the Commissioner of the U.S. Food and Drug Administration (FDA), and in consultation with ONC and the Chairman of the Federal Communications Commission, to develop a report that contains a proposed strategy and recommendations on an appropriate, risk-based regulatory framework for health IT, including medical mobile applications, that promotes innovation, protects patient safety, and avoids regulatory duplication. The Health IT Policy Committee formed a FDASIA workgroup and issued recommendations to ONC, FDA, and FCC as of the September 4th, 2013 HIT Policy Committee meeting.

HIPAA

The Health Insurance Portability and Accountability Act (HIPAA) of 1996 protects health insurance coverage for workers and their families when they change or lose their jobs, requires the establishment of national standards for electronic healthcare transactions, and requires establishment of national identifiers for providers, health insurance plans, and employers.

The HHS Office for Civil Rights administers the HIPAA Privacy and Security Rules. The HIPAA Privacy Rule describes what information is protected and how protected information can be used and disclosed. The HIPAA Security Rule describes who is covered by the HIPAA privacy protections and what safeguards must be in place to ensure appropriate protection of electronic protected health information.

The Centers for Medicare and Medicaid Services (CMS) administer and enforce the HIPAA Administrative Simplification Rules, including the Transactions and Code Set Standards, Employer Identifier Standard, and National Provider Identifier Standard. The HIPAA Enforcement Rule provides standards for the enforcement of all the Administrative Simplification Rules.

Affordable Care Act

The Affordable Care Act (ACA) of 2010 establishes comprehensive healthcare insurance reforms that aim to increase access to healthcare, improve quality and lower healthcare costs, and provide new consumer protections.

Chapter 44

HIPAA Privacy Rule's Right of Access and Health Information Technology

Since its inception, the Health Insurance Portability and Accountability Act (HIPAA) Privacy Rule's right of an individual to access protected health information (PHI) about him or her held by a covered entity has operated in a primarily paper-based environment. While it has been common for covered entities to create, maintain, and exchange PHI in paper form, an increasing number of covered entities are beginning to utilize new forms of health information technology (health IT), which often involve the transition of PHI from paper to electronic form. Many healthcare providers, for example, are adopting comprehensive electronic health records (EHRs) to enhance the quality and efficiency of care they deliver. Health IT also may create mechanisms by which individuals can electronically request access to their PHI and by which covered entities can respond by providing or denying access electronically.

An individual's right to access his or her PHI is a critical aspect of the Privacy Rule, the application of which naturally extends to an electronic environment. The Privacy Rule establishes, with limited

This chapter includes text excerpted from "The HIPAA Privacy Rule's Right of Access and Health Information Technology," U.S. Department of Health and Human Services (HHS), December 16, 2008. Reviewed December 2017.

exceptions, an enforceable means by which individuals have a right to review or obtain copies of their PHI, to the extent it is maintained in the designated record set(s) of a covered entity. The Privacy Rule's specific, yet flexible, standards also address individuals' requests for access and timely action by the covered entity, including the provision of access, denial of access, and documentation.

Health IT has the potential to facilitate the Privacy Rule's right of access from both an individual's and a covered entity's perspective. Because the right of access operates regardless of the format of the PHI, its application in an electronic environment is similar to that in a paper-based environment. Several provisions, however, such as those related to requests for access, timely action, verification, form or format of access, and denial of access, may apply slightly differently and, thus, require additional consideration. The discussion that follows addresses an individual's right to request access electronically, a covered entity's electronic provision or denial of access and other specific applications of the Privacy Rule that will assist covered entities in tailoring their compliance appropriately.

The guidance also is meant to serve as a stepping stone for covered entities that are considering how an individual's access rights may be fulfilled within an electronic health information exchange environment. To that end, the guidance demonstrates how the Privacy Rule's access standard provides a strong foundation from which covered entities can develop policies and procedures that also meet several of the objectives enumerated in the Individual Access Principle identified within The Nationwide Privacy and Security Framework for Electronic Exchange of Individually Identifiable Health Information.

Requests for Access

The Privacy Rule allows covered entities to require that individuals make requests for access in writing, provided they inform individuals of such a requirement. In addition, the Privacy Rule has always considered electronic documents to qualify as written documents. Thus, the Privacy Rule supports covered entities' offering individuals the option of using electronic means (e.g., e-mail, web portal) to make requests for access.

Timely Action

The Privacy Rule requires covered entities to respond to requests for access in a timely manner. Except as otherwise specified, the Privacy

Rule requires the individual be notified of the decision within 30 days of the covered entity's receipt of the request. While the Privacy Rule establishes 30 days as an outside limit, it does not preclude covered entities from responding sooner. Indeed, a covered entity may have the capacity through the use of some electronic systems to provide automated access to an individual's PHI or respond to requests with immediate access, 24 hours a day. Not all electronic systems, however, may allow for the provision of immediate access, and the covered entity's response time-frame will normally depend, in part, on its system capacity.

As in a paper-based system, other factors also will impact a covered entity's response time in an electronic environment. For example, the Privacy Rule's 30-day parameter was originally conceptualized to allow covered entities sufficient time to accommodate normal business functions (e.g., interpretation of test results), as well as those unusual circumstances that might delay a response (e.g., reporting suspected child abuse). Similar allowances may be necessary in an electronic health information environment as well.

As a practical matter, individuals might expect, when making a request of a technologically sophisticated covered entity, that their requests could be responded to instantaneously or well before the current required time-frame. This might be the case, for example, when access is provided through a direct view or portal into a healthcare provider's EHR. Providing more timely access than the Privacy Rule requires may be a means by which covered entities distinguish themselves within the market.

Provision of Access

Who May Exercise the Right of Access?

Individuals and Personal Representatives. While the Privacy Rule's right of access belongs primarily to the individual who is the subject of the PHI, the Privacy Rule also generally requires that persons who are legally authorized to act on behalf of the individual regarding healthcare matters be granted the same right of access. The Privacy Rule defers to state law to determine when a person has the legal authority to act on behalf of an individual with regard to healthcare matters. Healthcare powers of attorney and parental rights, for example, are two legal bases by which state law may be determinative of a person's authority to act on behalf of an individual.

The Privacy Rule's personal representative requirement ensures that certain people will have access to an individual's PHI when the individual is incapacitated or otherwise unable to exercise the right of access on his or her own behalf. The Privacy Rule would require that covered entities grant personal representatives with the right of access on behalf of an individual in an electronic environment, just as they do today with regard to paper-based information. Covered entities will want to make sure, however, that they have the capacity to identify, authenticate, and properly respond to requests from these individuals, whether electronically or otherwise, as the Privacy Rule requires.

Verification. The Privacy Rule requires covered entities to develop and implement reasonable policies and procedures to verify the identity of any person who requests PHI, as well as the authority of the person to have access to the information, if the identity or authority of the person is not already known. These verification requirements apply to individuals who request access to their PHI that is maintained in a designated record set. The Privacy Rule refrains from defining specific or technical verification requirements and largely defers to the covered entity's professional judgment and industry standards to determine what is reasonable and appropriate under the circumstances.

Verification may be obtained either orally or in writing (which may be satisfied electronically), so long as the requisite documentation, statements or representations are obtained where required by a specific Privacy Rule disclosure provision, and that the appropriate steps are ultimately taken to verify the identity and authority of individuals or personal representatives who are otherwise unknown. Therefore, covered entities that receive and/or respond to access requests electronically should revisit their verification and documentation policies and procedures to ensure that they are reasonable in light of the electronic environment within which they are operating.

Content—Designated Record Sets

An individual's right of access generally applies to the information that exists within a covered entity's designated record set(s), including:

1. a healthcare provider's medical and billing records,

2. a health plan's enrollment, payment, claims adjudication, and case or medical management record systems, and

3. any information used, in whole or in part, by or for the covered entity to make decisions about individuals. A record is any

item, collection, or grouping of information that includes PHI and is maintained, collected, used, or disseminated by or for the covered entity.

Covered entities that use electronic records (e.g., EHRs or electronic claims systems) will want to remain cognizant that the right of access applies regardless of the information's format. The term "designated record set," therefore, cannot be limited to information contained in an electronic record, but also will include any nonduplicative, electronic or paper-based information that meets the term's definition. While overlap may initially exist between electronic and paper-based record sets, covered entities will likely find their access-related obligations to be less time and labor intensive the more PHI they convert to being electronic.

Furthermore, a covered entity that utilizes a business associate to maintain or otherwise operate its electronic records will want to ensure the business associate is obligated to share nonduplicative information pursuant to electronic access requests. The same would be true if a health information organization (HIO), as a business associate, maintains an electronic repository of some or all of a covered entity's PHI.

Form or Format of Access Provided

The Privacy Rule requires covered entities to provide access to the PHI in the form or format requested by the individual, if it is readily producible in such form or format. If the PHI is not readily producible in the form or format requested, access must be provided in a readable hard copy form, or in the alternative, some other form or format as agreed to by the covered entity and the individual. The covered entity also may provide the individual with a summary of the PHI or may provide an explanation of the PHI which has been provided, so long as the individual agrees to the alternative form and associated fees.

To the extent individuals request that access to their PHI be provided in an electronic form or format, covered entities' utilization of electronic records will likely increase the amount of PHI that is "readily producible" in electronic form, thereby benefiting both the requesting individual, as well as the covered entity:

Electronic access may provide individuals with more timely access to more information in a more convenient manner. For example:

- Electronic copies of PHI may be downloaded to USB thumbdrives or copied to compact discs relatively quickly and may provide individuals with a more convenient means of transporting and maintaining the information.

- EHRs may enable covered entities to offer individuals an immediate and ongoing view into the covered entity's designated record set(s), either through a personal health record (PHR) or otherwise, while limiting the time, expense, and labor that may be required otherwise in order to provide access to the individual.

Electronic access also may be a means by which covered entities can limit the time, resources, and other expenses required to provide the individual with access.

- Electronic copies of PHI that are downloaded to USB thumbdrives or copied to compact discs may require less labor and overhead than access to paper records would require.

- Covered entities may find that providing individuals with electronic access to PHI could save them time and resources by limiting, if not eliminating, the need to provide hard copies of the information or some other, more expensive, form or format.

- Providing such "readily producible" electronic access may have the secondary effect of enhancing their communication with individuals, which may in turn, lead to improved quality of care and strengthened consumer satisfaction.

The right of access also affords covered entities the option of making alternative agreements with individuals as to the form or format of access provided. If, for example, a covered entity's default administrative safeguards policies and procedures limit the provision of electronic access to standalone devices and secure, web-based portals, and an individual requests access via e-mail, the Privacy Rule would permit alternative agreements that satisfy both parties, so long as reasonable safeguards are otherwise in place.

To the extent that individuals request access to their PHI in hardcopy form, the covered entity must provide such access, even if the information is stored in an electronic record.

Denial of Access

Grounds for Denial

The Privacy Rule contemplates circumstances under which covered entities may deny an individual access to PHI and distinguishes those grounds for denial which are reviewable from those which are not.

Unreviewable grounds for denial are situations involving:

1. psychotherapy notes, information compiled for use in legal proceedings, and certain information held by clinical laboratories;

2. certain requests that are made by inmates of correctional institutions;

3. information created or obtained during research that includes treatment if certain conditions are met;

4. denials permitted by the Privacy Act; and

5. information obtained from nonhealthcare providers pursuant to promises of confidentiality.

Reviewable grounds for denial are:

1. disclosures which would cause endangerment of the individual or another person;

2. situations where the PHI refers to another and disclosure is likely to cause substantial harm; and

3. requests made by a personal representative where disclosure is likely to cause substantial harm.

Implementation of Denial

The Privacy Rule further requires that denials of access be timely, written, provided to individuals in plain language, with a description of the basis for denial, and if applicable, contain statements of the individual's rights to have the decision reviewed and how to request such a review. In addition, the notice of denial must inform the individual of how complaints may be filed with the covered entity or the Secretary of HHS. If access to some of the PHI is denied, the covered entity must, to the extent possible, give the individual access to any other PHI requested, after excluding the PHI to which the covered entity has a ground to deny access.

A covered entity may satisfy the Privacy Rule's writing requirement for denials electronically, though its denial still must be based on the grounds identified by the Privacy Rule, and must comply with each of the Privacy Rule's procedural requirements. In cases where the covered entity is able to receive and process a request for access by the individual electronically and provide access in an electronic format, the denial of the request, in whole or in part, may also be done electronically. As emphasized above, the form of the denial does not change the covered entity's obligations regarding the basis for the denial or the content of the notification to the individual. However, where the covered entity provides individuals with electronic access to some or all of their health information, through a PHR or similar means, and the access is available to the individual at any time and without a request, it becomes more difficult to determine whether a denial of access has occurred and when notice to the individual is required.

For example, the requirements in the Privacy Rule are flexible enough to permit a covered entity to notify the individual in advance of the types of PHI to which it intends to deny access and for which the Privacy Rule does not provide a right of review. Such advance notification would not be appropriate, however, for other types of PHI to which a covered entity may deny access because the denial must be based on the specific exercise of professional judgment by a licensed healthcare professional and are subject to the individual's right to request a review of the denial by another licensed healthcare professional. In these cases, the individual must be aware of the fact that he or she has been denied access to certain information for which the individual has a right to request a review. The covered entity's policies and procedures for the provision of electronic access must appropriately provide for these individualized grounds for denial of access.

Chapter 45

Personal Health Records (PHRs) and the HIPAA Privacy Rule

A personal health record (PHR) is an emerging health information technology that individuals can use to engage in their own healthcare to improve the quality and efficiency of that care. In this rapidly developing market, there are several types of PHRs available to individuals with varying functionalities. Some PHRs are offered by healthcare providers and health plans covered by the Health Insurance Portability and Accountability Act of 1996 (HIPAA) Privacy Rule, known as HIPAA-covered entities. The HIPAA Privacy Rule applies to these PHRs and protects the privacy of the information in them. Alternatively, some PHRs are not offered by HIPAA-covered entities, and, in these cases, it is the privacy policies of the PHR vendor as well as any other applicable laws, which will govern how information in the PHR is protected. This document describes how the Privacy Rule may apply to and supports the use of PHRs.

What Is a PHR?

There is currently no universal definition of a PHR, although several relatively similar definitions exist within the industry. In general,

This chapter includes text excerpted from "Personal Health Records and the HIPAA Privacy Rule," U.S. Department of Health and Human Services (HHS), December 16, 2008. Reviewed December 2017.

a PHR is an electronic record of an individual's health information by which the individual controls access to the information and may have the ability to manage, track, and participate in his or her own healthcare. A PHR should not be confused with an electronic health record (EHR). An EHR is held and maintained by a healthcare provider and may contain all the information that once existed in a patient's paper medical record, but in electronic form.

PHRs universally focus on providing individuals with the ability to manage their health information and to control, to varying extents, who can access that health information. A PHR has the potential to provide individuals with a way to create a longitudinal health history and may include common information such as medical diagnoses, medications, and test results. Most PHRs also provide individuals with the capability to control who can access the health information in the PHR, and because PHRs are electronic and generally accessible over the Internet, individuals have the flexibility to view their health information at any time and from any computer at any location. The accessibility of health information in a PHR may facilitate appropriate and improved treatment for conditions or emergencies that occur away from an individual's usual healthcare provider. Additionally, the ability to access one's own health information in a PHR may assist individuals in identifying potential errors or mistakes in their information.

Depending on the type of PHR, individuals also may be able to input family histories and emergency contact information, to track and chart their own health information and the health information of their children or others whose care they manage, to schedule and receive reminders about upcoming appointments or procedures, to research medical conditions, to renew prescriptions, and to communicate directly with their healthcare providers through secure messaging systems. The PHR also may function as a way for both individuals and healthcare providers to streamline the administrative processes involved in transferring patient records or for coordinating patient care.

PHRs Offered by HIPAA-Covered Entities

PHRs offered by HIPAA-covered entities, such as healthcare providers or health plans, generally link individuals to, and allow them to view, some or all of the health records maintained about them within the covered entity. In many cases, an individual may not be given access to the entirety of his or her health record held by the healthcare provider or health plan and may only have the ability to view and not update or edit the information that is assembled by the healthcare provider or health plan. These PHRs also may allow individuals to add their own information into their PHRs and to update or edit this self-entered information. Many PHRs will include notations as to the sources of information in the PHR, whether it be self-entered by the individual or entered by the healthcare provider or health plan. The individual may be able to control who else has access to the information in the PHR, such a spouse, family member, or another healthcare provider.

A PHR offered by a healthcare provider or health plan may not be a comprehensive record of the individual's healthcare, because it may not be automatically updated with information from all healthcare providers that treat the individual or health plans that cover the individual. However, in many cases, individuals can request copies of their health information from other healthcare providers or health plans and can update their PHRs with this information to ensure that their PHRs are up-to-date and as comprehensive as possible. Alternatively, if the functionality exists, individuals may authorize other healthcare providers or health plans to update the individual's information into the individual's PHR directly. In addition, a PHR offered by a covered entity may not be portable, so individuals may not be able to take their PHR with them when they switch healthcare providers or health plans. In these cases, as above, individuals who want comprehensive records may have to retrieve information from their prior PHR or directly from their healthcare provider or health plan and input the information directly into any PHR.

PHRs Not Offered by HIPAA-Covered Entities

The Privacy Rule does not apply to PHRs that are not offered by health plans or healthcare providers that are covered by the Privacy Rule. For example, PHRs may be offered by employers (separate from the employer's group health plan) or by PHR vendors directly to individuals. These types of PHRs are governed by the privacy policies of the entity that offers them, and in certain cases, may be governed by laws other than the Privacy Rule. However, the Privacy Rule still regulates how an individual's health information held by a HIPAA-covered entity enters the PHR.

The HIPAA Privacy Rule's Application to PHRs Offered by Covered Entities

The Privacy Rule protects the privacy of certain individually identifiable health information, in own as protected health information (PHI), created or maintained by covered entities. Covered entities include health plans and those healthcare providers that transmit any health information in electronic form in connection with certain standard transactions, such as healthcare claims. The Privacy Rule governs how these covered entities may use and disclose an individual's PHI and grants individuals certain rights regarding their health information. PHRs that are offered by a covered entity will contain PHI and, thus, the covered entity must appropriately safeguard this information as required by the Privacy Rule.

The Use and Disclosure of Protected Health Information

Covered entities may not use or disclose an individual's PHI except as the Privacy Rule expressly permits or requires, or with an individual's written authorization. The Privacy Rule's use and disclosure provisions were designed with the typical business or clinical healthcare record in mind. Thus, the Privacy Rule generally allows covered entities to use and disclose a individual's PHI for treatment, payment of healthcare, and healthcare operations (certain functions that support treatment and payment). Also, in recognition that there are certain legitimate and important additional uses of an individual's health information, the Privacy Rule allows a covered entity to disclose, subject to conditions, individual's PHI for certain other purposes, such as research and public health.

With respect to offering and maintaining a PHR, a covered entity is generally permitted by the Privacy Rule to use and disclose an individual's PHI for purposes of providing this service to the individual, as well as communicating with the individual through the use of a PHR. With respect to PHI within the PHR, a covered entity offering a PHR may establish privacy policies that restrict its uses and disclosures of such information beyond what is required by the Privacy Rule. Because the fundamental purpose of a PHR is to give individuals more control over, and access to, their health information, covered entities are encouraged to reassess what uses and disclosures of individuals' information in the PHR may be appropriate, and to give individual greater control over the information in their PHRs.

This may include, for example, allowing an individual to control not only access to the information in the PHR by third parties, but even by the covered entity itself. However, covered entities should be aware of the circumstances in which they may need to access or disclose information within an individual's PHR to comply with other legal obligations, and should make these circumstances clear to the individual.

Individual Rights

The Privacy Rule grants individuals several rights with respect to their own health information, such as the right to view and obtain a copy of much of their health information and to have corrections made to such information. Because PHRs provide individuals with access to their health information and can facilitate communication between individuals and their healthcare providers or health plans, PHRs may be useful mechanisms for covered entities to facilitate providing individuals with their HIPAA rights.

Access

The Privacy Rule gives individuals a right of access to inspect and obtain a copy of their PHI in a designed record set held by a covered entity. A designated record set is the medical records, billing records, enrollment and claims records, and other information used by the covered entity to make decisions about the individual. A PHR offered by a HIPAA-covered entity may allow individuals to view all or part of their PHI held by a covered entity and to download and print this information. Thus, depending on the breadth and usefulness of the information to which the individual has access, a PHR could eliminate or reduce the need for individuals to otherwise request access to their complete designated record set held by the HIPAA-covered entity.

However, access to health information through a PHR would not replace an individual's right to obtain access to health information in his or her designated record set that is not available through the PHR and to which he or she is entitled under the Privacy Rule. Thus, covered entities providing the individual with access to only a portion of the individual's health information in a designated record set through a PHR should make clear the individual's right to obtain access to the information in the designated record set that is not available through PHR. Also, individuals always retain the right to a paper copy of the individual's health information in the designated record set held by the covered entity.

In addition, the Privacy Rule requires a covered entity to have a mechanism to provide an individual's personal representatives with access to the individual's PHI and, as with access provided to the individual, a PHR may be a way to eliminate or reduce the need for personal representatives otherwise request access to the complete designated record set about the individual. Additionally, covered entities are not precluded from setting up a PHR system that allows individuals to designate family members or other persons to have access to the information in their PHRs.

Amendment

The Privacy Rule gives individuals the right to have amendments or corrections made to the PHI in their health records or other designated record set held by a covered entity. See 45 C.F.R. 164.526. PHRs that replicate some or all of the information in the health record may be helpful mechanisms for individuals to identify potential errors in their health information and to request that the covered entity correct the information. If there is a mistake, the covered entity can correct or append additional information to the individual's health information held in the covered entity's health records system and can update the PHR with the corrected information. The individual control inherent in PHRs also may allow individuals to revise and update some information, such as that information they themselves have entered in their PHRs.

Notice of Privacy Practices

The Privacy Rule requires covered entities to provide individuals with a notice of privacy practices (NPP) outlining individuals' rights with respect to their health information and how the covered entity may use and disclose this information. The PHR may be a useful mechanism for a covered entity to distribute its HIPAA NPP, in addition to the other distribution methods required by the Privacy Rule. Also, a covered entity that offers a PHR to individuals is encouraged to consider highlighting its privacy practices with respect to the PHR explicitly in its HIPAA NPP, particularly to the extent such practices provide greater restrictions on the use and disclosure of health information compared to the covered entity's policies generally with respect to PHI. Alternatively, covered entities may consider creating a separate and more detailed NPP specific to PHRs that outlines the privacy practices and highlights the extent to which individuals can control information in their PHRs. Making available to individuals specific information about the privacy protections and controls over information in a PHR may build trust in, and help promote use of, PHRs by individuals.

Accounting of Disclosures

The Privacy Rule gives individuals the right to receive an accounting of certain disclosures of their PHI made by a covered entity for the six years prior to the request for the accounting, so that individuals are aware of how their information has been shared. See 45 C.F.R. 164.528. However, because disclosures from the PHR will generally be to the individual or for limited other purposes, such as for administering the PHR, disclosures of information from a PHR generally would not be subject to the HIPAA accounting requirement. However, consistent with the intent of the accounting for disclosures, covered entities may want to consider setting up a functionality within a PHR that provides individuals with the ability to view a log of who accessed their PHR.

Chapter 46

Privacy, Security, and Electronic Health Records (EHRs)

Your healthcare provider may be moving from paper records to electronic health records (EHRs) or may be using EHRs already. EHRs allow providers to use information more effectively to improve the quality and efficiency of your care, but EHRs will not change the privacy protections or security safeguards that apply to your health information.

Most of us feel that our health information is private and should be protected. That is why there is a federal law that sets rules for healthcare providers and health insurance companies about who can look at and receive our health information. This law, called the Health Insurance Portability and Accountability Act of 1996 (HIPAA), gives you rights over your health information, including the right to get a

This chapter contains text excerpted from the following sources: Text in this chapter begins with excerpts from "Privacy, Security, and Electronic Health Records," U.S. Department of Health and Human Services (HHS), March 17, 2013. Reviewed December 2017; Text under the heading "Your Health Information Privacy Rights" is excerpted from "Your Health Information Privacy Rights," U.S. Department of Health and Human Services (HHS), February 6, 2012. Reviewed December 2017.

copy of your information, make sure it is correct, and know who has seen it.

EHRs and Your Health Information

EHRs are electronic versions of the paper charts in your doctor's or other healthcare provider's office. An EHR may include your medical history, notes, and other information about your health including your symptoms, diagnoses, medications, lab results, vital signs, immunizations, and reports from diagnostic tests such as X-rays. Providers are working with other doctors, hospitals, and health plans to find ways to share that information. The information in EHRs can be shared with other organizations involved in your care if the computer systems are set up to talk to each other. Information in these records should only be shared for purposes authorized by law or by you. You have privacy rights whether your information is stored as a paper record or stored in an electronic form. The same federal laws that already protect your health information also apply to information in EHRs.

Keeping Your Electronic Health Information Secure

Most of us feel that our health information is private and should be protected. The federal government put in place the Health Insurance Portability and Accountability Act of 1996 (HIPAA) Privacy Rule to ensure you have rights over your own health information, no matter what form it is in. The government also created the HIPAA Security Rule to require specific protections to safeguard your electronic health information. A few possible measures that can be built in to EHR systems may include:

- "Access control" tools like passwords and PIN numbers, to help limit access to your information to authorized individuals.

- "Encrypting" your stored information. That means your health information cannot be read or understood except by those using a system that can "decrypt" it with a "key."

- An "audit trail" feature, which records who accessed your information, what changes were made and when.

Finally, federal law requires doctors, hospitals, and other healthcare providers to notify you of a "breach." The law also requires the healthcare provider to notify the Secretary of Health and Human Services.

If a breach affects more than 500 residents of a state or jurisdiction, the healthcare provider must also notify prominent media outlets serving the state or jurisdiction. This requirement helps patients know if something has gone wrong with the protection of their information and helps keep providers accountable for EHR protection.

Your Health Information Privacy Rights

Most of us feel that our health information is private and should be protected. That is why there is a federal law that sets rules for healthcare providers and health insurance companies about who can look at and receive our health information. This law, called the Health Insurance Portability and Accountability Act of 1996 (HIPAA), gives you rights over your health information, including the right to get a copy of your information, make sure it is correct, and know who has seen it.

Get It

You can ask to see or get a copy of your medical record and other health information. If you want a copy, you may have to put your request in writing and pay for the cost of copying and mailing. In most cases, your copies must be given to you within 30 days.

Check It

You can ask to change any wrong information in your file or add information to your file if you think something is missing or incomplete. For example, if you and your hospital agree that your file has the wrong result for a test, the hospital must change it. Even if the hospital believes the test result is correct, you still have the right to have your disagreement noted in your file. In most cases, the file should be updated within 60 days.

Know Who Has Seen It

By law, your health information can be used and shared for specific reasons not directly related to your care, like making sure doctors give good care, making sure nursing homes are clean and safe, reporting when the flu is in your area, or reporting as required by state or federal law. In many of these cases, you can find out who has seen your health information. You can:

- **Learn how your health information is used and shared by your doctor or health insurer.** Generally, your health information cannot be used for purposes not directly related to your care without your permission. For example, your doctor cannot give it to your employer, or share it for things like marketing and advertising, without your written authorization. You probably received a notice telling you how your health information may be used on your first visit to a new healthcare provider or when you got new health insurance, but you can ask for another copy anytime.

- **Let your providers or health insurance companies know if there is information you do not want to share.** You can ask that your health information not be shared with certain people, groups, or companies. If you go to a clinic, for example, you can ask the doctor not to share your medical records with other doctors or nurses at the clinic. You can ask for other kinds of restrictions, but they do not always have to agree to do what you ask, particularly if it could affect your care. Finally, you can also ask your healthcare provider or pharmacy not to tell your health insurance company about care you receive or drugs you take, if you pay for the care or drugs in full and the provider or pharmacy does not need to get paid by your insurance company.

- **Ask to be reached somewhere other than home.** You can make reasonable requests to be contacted at different places or in a different way. For example, you can ask to have a nurse call you at your office instead of your home or to send mail to you in an envelope instead of on a postcard. If you think your rights are being denied or your health information is not being protected, you have the right to file a complaint with your provider, health insurer, or the U.S. Department of Health and Human Services (HHS).

Chapter 47

Cloning and Law

What Is Cloning?

The term cloning describes a number of different processes that can be used to produce genetically identical copies of a biological entity. The copied material, which has the same genetic makeup as the original, is referred to as a clone.

Researchers have cloned a wide range of biological materials, including genes, cells, tissues and even entire organisms, such as a sheep.

Do Clones Ever Occur Naturally?

Yes. In nature, some plants and single-celled organisms, such as bacteria, produce genetically identical offspring through a process called asexual reproduction. In asexual reproduction, a new individual is generated from a copy of a single cell from the parent organism.

Natural clones, also known as identical twins, occur in humans and other mammals. These twins are produced when a fertilized egg splits, creating two or more embryos that carry almost identical

---

This chapter contains text excerpted from the following sources: Text beginning with the heading "What Is Cloning?" is excerpted from "Cloning," National Human Genome Research Institute (NHGRI), March 21, 2017; Text under the heading "Human Cloning Prohibition Act of 2105" is excerpted from "H.R.3498 — Human Cloning Prohibition Act of 2105 [sic]," U.S. Library of Congress (LOC), October 5, 2015.

deoxyribonucleic acid (DNA). Identical twins have nearly the same genetic makeup as each other, but they are genetically different from either parent.

What Are the Types of Artificial Cloning?

There are three different types of artificial cloning: gene cloning, reproductive cloning, and therapeutic cloning.

Gene cloning produces copies of genes or segments of DNA (deoxyribonucleic acid). Reproductive cloning produces copies of whole animals. Therapeutic cloning produces embryonic stem cells for experiments aimed at creating tissues to replace injured or diseased tissues.

Gene cloning, also known as DNA cloning, is a very different process from reproductive and therapeutic cloning. Reproductive and therapeutic cloning share many of the same techniques, but are done for different purposes.

What Sort of Cloning Research Is Going on at NHGRI?

Gene cloning is the most common type of cloning done by researchers at the National Human Genome Research Institute (NHGRI). NHGRI researchers have not cloned any mammals and NHGRI does not clone humans.

How Are Genes Cloned?

Researchers routinely use cloning techniques to make copies of genes that they wish to study. The procedure consists of inserting a gene from one organism, often referred to as "foreign DNA," into the genetic material of a carrier called a vector. Examples of vectors include bacteria, yeast cells, viruses or plasmids, which are small DNA circles carried by bacteria. After the gene is inserted, the vector is placed in laboratory conditions that prompt it to multiply, resulting in the gene being copied many times over.

Have Humans Been Cloned?

Despite several highly publicized claims, human cloning still appears to be fiction. There currently is no solid scientific evidence that anyone has cloned human embryos.

In 1998, scientists in South Korea claimed to have successfully cloned a human embryo, but said the experiment was interrupted very early when the clone was just a group of four cells. In 2002, Clonaid, part of a religious group that believes humans were created by extraterrestrials, held a news conference to announce the birth of what it claimed to be the first cloned human, a girl named Eve. However, despite repeated requests by the research community and the news media, Clonaid never provided any evidence to confirm the existence of this clone or the other 12 human clones it purportedly created.

In 2004, a group led by Woo-Suk Hwang of Seoul National University in South Korea published a paper in the journal Science in which it claimed to have created a cloned human embryo in a test tube. However, an independent scientific committee later found no proof to support the claim and, in January 2006, Science announced that Hwang's paper had been retracted.

From a technical perspective, cloning humans and other primates is more difficult than in other mammals. One reason is that two proteins essential to cell division, known as spindle proteins, are located very close to the chromosomes in primate eggs. Consequently, removal of the egg's nucleus to make room for the donor nucleus also removes the spindle proteins, interfering with cell division. In other mammals, such as cats, rabbits, and mice, the two spindle proteins are spread throughout the egg. So, removal of the egg's nucleus does not result in loss of spindle proteins. In addition, some dyes and the ultraviolet light used to remove the egg's nucleus can damage the primate cell and prevent it from growing.

Human Cloning Prohibition Act of 2105 [sic]

This bill amends the federal criminal code to prohibit human cloning for reproductive and research purposes. Specifically, the bill makes it a crime for any public or private person or entity to:

- perform, attempt to perform, or participate in an attempt to perform human cloning; or

- ship, receive, or import a product of human cloning for any purpose.

It defines "human cloning" as asexual reproduction by replacing a fertilized or unfertilized egg nucleus with a human somatic (body) cell nucleus to produce a living organism with a human or predominantly human genetic constitution.

A person or entity convicted of a human cloning offense is subject to a fine, up to 10 years in prison, or both. A person or entity who profits from such offense is also subject to a civil penalty of at least $1,000,000.

This bill does not restrict scientific research using nuclear transfer or other cloning techniques to produce molecules, DNA, cells other than human embryos, tissues, organs, plants, or animals other than humans.

Part Eight

Future of Health Technology

Chapter 48

Artificial Brains

For every thought or behavior, the brain erupts in a riot of activity, as thousands of cells communicate via electrical and chemical signals. Each nerve cell influences others within an intricate, interconnected neural network. And connections between brain cells change over time in response to our environment.

Despite supercomputer advances, the human brain remains the most flexible, efficient information processing device in the world. Its exceptional performance inspires researchers to study and imitate it as an ideal of computing power.

Artificial Neural Networks

Computer models built to replicate how the brain processes, memorizes, and/or retrieves information are called artificial neural networks. For decades, engineers and computer scientists have used artificial neural networks as an effective tool in many real-world problems involving tasks such as classification, estimation, and control.

However, artificial neural networks do not take into consideration some of the basic characteristics of the human brain such as signal transmission delays between neurons, membrane potentials, and synaptic currents.

A new generation of neural network models—called spiking neural networks—are designed to better model the dynamics of the brain,

This chapter includes text excerpted from "Artificial Brains Learn to Adapt," National Science Foundation (NSF), May 15, 2014. Reviewed December 2017.

where neurons initiate signals to other neurons in their networks with a rapid spike in cell voltage. In modeling biological neurons, spiking neural networks may have the potential to mimick brain activities in simulations, enabling researchers to investigate neural networks in a biological context.

With funding from the National Science Foundation (NSF), Silvia Ferrari of the Laboratory for Intelligent Systems and Controls at Duke University uses a new variation of spiking neural networks to better replicate the behavioral learning processes of mammalian brains.

Behavioral learning involves the use of sensory feedback, such as vision, touch, and sound, to improve motor performance and enable people to respond and quickly adapt to their changing environment.

"Although existing engineering systems are very effective at controlling dynamics, they are not yet capable of handling unpredicted damages and failures handled by biological brains," Ferrari said.

How to Teach an Artificial Brain

Ferrari's team is applying the spiking neural network model of learning on the fly to complex, critical engineering systems, such as aircraft and power plants, with the goal of making them safer, more cost-efficient and easier to operate.

The team has constructed an algorithm that teaches spiking neural networks which information is relevant and how important each factor is to the overall goal. Using computer simulations, they've demonstrated the algorithm on aircraft flight control and robot navigation.

They started, however, with an insect.

"Our method has been tested by training a virtual insect to navigate in an unknown terrain and find foods," said Xu Zhang, a Ph.D. candidate who works on training the spiking neural network. "The nervous system was modeled by a large spiking neural network with unknown and random synaptic connections among those neurons."

Having tested their algorithm in computer simulations, they now are in the process of testing it biologically.

To do so, they will use lab-grown brain cells genetically altered to respond to certain types of light. This technique, called optogenetics, allows researchers to control how nerve cells communicate. When the light pattern changes, the neural activity changes.

The researchers hope to observe that the living neural network adapts over time to the light patterns and therefore have the ability to store and retrieve sensory information, just as human neuronal networks do.

Large-Scale Applications of Small-Scale Findings

Uncovering the fundamental mechanisms responsible for the brain's learning processes can potentially yield insights into how humans learn—and make an everyday difference in people's lives.

Such insights may advance the development of certain artificial devices that can substitute for certain motor, sensory, or cognitive abilities, particularly prosthetics that respond to feedback from the user and the environment. People with Parkinson disease and epilepsy have already benefited from these types of devices.

"One of the most significant challenges in reverse-engineering the brain is to close the knowledge gap that exists between our understanding of biophysical models of neuron-level activity and the synaptic plasticity mechanisms that drive meaningful learning," said Greg Foderaro, a postdoctoral fellow involved the research.

"We believe that by considering the networks at several levels—from computation to cell cultures to brains—we can greatly expand our understanding of the system of sensory and motor functions, as well as making a large step towards understanding the brain as a whole."

Chapter 49

Computational Modeling

What Is Computational Modeling?

Computational modeling is the use of computers to simulate and study the behavior of complex systems using mathematics, physics, and computer science. A computational model contains numerous variables that characterize the system being studied. Simulation is done by adjusting each of these variables alone or in combination and observing how the changes affect the outcomes. The results of model simulations help researchers make predictions about what will happen in the real system that is being studied in response to changing conditions. Modeling can expedite research by allowing scientists to conduct thousands of simulated experiments by computer in order to identify the actual physical experiments that are most likely to help the researcher find the solution to the problem being studied.

A key feature of today's computational models is that they are able to study a biological system at multiple levels, including molecular processes, cell-to-cell interactions, and how those interactions result in changes at the tissue and organ level. The ability to study a system at these multiple levels is known as multiscale modeling.

This chapter includes text excerpted from "Science Education—Computational Modeling," National Institute of Biomedical Imaging and Bioengineering (NIBIB), September 2016.

How Can Computational Modeling Accelerate Discovery?

To gain a better understanding of how computer modeling works, let's think about baking a cake that has 20 ingredients. If you want to know how each ingredient contributes to the outcome of the cake, one option would be to bake 20 cakes and leave out a different ingredient each time. Such an approach would be extremely time-consuming. Alternatively, you could enter all 20 ingredients into a computer model, explaining to the computer what each ingredient does and how it interacts with other ingredients. You could then run a simulation in which a different ingredient is left out each time. In a matter of seconds, the computer could tell you how each of the 20 cakes would likely turn out if baked in real life.

Let's say you now want to know how changing the amount of each ingredient will affect the cake. In your computer model, you could adjust the amounts of each of the 20 ingredients any number of times until the outcome of your simulation is a cake that suits your needs (e.g., fluffy, sticky, soft, hard, etc.). In real-life, you would need to bake 190 cakes to find out the results of changing any 2 ingredients; 1,140 cakes to find the results of changing any 3 ingredients; and 4,845 cakes to find the results of changing any 4 ingredients. The power of computational modeling is that it allows scientists and engineers to simulate variations more efficiently by computer, saving time, money, and materials.

What Are Some Examples of Computational Modeling and How It Can Be Used to Study Complex Systems?

Computational modeling is used to study a wide range of complex systems. Some examples include:

- **Forecasting the weather.** Weather forecasting uses computer models that analyze and make predictions based on numerous atmospheric factors. This is important for many reasons including protecting life, property, and crops, and helping utility companies plan for increases in power demand, especially when extreme climate shifts are expected.

- **Building better airplanes.** Flight simulators recreate aircraft flight using the complex equations that govern how aircraft fly and the reaction of the aircraft to external environmental factors such as turbulence, air density, and precipitation. In addition to being used to train pilots, flight simulators are used for the design of aircraft and research into how aircraft might be affected by different conditions.

- **Studying earthquakes.** Computational modeling is used in the study of earthquakes, with the goal of saving lives, buildings, and other types of infrastructure. Computer simulations model how the construction, composition, and motion of structures, and the surfaces on which they are built, interact to affect what happens during an earthquake.

How Can Computational Modeling Improve Medical Care and/or Biomedical Research?

- Researchers are developing models of the mechanics of blood vessels, blood flow, and heart valves. These models can then be used in a number of ways, including optimizing the design of implanted devices such as artificial heart valves and coronary artery stents. Computational models also aid in the creation of decision tools for doctors that can provide guidance for the treatment of cardiovascular disease, based on detailed analysis of specific characteristics of each patient.

- Computer models of the human cornea can help simulate laser eye surgery and refine the technique. They are also used for virtual training of physicians in how to perform the procedure.

- Researchers use computational modeling to help design drugs, early in the development process, that will be the safest for patients. Identifying which drugs are the least likely to have adverse side effects also has the potential to reduce the many years needed to bring a promising candidate drug from the experimental stage to winning approval as a safe and effective medication.

What Are NIBIB-Funded Researchers Developing in the Area of Computational Modeling?

- **Improving healing of chronic wounds.** Chronic skin wounds, especially in people suffering from conditions such as diabetes and obesity, are a significant health and economic problem in the United States and worldwide. Healing requires recruitment of new skin fibroblasts into the wound region, which is directed by a protein called platelet-derived growth factor (PDGF). Although much is known about the signals that activate PDGF, little is known about how different concentrations of PDGF are distributed throughout the wound site and how this orchestrates the movement of fibroblasts into the wound to promote healing. National Institute of Biomedical Imaging and Bioengineering (NIBIB)-funded scientists are developing a computer model that incorporates a wealth of experimental data about the signals that activate PDGF. The model will be used to understand and predict the key triggers of the healing process at multiple levels, including self-assembly of contractile proteins, cell migration, and cell to cell interactions to form new tissue. The model will be used to identify, test, and refine wound-healing approaches for patients with persistent chronic wounds.

- **Reducing osteoarthritis following knee surgery.** Anterior cruciate ligament (ACL) tears are a common knee injury. ACL reconstructive surgeries are often successful at improving joint stability, but patients have a high risk for developing early onset osteoarthritis (OA). Researchers are working to understand why OA develops in these patients, and the best treatment strategy to lower the risk. They are creating a new multi-scale computational model to examine the mechanics of walking in terms of muscle, bone, and soft tissues. The model will be used to test key surgical variables affecting cartilage stresses after ACL reconstruction that are believed to increase osteoarthritic changes to the joint, which include graft stiffness, and the angle of ACL attachment to the bones. The model will then examine the influence of surgical procedures on knee mechanics using MRI. The studies aim to identify clinical and surgical protocols that can best reduce the risk for early onset OA following ligament injury and surgical repair.

- **Multiscale modeling of microbial biofilms for improved treatment of antibiotic resistant infections.** The majority of naturally occurring bacteria grow as biofilms—large numbers of bacteria that self-organize into three-dimensional structures— which often renders them resistant to antibiotic treatments. Although they represent the vast majority of microbial life on the planet, the basic structural and biochemical characteristics of biofilms are still poorly understood. Scientists are combining computational and experimental tools to address the challenge of characterizing, predicting, and treating these complex systems. The goal is to develop an experimentally driven computer model that generates accurate predictions of biofilm behavior. The predictions will be used to develop novel ways for treating resistant biofilms found on the surfaces of implanted medical devices, such as urinary and venous catheters, breast implants, and pacemakers.

Computer Modeling to Design Opioid Alternatives

Researchers funded by National Institute on Drug Abuse (NIDA) founded a new compound called PZM21 that could serve as an alternative to regular opioids. The molecule, identified after evaluating more than 1 million structural configurations using computer modeling, offers pain relief with longer effects and displays fewer addictive characteristics and side effects compared to a regular opioid such as morphine.

(Source: "Designing More Effective Opioids," National Institutes of Health (NIH).)

Chapter 50

Stem Cell Research

What Are Stem Cells, and Why Are They Important?

Stem cells have the remarkable potential to develop into many different cell types in the body during early life and growth. In addition, in many tissues they serve as a sort of internal repair system, dividing essentially without limit to replenish other cells as long as the person or animal is still alive. When a stem cell divides, each new cell has the potential either to remain a stem cell or become another type of cell with a more specialized function, such as a muscle cell, a red blood cell, or a brain cell.

Stem cells are distinguished from other cell types by two important characteristics. First, they are unspecialized cells capable of renewing themselves through cell division, sometimes after long periods of inactivity. Second, under certain physiologic or experimental conditions, they can be induced to become tissue- or organ-specific cells with special functions. In some organs, such as the gut and bone marrow, stem cells regularly divide to repair and replace worn out or damaged tissues. In other organs, however, such as the pancreas and the heart, stem cells only divide under special conditions.

This chapter contains text excerpted from the following sources: Text beginning with the heading "What Are Stem Cells, and Why Are They Important?" is excerpted from "Stem Cell Basics VII," National Institutes of Health (NIH), October 17, 2017; Text under the heading "Fixing Flawed Body Parts" is excerpted from "Fixing Flawed Body Parts," *NIH News in Health*, National Institutes of Health (NIH), February 2015.

447

Until recently, scientists primarily worked with two kinds of stem cells from animals and humans: embryonic stem cells and nonembryonic "somatic" or "adult" stem cells. The functions and characteristics of these cells will be explained in this document. Scientists discovered ways to derive embryonic stem cells from early mouse embryos more than 30 years ago, in 1981. The detailed study of the biology of mouse stem cells led to the discovery, in 1998, of a method to derive stem cells from human embryos and grow the cells in the laboratory. These cells are called human embryonic stem cells. The embryos used in these studies were created for reproductive purposes through *in vitro* fertilization procedures. When they were no longer needed for that purpose, they were donated for research with the informed consent of the donor. In 2006, researchers made another breakthrough by identifying conditions that would allow some specialized adult cells to be "reprogrammed" genetically to assume a stem cell-like state. This new type of stem cell, called induced pluripotent stem cells (iPSCs), will be discussed in a later section of this document.

Stem cells are important for living organisms for many reasons. In the 3- to 5-day-old embryo, called a blastocyst, the inner cells give rise to the entire body of the organism, including all of the many specialized cell types and organs such as the heart, lungs, skin, sperm, eggs, and other tissues. In some adult tissues, such as bone marrow, muscle, and brain, discrete populations of adult stem cells generate replacements for cells that are lost through normal wear and tear, injury, or disease.

Given their unique regenerative abilities, stem cells offer new potentials for treating diseases such as diabetes, and heart disease. However, much work remains to be done in the laboratory and the clinic to understand how to use these cells for cell-based therapies to treat disease, which is also referred to as regenerative or reparative medicine.

Laboratory studies of stem cells enable scientists to learn about the cells' essential properties and what makes them different from specialized cell types. Scientists are already using stem cells in the laboratory to screen new drugs and to develop model systems to study normal growth and identify the causes of birth defects.

Research on stem cells continues to advance knowledge about how an organism develops from a single cell and how healthy cells replace damaged cells in adult organisms. Stem cell research is one of the most fascinating areas of contemporary biology, but, as with many expanding fields of scientific inquiry, research on stem cells raises scientific questions as rapidly as it generates new discoveries.

What Are the Unique Properties of All Stem Cells?

Stem cells differ from other kinds of cells in the body. All stem cells—regardless of their source—have three general properties:

- they are capable of dividing and renewing themselves for long periods;

- they are unspecialized; and

- they can give rise to specialized cell types.

Stem cells are capable of dividing and renewing themselves for long periods. Unlike muscle cells, blood cells, or nerve cells—which do not normally replicate themselves—stem cells may replicate many times, or proliferate. A starting population of stem cells that proliferates for many months in the laboratory can yield millions of cells. If the resulting cells continue to be unspecialized, like the parent stem cells, the cells are said to be capable of long term self-renewal.

Scientists are trying to understand two fundamental properties of stem cells that relate to their long-term self-renewal:

1. Why can embryonic stem cells proliferate for a year or more in the laboratory without differentiating, but most adult stem cells cannot; and

2. What are the factors in living organisms that normally regulate stem cell proliferation and self-renewal?

Discovering the answers to these questions may make it possible to understand how cell proliferation is regulated during normal embryonic development or during the abnormal cell division that leads to cancer. Such information would also enable scientists to grow embryonic and nonembryonic stem cells more efficiently in the laboratory.

The specific factors and conditions that allow stem cells to remain unspecialized are of great interest to scientists. It has taken scientists many years of trial and error to learn to derive and maintain stem cells in the laboratory without them spontaneously differentiating into specific cell types. For example, it took two decades to learn how to grow human embryonic stem cells in the laboratory following the development of conditions for growing mouse stem cells. Likewise, scientists must first understand the signals that enable a nonembryonic (adult) stem cell population to proliferate and remain unspecialized before they will be able to grow large numbers of unspecialized adult stem cells in the laboratory.

Stem cells are unspecialized. One of the fundamental properties of a stem cell is that it does not have any tissue-specific structures that allow it to perform specialized functions. For example, a stem cell cannot work with its neighbors to pump blood through the body (like a heart muscle cell), and it cannot carry oxygen molecules through the bloodstream (like a red blood cell). However, unspecialized stem cells can give rise to specialized cells, including heart muscle cells, blood cells, or nerve cells.

Stem cells can give rise to specialized cells. When unspecialized stem cells give rise to specialized cells, the process is called differentiation. While differentiating, the cell usually goes through several stages, becoming more specialized at each step. Scientists are just beginning to understand the signals inside and outside cells that trigger each step of the differentiation process. The internal signals are controlled by a cell's genes, which are interspersed across long strands of deoxyribonucleic acid (DNA) and carry coded instructions for all cellular structures and functions. The external signals for cell differentiation include chemicals secreted by other cells, physical contact with neighboring cells, and certain molecules in the microenvironment. The interaction of signals during differentiation causes the cell's DNA to acquire epigenetic marks that restrict DNA expression in the cell and can be passed on through cell division.

Many questions about stem cell differentiation remain. For example, are the internal and external signals for cell differentiation similar for all kinds of stem cells? Can specific sets of signals be identified that promote differentiation into specific cell types? Addressing these questions may lead scientists to find new ways to control stem cell differentiation in the laboratory, thereby growing cells or tissues that can be used for specific purposes such as cell-based therapies or drug screening.

Adult stem cells typically generate the cell types of the tissue in which they reside. For example, a blood-forming adult stem cell in the bone marrow normally gives rise to the many types of blood cells. It is generally accepted that a blood-forming cell in the bone marrow—which is called a hematopoietic stem cell—cannot give rise to the cells of a very different tissue, such as nerve cells in the brain. Experiments over the last several years have purported to show that stem cells from one tissue may give rise to cell types of a completely different tissue. This remains an area of great debate within the research community. This controversy demonstrates the challenges of studying adult stem cells and suggests that additional research using adult stem cells is necessary to understand their full potential as future therapies.

What Are Embryonic Stem Cells?

What Stages of Early Embryonic Development Are Important for Generating Embryonic Stem Cells?

Embryonic stem cells, as their name suggests, are derived from embryos. Most embryonic stem cells are derived from embryos that develop from eggs that have been fertilized *in vitro*—in an *in vitro* fertilization clinic—and then donated for research purposes with informed consent of the donors. They are not derived from eggs fertilized in a woman's body.

How Are Embryonic Stem Cells Grown in the Laboratory?

Growing cells in the laboratory is known as cell culture. Human embryonic stem cells (hESCs) are generated by transferring cells from a preimplantation-stage embryo into a plastic laboratory culture dish that contains a nutrient broth known as culture medium. The cells divide and spread over the surface of the dish. In the original protocol, the inner surface of the culture dish was coated with mouse embryonic skin cells specially treated so they will not divide. This coating layer of cells is called a feeder layer. The mouse cells in the bottom of the culture dish provide the cells a sticky surface to which they can attach. Also, the feeder cells release nutrients into the culture medium. Researchers have now devised ways to grow embryonic stem cells without mouse feeder cells. This is a significant scientific advance because of the risk that viruses or other macromolecules in the mouse cells may be transmitted to the human cells.

The process of generating an embryonic stem cell line is somewhat inefficient, so lines are not produced each time cells from the preimplantation-stage embryo are placed into a culture dish. However, if the plated cells survive, divide, and multiply enough to crowd the dish, they are removed gently and plated into several fresh culture dishes. The process of replating or subculturing the cells is repeated many times and for many months. Each cycle of subculturing the cells is referred to as a passage. Once the cell line is established, the original cells yield millions of embryonic stem cells. Embryonic stem cells that have proliferated in cell culture for six or more months without differentiating, are pluripotent, and appear genetically normal are referred to as an embryonic stem cell line. At any stage in the process, batches of cells can be frozen and shipped to other laboratories for further culture and experimentation.

451

What Laboratory Tests Are Used to Identify Embryonic Stem Cells?

At various points during the process of generating embryonic stem cell lines, scientists test the cells to see whether they exhibit the fundamental properties that make them embryonic stem cells. This process is called characterization.

Scientists who study human embryonic stem cells have not yet agreed on a standard battery of tests that measure the cells' fundamental properties. However, laboratories that grow human embryonic stem cell lines use several kinds of tests, including:

- Growing and subculturing the stem cells for many months. This ensures that the cells are capable of long-term growth and self-renewal. Scientists inspect the cultures through a microscope to see that the cells look healthy and remain undifferentiated.

- Using specific techniques to determine the presence of transcription factors that are typically produced by undifferentiated cells. Two of the most important transcription factors are Nanog and Oct4. Transcription factors help turn genes on and off at the right time, which is an important part of the processes of cell differentiation and embryonic development. In this case, both Oct4 and Nanog are associated with maintaining the stem cells in an undifferentiated state, capable of self-renewal.

- Using specific techniques to determine the presence of particular cell surface markers that are typically produced by undifferentiated cells.

- Examining the chromosomes under a microscope. This is a method to assess whether the chromosomes are damaged or if the number of chromosomes has changed. It does not detect genetic mutations in the cells.

- Determining whether the cells can be regrown, or subcultured, after freezing, thawing, and replating.

- Testing whether the human embryonic stem cells are pluripotent by:

  1. allowing the cells to differentiate spontaneously in cell culture;

  2. manipulating the cells so they will differentiate to form cells characteristic of the three germ layers; or

3. injecting the cells into a mouse with a suppressed immune system to test for the formation of a benign tumor called a teratoma.

Since the mouse's immune system is suppressed, the injected human stem cells are not rejected by the mouse immune system and scientists can observe growth and differentiation of the human stem cells. Teratomas typically contain a mixture of many differentiated or partly differentiated cell types—an indication that the embryonic stem cells are capable of differentiating into multiple cell types.

How Are Embryonic Stem Cells Stimulated to Differentiate?

As long as the embryonic stem cells in culture are grown under appropriate conditions, they can remain undifferentiated (unspecialized). But if cells are allowed to clump together to form embryoid bodies, they begin to differentiate spontaneously. They can form muscle cells, nerve cells, and many other cell types. Although spontaneous differentiation is a good indication that a culture of embryonic stem cells is healthy, the process is uncontrolled and therefore an inefficient strategy to produce cultures of specific cell types.

So, to generate cultures of specific types of differentiated cells— heart muscle cells, blood cells, or nerve cells, for example—scientists try to control the differentiation of embryonic stem cells. They change the chemical composition of the culture medium, alter the surface of the culture dish, or modify the cells by inserting specific genes. Through years of experimentation, scientists have established some basic protocols or "recipes" for the directed differentiation of embryonic stem cells into some specific cell types.

If scientists can reliably direct the differentiation of embryonic stem cells into specific cell types, they may be able to use the resulting, differentiated cells to treat certain diseases in the future. Diseases that might be treated by transplanting cells generated from human embryonic stem cells include diabetes, traumatic spinal cord injury, Duchenne's muscular dystrophy, heart disease, and vision and hearing loss.

What Are Adult Stem Cells?

An adult stem cell is thought to be an undifferentiated cell, found among differentiated cells in a tissue or organ. The adult stem cell can renew itself and can differentiate to yield some or all of the major specialized cell types of the tissue or organ. The primary roles of adult stem cells in a living organism are to maintain and repair the tissue in which they are found. Scientists also use the term somatic stem cell instead of adult stem cell, where somatic refers to cells of the body (not the germ cells, sperm or eggs). Unlike embryonic stem cells, which are defined by their origin (cells from the preimplantation-stage embryo), the origin of adult stem cells in some mature tissues is still under investigation.

Research on adult stem cells has generated a great deal of excitement. Scientists have found adult stem cells in many more tissues than they once thought possible. This finding has led researchers and clinicians to ask whether adult stem cells could be used for transplants. In fact, adult hematopoietic, or blood-forming, stem cells from bone marrow have been used in transplants for more than 40 years. Scientists now have evidence that stem cells exist in the brain and the heart, two locations where adult stem cells were not at first expected to reside. If the differentiation of adult stem cells can be controlled in the laboratory, these cells may become the basis of transplantation-based therapies.

The history of research on adult stem cells began more than 60 years ago. In the 1950s, researchers discovered that the bone marrow contains at least two kinds of stem cells. One population, called hematopoietic stem cells, forms all the types of blood cells in the body. A second population, called bone marrow stromal stem cells (also called mesenchymal stem cells, or skeletal stem cells by some), were discovered a few years later. These nonhematopoietic stem cells make up a small proportion of the stromal cell population in the bone marrow and can generate bone, cartilage, and fat cells that support the formation of blood and fibrous connective tissue.

In the 1960s, scientists who were studying rats discovered two regions of the brain that contained dividing cells that ultimately become nerve cells. Despite these reports, most scientists believed that the adult brain could not generate new nerve cells. It was not until the 1990s that scientists agreed that the adult brain does contain stem cells that are able to generate the brain's three major cell types—astrocytes and oligodendrocytes, which are non-neuronal cells, and neurons, or nerve cells.

Where Are Adult Stem Cells Found, and What Do They Normally Do?

Adult stem cells have been identified in many organs and tissues, including brain, bone marrow, peripheral blood, blood vessels, skeletal muscle, skin, teeth, heart, gut, liver, ovarian epithelium, and testis.

They are thought to reside in a specific area of each tissue (called a "stem cell niche"). In many tissues, current evidence suggests that some types of stem cells are pericytes, cells that compose the outermost layer of small blood vessels. Stem cells may remain quiescent (nondividing) for long periods of time until they are activated by a normal need for more cells to maintain tissues, or by disease or tissue injury.

Typically, there is a very small number of stem cells in each tissue and, once removed from the body, their capacity to divide is limited, making generation of large quantities of stem cells difficult. Scientists in many laboratories are trying to find better ways to grow large quantities of adult stem cells in cell culture and to manipulate them to generate specific cell types so they can be used to treat injury or disease. Some examples of potential treatments include regenerating bone using cells derived from bone marrow stroma, developing insulin-producing cells for type 1 diabetes, and repairing damaged heart muscle following a heart attack with cardiac muscle cells.

What Tests Are Used to Identify Adult Stem Cells?

Scientists often use one or more of the following methods to identify adult stem cells:

1. Label the cells in a living tissue with molecular markers and then determine the specialized cell types they generate;

2. Remove the cells from a living animal, label them in cell culture, and transplant them back into another animal to determine whether the cells replace (or "repopulate") their tissue of origin.

Importantly, scientists must demonstrate that a single adult stem cell can generate a line of genetically identical cells that then gives rise to all the appropriate differentiated cell types of the tissue. To confirm experimentally that a putative adult stem cell is indeed a stem cell, scientists tend to show either that the cell can give rise to these genetically identical cells in culture, and/or that a purified population of these candidate stem cells can repopulate or reform the tissue after transplant into an animal.

What Is Known about Adult Stem Cell Differentiation?

As indicated above, scientists have reported that adult stem cells occur in many tissues and that they enter normal differentiation pathways to form the specialized cell types of the tissue in which they reside.

Normal differentiation pathways of adult stem cells. In a living animal, adult stem cells are available to divide for a long period, when needed, and can give rise to mature cell types that have characteristic shapes and specialized structures and functions of a particular tissue. The following are examples of differentiation pathways of adult stem cells that have been demonstrated *in vitro* or *in vivo*.

- Hematopoietic stem cells give rise to all the types of blood cells: red blood cells, B lymphocytes, T lymphocytes, natural killer cells, neutrophils, basophils, eosinophils, monocytes, and macrophages.

- Mesenchymal stem cells have been reported to be present in many tissues. Those from bone marrow (bone marrow stromal stem cells, skeletal stem cells) give rise to a variety of cell types: bone cells (osteoblasts and osteocytes), cartilage cells (chondrocytes), fat cells (adipocytes), and stromal cells that support blood formation. However, it is not yet clear how similar or dissimilar mesenchymal cells derived from nonbone marrow sources are to those from bone marrow stroma.

- Neural stem cells in the brain give rise to its three major cell types: nerve cells (neurons) and two categories of non-neuronal cells—astrocytes and oligodendrocytes.

- Epithelial stem cells in the lining of the digestive tract occur in deep crypts and give rise to several cell types: absorptive cells, goblet cells, Paneth cells, and enteroendocrine cells.

- Skin stem cells occur in the basal layer of the epidermis and at the base of hair follicles. The epidermal stem cells give rise to keratinocytes, which migrate to the surface of the skin and form a protective layer. The follicular stem cells can give rise to both the hair follicle and to the epidermis.

Transdifferentiation. A number of experiments have reported that certain adult stem cell types can differentiate into cell types seen in organs or tissues other than those expected from the cells' predicted lineage (i.e., brain stem cells that differentiate into blood cells or blood-forming cells that differentiate into cardiac muscle cells, and so forth). This reported phenomenon is called transdifferentiation.

Although isolated instances of transdifferentiation have been observed in some vertebrate species, whether this phenomenon actually occurs in humans is under debate by the scientific community. Instead of transdifferentiation, the observed instances may involve fusion of a donor cell with a recipient cell. Another possibility is that transplanted stem cells are secreting factors that encourage the recipient's own stem cells to begin the repair process. Even when transdifferentiation has been detected, only a very small percentage of cells undergo the process.

In a variation of transdifferentiation experiments, scientists have recently demonstrated that certain adult cell types can be "reprogrammed" into other cell types *in vivo* using a well-controlled process of genetic modification. This strategy may offer a way to reprogram available cells into other cell types that have been lost or damaged due to disease. For example, one recent experiment shows how pancreatic beta cells, the insulin-producing cells that are lost or damaged in diabetes, could possibly be created by reprogramming other pancreatic cells. By "restarting" expression of three critical beta cell genes in differentiated adult pancreatic exocrine cells, researchers were able to create beta cell-like cells that can secrete insulin. The reprogrammed cells were similar to beta cells in appearance, size, and shape; expressed genes characteristic of beta cells; and were able to partially restore blood sugar regulation in mice whose own beta cells had been chemically destroyed. While not transdifferentiation by definition, this method for reprogramming adult cells may be used as a model for directly reprogramming other adult cell types.

In addition to reprogramming cells to become a specific cell type, it is now possible to reprogram adult somatic cells to become like embryonic stem cells (induced pluripotent stem cells, iPSCs) through the introduction of embryonic genes. Thus, a source of cells can be generated that are specific to the donor, thereby increasing the chance of compatibility if such cells were to be used for tissue regeneration. However, like embryonic stem cells, determination of the methods by which iPSCs can be completely and reproducibly committed to appropriate cell lineages is still under investigation.

What Are the Key Questions about Adult Stem Cells?

Many important questions about adult stem cells remain to be answered. They include:

- How many kinds of adult stem cells exist, and in which tissues do they exist?

- How do adult stem cells evolve during development and how are they maintained in the adult? Are they "leftover" embryonic stem cells, or do they arise in some other way?

- Why do stem cells remain in an undifferentiated state when all the cells around them have differentiated? What are the characteristics of their "niche" that controls their behavior?

- Do adult stem cells have the capacity to transdifferentiate, and is it possible to control this process to improve its reliability and efficiency?

- If the beneficial effect of adult stem cell transplantation is a trophic effect, what are the mechanisms? Is donor cell-recipient cell contact required, secretion of factors by the donor cell, or both?

- What are the factors that control adult stem cell proliferation and differentiation?

- What are the factors that stimulate stem cells to relocate to sites of injury or damage, and how can this process be enhanced for better healing?

What Are the Similarities and Differences between Embryonic and Adult Stem Cells?

Human embryonic and adult stem cells each have advantages and disadvantages regarding potential use for cell-based regenerative therapies. One major difference between adult and embryonic stem cells is their different abilities in the number and type of differentiated cell types they can become. Embryonic stem cells can become all cell types of the body because they are pluripotent. Adult stem cells are thought to be limited to differentiating into different cell types of their tissue of origin.

Embryonic stem cells can be grown relatively easily in culture. Adult stem cells are rare in mature tissues, so isolating these cells from an adult tissue is challenging, and methods to expand their numbers in cell culture have not yet been worked out. This is an important distinction, as large numbers of cells are needed for stem cell replacement therapies.

Scientists believe that tissues derived from embryonic and adult stem cells may differ in the likelihood of being rejected after transplantation. It's not yet known for certain whether tissues derived from embryonic stem cells would cause transplant rejection, since relatively few clinical trials have tested the safety of transplanted cells derived from hESCS.

Adult stem cells, and tissues derived from them, are currently believed less likely to initiate rejection after transplantation. This is because a patient's own cells could be expanded in culture, coaxed into assuming a specific cell type (differentiation), and then reintroduced into the patient. The use of adult stem cells and tissues derived from the patient's own adult stem cells would mean that the cells are less likely to be rejected by the immune system. This represents a significant advantage, as immune rejection can be circumvented only by continuous administration of immunosuppressive drugs, and the drugs themselves may cause deleterious side effects.

What Are Induced Pluripotent Stem Cells?

Induced pluripotent stem cells (iPSCs) are adult cells that have been genetically reprogrammed to an embryonic stem cell-like state by being forced to express genes and factors important for maintaining the defining properties of embryonic stem cells. Although these cells meet the defining criteria for pluripotent stem cells, it is not known if iPSCs and embryonic stem cells differ in clinically significant ways. Mouse iPSCs were first reported in 2006, and human iPSCs were first reported in late 2007. Mouse iPSCs demonstrate important characteristics of pluripotent stem cells, including expressing stem cell markers, forming tumors containing cells from all three germ layers, and being able to contribute to many different tissues when injected into mouse embryos at a very early stage in development. Human iPSCs also express stem cell markers and are capable of generating cells characteristic of all three germ layers.

Although additional research is needed, iPSCs are already useful tools for drug development and modeling of diseases, and scientists hope to use them in transplantation medicine. Viruses are currently used to introduce the reprogramming factors into adult cells, and this process must be carefully controlled and tested before the technique can lead to useful treatment for humans. In animal studies, the virus used to introduce the stem cell factors sometimes causes cancers. Researchers are currently investigating nonviral delivery strategies. In any case, this breakthrough discovery has created a powerful new way to "de-differentiate" cells whose developmental fates had been previously assumed to be determined. In addition, tissues derived from iPSCs will be a nearly identical match to the cell donor and thus probably avoid rejection by the immune system. The iPSC strategy creates pluripotent stem cells that, together with studies of other types of pluripotent stem cells, will help researchers learn how to reprogram cells to repair damaged tissues in the human body.

What Are the Potential Uses of Human Stem Cells and the Obstacles That Must Be Overcome before These Potential Uses Will Be Realized?

There are many ways in which human stem cells can be used in research and the clinic. Studies of human embryonic stem cells will yield information about the complex events that occur during human development. A primary goal of this work is to identify how undifferentiated stem cells become the differentiated cells that form the tissues and organs. Scientists know that turning genes on and off is central to this process. Some of the most serious medical conditions, such as cancer and birth defects, are due to abnormal cell division and differentiation. A more complete understanding of the genetic and molecular controls of these processes may yield information about how such diseases arise and suggest new strategies for therapy. Predictably controlling cell proliferation and differentiation requires additional basic research on the molecular and genetic signals that regulate cell division and specialization. While recent developments with iPS cells suggest some of the specific factors that may be involved, techniques must be devised to introduce these factors safely into the cells and control the processes that are induced by these factors.

Human stem cells are currently being used to test new drugs. New medications are tested for safety on differentiated cells generated from human pluripotent cell lines. Other kinds of cell lines have a long history of being used in this way. Cancer cell lines, for example, are used to screen potential antitumor drugs. The availability of pluripotent stem cells would allow drug testing in a wider range of cell types. However, to screen drugs effectively, the conditions must be identical when comparing different drugs. Therefore, scientists must be able to precisely control the differentiation of stem cells into the specific cell type on which drugs will be tested. For some cell types and tissues, current knowledge of the signals controlling differentiation falls short of being able to mimic these conditions precisely to generate pure populations of differentiated cells for each drug being tested.

Perhaps the most important potential application of human stem cells is the generation of cells and tissues that could be used for cell-based therapies. Today, donated organs and tissues are often used to replace ailing or destroyed tissue, but the need for transplantable tissues and organs far outweighs the available supply. Stem cells, directed to differentiate into specific cell types, offer the possibility of a renewable source of replacement cells and tissues to treat diseases including macular degeneration, spinal cord injury, stroke, burns, heart disease, diabetes, osteoarthritis, and rheumatoid arthritis.

For example, it may become possible to generate healthy heart muscle cells in the laboratory and then transplant those cells into patients with chronic heart disease. Preliminary research in mice and other animals indicates that bone marrow stromal cells, transplanted into a damaged heart, can have beneficial effects. Whether these cells can generate heart muscle cells or stimulate the growth of new blood vessels that repopulate the heart tissue, or help via some other mechanism is actively under investigation. For example, injected cells may accomplish repair by secreting growth factors, rather than actually incorporating into the heart. Promising results from animal studies have served as the basis for a small number of exploratory studies in humans. Other recent studies in cell culture systems indicate that it may be possible to direct the differentiation of embryonic stem cells or adult bone marrow cells into heart muscle cells.

In people who suffer from type 1 diabetes, the cells of the pancreas that normally produce insulin are destroyed by the patient's own immune system. New studies indicate that it may be possible to direct the differentiation of human embryonic stem cells in cell culture to form insulin-producing cells that eventually could be used in transplantation therapy for persons with diabetes.

To realize the promise of novel cell-based therapies for such pervasive and debilitating diseases, scientists must be able to manipulate stem cells so that they possess the necessary characteristics for successful differentiation, transplantation, and engraftment. The following is a list of steps in successful cell-based treatments that scientists will have to learn to control to bring such treatments to the clinic. To be useful for transplant purposes, stem cells must be reproducibly made to:

- Proliferate extensively and generate sufficient quantities of cells for making tissue.

- Differentiate into the desired cell type(s).

- Survive in the recipient after transplant.

- Integrate into the surrounding tissue after transplant.

461

- Function appropriately for the duration of the recipient's life.

- Avoid harming the recipient in any way.

Also, to avoid the problem of immune rejection, scientists are experimenting with different research strategies to generate tissues that will not be rejected.

To summarize, stem cells offer exciting promise for future therapies, but significant technical hurdles remain that will only be overcome through years of intensive research.

Stem Cells for the Future Treatment of Heart Disease

Cardiovascular disease (CVD), which includes hypertension, coronary heart disease, stroke, and congestive heart failure, has ranked as the number one cause of death in the United States every year since 1900 except 1918, when the nation struggled with an influenza epidemic. Nearly 2,600 Americans die of CVD each day, roughly one person every 34 seconds. Given the aging of the population and the relatively dramatic recent increases in the prevalence of cardiovascular risk factors such as obesity and type 2 diabetes, CVD will be a significant health concern well into the 21st century.

Cardiovascular disease can deprive heart tissue of oxygen, thereby killing cardiac muscle cells (cardiomyocytes). This loss triggers a cascade of detrimental events, including formation of scar tissue, an overload of blood flow and pressure capacity, the overstretching of viable cardiac cells attempting to sustain cardiac output, leading to heart failure, and eventual death. Restoring damaged heart muscle tissue, through repair or regeneration, is therefore a potentially new strategy to treat heart failure.

The use of embryonic and adult-derived stem cells for cardiac repair is an active area of research. A number of stem cell types, including embryonic stem (ES) cells, cardiac stem cells that naturally reside within the heart, myoblasts (muscle stem cells), adult bone marrow-derived cells including mesenchymal cells (bone marrow-derived cells that give rise to tissues such as muscle, bone, tendons, ligaments, and adipose tissue), endothelial progenitor cells (cells that give rise to the endothelium, the interior lining of blood vessels), and umbilical cord blood cells, have been investigated as possible sources for regenerating damaged heart tissue. All have been explored in mouse or rat models, and some have been tested in larger animal models, such as pigs.

A few small studies have also been carried out in humans, usually in patients who are undergoing open-heart surgery. Several of these have demonstrated that stem cells that are injected into the circulation or directly into the injured heart tissue appear to improve cardiac function and/or induce the formation of new capillaries. The mechanism for this repair remains controversial, and the stem cells likely regenerate heart tissue through several pathways. However, the stem cell populations that have been tested in these experiments vary widely, as do the conditions of their purification and application. Although much more research is needed to assess the safety and improve the efficacy of this approach, these preliminary clinical experiments show how stem cells may one day be used to repair damaged heart tissue, thereby reducing the burden of cardiovascular disease.

Fixing Flawed Body Parts

How can you mend a broken heart? Or repair a damaged liver, kidney, or knee? National Institutes of Health (NIH)-funded scientists are exploring innovative ways to fix faulty organs and tissues or even grow new ones. This type of research is called tissue engineering. Exciting advances continue to emerge in this fast-moving field.

Tissue engineering could allow doctors to repair or replace worn-out tissues and organs with living, working parts. Most important, tissue engineering might help some of the 120,000 people on the waitlist to receive donated kidneys, livers, or other organs.

Doctors have long used tissue-engineered skin to heal severe burns or other injuries. But most tissue engineering methods are still experimental. They've been tested only in laboratory dishes and sometimes in animals, but only a few new approaches have been tested in people. Several clinical studies (involving human volunteers) are in the early stages of testing newly developed tissues.

"With this approach, scientists are combining engineering and biology to restore a damaged organ or tissue, whether it's been damaged by disease or injury or something else," says Dr. Martha Lundberg, an NIH expert in heart-related tissue engineering.

Some scientists are creating special net-like structures, or scaffolds, in desired shapes and then coaxing cells to grow within them. Some use a mixture of natural substances called growth factors, which direct cells to grow and develop in certain ways.

"Other scientists are using different 3-D bioprinting technologies—some are like fancy inkjet printers—to create new tissues or organs," Lundberg says. They've printed 3-D kidneys and other organs that look like the real thing. But while most of these printed body parts have the right shape, they're not fully functional.

"Scientists haven't yet figured out how to print an organ that includes the correct blood vessel patterns, nerve connections, and other components that come together in a mature organ," Lundberg says. "When creating a new organ, if it can perform the right job and functions, it may not need to look like the real thing."

Many tissue engineering methods use stem cells, which can be nudged to turn into different cell types. One research team guided human stem cells to become a 3-D structure that can respond to light. The method might one day lead to new therapies for eye disorders. Other stem cell approaches may lead to improved treatment for spinal cord injuries, diabetes, and more.

Another approach, called decellularization, involves removing all the cells from an organ. What's left behind is a thin, pale framework that contains the organ's natural structural proteins, including the pathways for tiny blood vessels and nerves. By infusing new cells into this mesh-like matrix, some researchers have successfully created working animal kidneys, livers, hearts, lungs, and other organs.

The decellularization technique was used by Dr. Martin Yarmush and his colleagues to create a functional rat liver that included a network of working blood vessels. Yarmush is a biomedical engineer at Rutgers University and the Massachusetts General Hospital. The engineered livers his team created were kept alive in the laboratory for days and functioned for several hours after transplantation into rats. The researchers are now working to help those transplanted livers survive even longer. They're also scaling up the methods to create a decellularized human liver that can be repopulated with functional cells.

"A parallel effort we are pursuing involves taking a donated organ that is not considered transplantable for a particular reason, and then using a reconditioning solution and perhaps even stem cells to revitalize the organ so it becomes transplantable," Yarmush says.

Other researchers are working to repair damaged body parts that are still in the body. At the University of Washington in Seattle, Dr. Charles Murry and colleagues are searching for ways to fix injured hearts. One of their latest studies used human stem cells to repair damaged hearts in monkeys. The stem cells were coaxed to become early-stage heart cells, which were then infused near the heart injury.

The new cells made their way into the damaged heart muscle and organized into muscle fibers in all of the treated monkeys. The infused stem cells replaced nearly half of the damaged heart tissue and began beating in sync with the heart. Still, the scientists note they need years of research before this type of therapy might be tried in people.

Some methods are already being tested in humans. Dr. Martha Murray, a surgeon at Boston Children's Hospital, is exploring new ways to heal a common knee injury known as a torn ACL (anterior cruciate ligament). Athletes who do a lot of twisting and turning, as in basketball or soccer, are at risk for damaging the ACL.

"Typical treatment today, called ACL reconstruction, works well, and it gets patients back to the playing field at a relatively high rate," Murray says. But the surgery involves removing a piece of tendon from elsewhere in the body and using that to replace the ACL. "So it involves making two injuries that the body has to heal from. And even with this treatment, patients still develop arthritis in the knee 15 to 20 years later," Murray adds. "We wanted to find a better therapy— something less invasive."

After testing several biomaterials, Murray's team found that stitching a bioengineered sponge between the torn ends of an injured ACL allows blood to clot and collect around the damaged ligament. Because blood naturally contains stem cells and growth factors, the blood-soaked sponge acts as a "bridge" that encourages ACL healing. The sponge is made of some of the same proteins normally found in ligaments, and it dissolves after a few weeks.

Studies in large animals showed that the bioengineered sponge was much less likely to lead to arthritis, and it healed ACL injuries as well as standard reconstruction surgery. The U.S. Food and Drug Administration (FDA) recently approved human safety testing of the sponge in 10 people with ACL injuries.

Metal, plastic, and other nonbiological devices can also replace or enhance malfunctioning body parts. One promising possibility still in development is an artificial kidney that could be implanted in the body and used in place of dialysis to treat end-stage kidney disease. Scientists are also studying a synthetic glue modeled after a natural adhesive that might help to repair tissues in the body.

Chapter 51

Medical Applications of 3D Printing

3D printers are used to manufacture a variety of medical devices, including those with complex geometry or features that match a patient's unique anatomy.

Some devices are printed from a standard design to make multiple identical copies of the same device. Other devices, called patient-matched or patient-specific devices, are created from a specific patient's imaging data.

Commercially available 3D printed medical devices include:

- Instrumentation (e.g., guides to assist with proper surgical placement of a device),

- Implants (e.g., cranial plates or hip joints), and

- External prostheses (e.g., hands).

Scientists are researching how to use the 3D printing process to manufacture living organs such as a heart or liver, but this research is in the early stages of development.

The 3D printing process can be accomplished using any of several different technologies. The choice of technology can depend on many factors including how the final product will be used and how easy the

This chapter includes text excerpted from "Medical Applications of 3D Printing," U.S. Food and Drug Administration (FDA), December 21, 2016.

printer is to use. The most common technology used for 3D printing medical devices is called powder bed fusion. Powder bed fusion is commonly used because it works with a variety of materials used in medical devices, such as titanium and nylon.

The powder bed fusion process builds a three-dimensional product from very fine metal or plastic powder, which is poured onto a platform and leveled carefully. A laser or electron beam then moves across the powder layer and melts the material it touches. Melted material fuses to the layer below it and to the powder around it to create a solid. Once a layer is completed, the platform moves down and one more layer of carefully leveled powder is placed on top.

The FDA has several 3D printers that help us better understand the capabilities of 3D printing of medical devices and the public health benefit of this technology. For example, the FDA has printers that use different printing technologies, including powder bed fusion, to evaluate what parts of the printing processes and workflows are critical to ensure quality of the finished medical device.

Patient-Matched Devices

While 3D printers are often used to create identical copies of the same device, they can also be used to create devices unique to a specific patient. Patient-matched (or patient-specific) devices are created specifically for the patient based on individual features, such as anatomy. They can be based on a template model that is matched to a patient using medical imaging. Patient-matching can be accomplished by techniques such as scaling of the device using one or more anatomic features from patient data.

The FDA regulates 3D-printed medical devices through the same pathways as traditional medical devices; therefore, they are evaluated according to the safety and effectiveness information submitted to us by the manufacturer. While traditionally manufactured medical devices come in discrete sizes, patient-matched devices can be made in a continuous range of shapes with predefined minimum and maximum specifications that we can use to review the devices in the same way as standard sized devices. For instance, the specification may define a minimum and maximum wall thickness or how sharp a curve can be to maintain device performance for its intended use.

There is a provision in federal law that exempts "custom" medical devices from FDA review, but patient-matched devices do not automatically meet all the requirements.

Other Uses of 3D Printing

The use of 3D printing is not limited to medical devices. Other industries and government departments are also interested in its use. For instance, the U.S. Department of Energy (DOE) is investing resources to study 3D printing, and how it can be used to reduce waste by using fewer raw materials and require fewer manufacturing steps. DOE has compiled information on how 3D printing works, the different types of printers and for what they are used.

3-D Placenta to Mimic Microbial Resistance

Researchers have developed a cell culture model derived from placental trophoblasts that are used as models to study placenta. The cells were placed inside a rotating bioreactor 3-D system to mimic an actual placental environment unlike a 2-D culture. The cells were introduced to various viruses and parasites like Toxoplasma gondii, to which they were resistant. Researchers propose to use this model to further identify how pathogens cross the placental barrier to cause certain diseases.

(Source: "3-D Cell Placenta Model Mimics Development, Microbial Resistance," National Institutes of Health (NIH).)

Chapter 52

Microneedle Patch for Flu Vaccination

A National Institutes of Health (NIH)-funded study led by a team at the Georgia Institute of Technology and Emory University has shown that an influenza vaccine can produce robust immune responses and be administered safely with an experimental patch of dissolving microneedles. The method is an alternative to needle-and-syringe immunization; with further development, it could eliminate the discomfort of an injection, as well as the inconvenience and expense of visiting a flu clinic.

"This bandage-strip sized patch of painless and dissolvable needles can transform how we get vaccinated," said Roderic I. Pettigrew, Ph.D., M.D., director of the National Institute of Biomedical Imaging and Bioengineering (NIBIB), which funded the study. "A particularly attractive feature is that this vaccination patch could be delivered in the mail and self-administered. In addition, this technology holds promise for delivering other vaccines in the future."

The researchers received funding through an NIBIB Quantum Grant and from the National Institute of Allergy and Infectious Diseases.

The study, published online June 27, 2017, in *The Lancet*, was led by Nadine Rouphael, M.D., associate professor of medicine, and Mark

This chapter includes text excerpted from "Researchers Develop Microneedle Patch for Flu Vaccination," National Institute of Biomedical Imaging and Bioengineering (NIBIB), June 27, 2017.

J. Mulligan, M.D., distinguished professor of medicine, Emory University School of Medicine, in collaboration with Mark R. Prausnitz, Ph.D., Regents Professor and J. Erskine Love Chair in Chemical and Biomolecular Engineering, Georgia Institute of Technology. A team led by Prausnitz designed the dime-sized patch of microneedles used in the study.

The vaccine patch consists of 100 solid, water-soluble needles that are just long enough to penetrate the skin. "The skin is an immune surveillance organ," Prausnitz said. "It's our interface with the outside world, so it's very well equipped to detect a pathogen and mount an immune response against it."

Adhesive helps the patch grip the skin during the administration of the vaccine, which is encapsulated in the needles and is released as the needle tips dissolve, within minutes. The patch is peeled away and discarded like a used bandage strip.

The researchers enrolled 100 adult participants, dividing them into four random groups: vaccination with microneedle patch given by a healthcare provider; vaccination with microneedle patch self-administered by the study participant; vaccination with intramuscular injection given by a healthcare provider; and placebo microneedle patch given by a healthcare provider. The researchers used an inactivated influenza vaccine formulated for the 2014–15 flu season to inoculate participants other than those in the placebo group.

The researchers found that vaccination with the microneedle patches was safe, with no serious related adverse events reported. Some participants developed local skin reactions to the patches, described as faint redness and mild itching that lasted 2-3 days.

The results also showed that antibody responses generated by the vaccine, as measured through analysis of blood samples, were similar in the groups vaccinated using patches and those receiving intramuscular injection, and these immune responses were still present after six months. More than 70 percent of patch recipients reported they would prefer patch vaccination over injection or intranasal vaccination for future vaccinations.

No significant difference was seen between the doses of vaccine delivered by the healthcare workers and the volunteers who self-administered the patches, showing that participants were able to correctly self-administer the patch. After vaccination, imaging of the used patches found that the microneedles had dissolved in the skin, suggesting that the used patches could be safely discarded as non-sharps waste. The vaccines remained potent in the patches without refrigeration for at least one year.

The prospective vaccine technology could offer economic and manufacturing advantages. The manufacturing cost for the patch is expected to be competitive with prefilled syringe costs. The patch, however, can dramatically reduce the cost of vaccination, since self-administration can eliminate the need to have health workers oversee the process. It can be easily packaged for transportation, requires no refrigeration, and is stable.

Prausnitz is cofounder of a company that is licensing the microneedle patch technology. He is an inventor on licensed patents and has ownership interest in companies developing microneedle products, including Micron Biomedical. These potential conflicts of interest have been disclosed and are overseen by Georgia Institute of Technology and Emory University.

The team plans to conduct further clinical trials to pursue its ultimate availability to patients. They also are working to develop microneedle patches for use with other vaccines, including measles, rubella, and polio.

Chapter 53

Photonic Dosimetry

Summary

As part of the NIST on a Chip program, the Photonic Dosimetry project is set to develop in-situ sub-micrometer ionizing-radiation dosimetry and calorimetry leading to new chip-based metrology for industrial and medical applications. Increased sensitivity, spatial resolution, optical readout and multiplexing capabilities could fill measurement gaps for industrial processing using electron and photon beams, enable new portable sensors, and quantify dose delivered to patients in radiation-treatment procedures.

Description

National Institute of Standards and Technology (NIST)'s goal is to facilitate the rapidly growing use of spatially localized radiation beams for precision medicine and for more efficient manufacturing. NIST is responding to industry requests to create measurement solutions for new applications. The sensors NIST is developing are also of great interest for use in harsh environments, such as space or energy-generation.

Presently, there is only limited traceability to national standards for measuring radiation dose at the very small length scales where industry is pushing, and NIST is investing in new technology to meet

---

This chapter includes text excerpted from "Photonic Dosimetry," National Institute of Standards and Technology (NIST), October 24, 2017.

this need. Now is a critical time for U.S. manufacturing in the large and growing markets for precise delivery of radiation for uses such as:

- Medical device sterilization by radiation, including low-energy electron and X-ray beams

- Food irradiation for safety and quality, including low-energy electron and X-ray beams

- Ionizing radiation medical therapy, including proton and ion therapy

To remain competitive in these fields, U.S. manufacturers are expanding capabilities in machine-based electron and ion beams, which are effective, efficient, and secure. However, the newer techniques such as low-energy electron irradiation and ion therapy deliver dose gradients over very short distances (microns), and therefore require high resolution absorbed-dose sensors for irradiation planning, validation, and quality assurance.

No sensors are currently able to meet all industrial and medical needs for these new techniques, but the NIST on a Chip program is researching a solution based on commercial silicon chip fabrication and telecommunications photonics technology. The goal of this program is not only to create a new sensor that is miniaturized for NIST calibrations, but to partner with industry to make the technology deployable in the field.

To this end, NIST has begun measuring the impact of ionizing radiation on the performance of silicon photonic devices. In the first round of testing, the team irradiated chips with up to 1 MGy dose—well beyond the dose required for many industrial applications, and several thousand times higher than most medical radiation treatment levels—with little to no damage to the photonic devices. These early results indicate that such photonic devices are robust enough to serve as an integral component in future calorimeter designs. Studies are ongoing of in-beam irradiation effects on photonic devices and material and device designs for ionizing radiation applications.

Part Nine

Additional Help and Information

Chapter 54

Glossary of Terms Related to Health Technology

angiography: A diagnostic X-ray imaging procedure used to see how blood flows through the blood vessels and organs of the body. This is done by injecting special dyes, known as contrast agents, into the blood vessel and using X-ray techniques such as fluoroscopy to monitor blood flow.

biocompatibility: A measure of how a biomaterial interacts in the body with the surrounding cells, tissues, and other factors.

bioengineering: The application of concepts and methods of engineering, biology, medicine, physiology, physics, materials science, chemistry, mathematics, and computer sciences to develop methods and technologies to solve health problems in humans.

bioinformatics: The branch of biology that is concerned with the acquisition, storage, display, and analysis of biological information.

biomaterial: Any matter, surface, or construct that interacts with biological systems. Biomaterials can be derived from nature or synthesized in the laboratory using metallic components, polymers, ceramics, or composite materials. Medical devices made of biomaterials are often used to replace or augment a natural function.

This glossary contains terms excerpted from documents produced by several sources deemed reliable.

biomedical imaging: The science and the branch of medicine concerned with the development and use of imaging devices and techniques to obtain internal anatomic images and to provide biochemical and physiological analysis of tissues and organs.

biomimetics: Using biological form and function seen in nature to inspire the design of solutions to engineering problems.

biosensors: A device that uses biological material, such as deoxyribonucleic acid (DNA), enzymes, and antibodies, to detect specific biological, chemical, or physical processes and then transmits or reports this data.

brain-computer interface (BCI): A system that uses the brain's electrical signals to allow individuals with limited mobility to learn to use their thoughts to move a computer cursor or other devices like a robotic arm or a wheelchair.

cardiovascular disease (CVD): It is also called heart disease is a class of diseases that involve the heart, the blood vessels (arteries, capillaries, and veins), or both.

Center for Devices and Radiological Health (CDRH): CDRH assures that patients and providers have timely and continued access to safe, effective, and high-quality medical devices and safe radiation-emitting products.

clinical decision support (CDS): An interactive software-based system designed to assist physicians and other health professionals as well as patients with diagnostic and treatment decisions and reminders.

computational modeling: A computational model contains numerous variables that characterize the system being studied. Simulation is done by adjusting these variables and observing how the changes affect the outcomes predicted by the model.

computed tomography (CT): A computerized X-ray imaging procedure in which a narrow beam of X-rays is aimed at a patient and quickly rotated around the body, producing signals that are processed by the machine's computer to generate cross-sectional images—or "slices"—of the body.

contrast agent: A substance used to enhance the imaged appearance of structures, processes or fluids within the body in biomedical imaging.

control group: The group of participants that receives standard treatment or a placebo. The control group may also be made up of healthy volunteers. Researchers compare results from the control group with results from the experimental group to find and learn from any differences.

drug delivery systems: Engineered technologies for the targeted delivery and/or controlled release of therapeutic agents.

elastography: A medical imaging technique that measures the elasticity or stiffness of a tissue. The technique captures snapshots of shear waves, a special type of sound wave, as they move through the tissue.

electronic health record (EHR): A real-time patient health record with access to evidence-based decision support tools that can be used to aid clinicians in decision making. The EHR can automate and streamline a clinician's workflow, ensuring that all clinical information is communicated.

electronic health record system (EHRS): An information technology system designed to store and manage electronic health records.

electronic medical record (EMR): An electronic record of health-related information on an individual that can be created, gathered, managed, and consulted by authorized clinicians and staff within one healthcare organization.

endoscope: A thin illuminated flexible or rigid tube-like optical system used to examine the interior of a hollow organ or body cavity by direct insertion.

exoskeleton: The external skeleton that supports and protects an animal's body in contrast to the bones of an internal skeleton.

fluorescence: The emission of light by a substance that has absorbed light or other electromagnetic radiation.

functional magnetic resonance imaging (fMRI): An MRI-based technique for measuring brain activity. It works by detecting the changes in blood oxygenation and flow that occur in response to neural activity—when a brain area is more active it consumes more oxygen and to meet this increased demand blood flow increases to the active area.

functionality: A set of capabilities associated with computer hardware, software or other electronic devices.

gamma ray: Electromagnetic radiation of the shortest wavelength and the highest energy.

health information exchange (HIE): The electronic movement of health-related information across organizations within a region, community, or hospital system and according to nationally recognized standards.

health information technology (HIT): The application of information processing involving both computer hardware and software that deals with the storage, retrieval, sharing, and use of healthcare information, data, and knowledge for communication and decision making.

HITECH Act: The Health Information Technology for Economic and Clinical Health Act, signed into law on February 17, 2009, as a part of the American Recovery and Reinvestment Act (ARRA), amended the Public Health Service Act to codify the Office of the National Coordinator for Health Information Technology (ONC), required the national coordinator to establish a governance mechanism for a nationwide health information network (NIHN), and required the national coordinator to establish a voluntary program to certify health IT.

image-guided robotic interventions: Medical procedures, primarily minimally invasive surgery, performed through a small incision or natural orifice using robotic tools operated remotely by a surgeon with visualization by devices such as cameras small enough to fit into a minimal incision.

implantable devices: Man-made medical devices implanted in the body to replace or augment biological functions.

***in vitro*:** In glass, as in a test tube. An *in vitro* test is one that is done in glass or plastic vessels in the laboratory. *In vitro* is the opposite of *in vivo*.

***in vivo*:** In the living organism. For example, an experiment that is done *in vivo* is done in the body of a living organism. *In vivo* is the opposite of *in vitro*.

induced pluripotent stem cell (iPSC): A stem cell that is formed by the introduction of stem cell inducing factors into a differentiated cell of the body, typically a skin cell.

informed consent: When a participant provides informed consent, it means that he or she has learned the key facts about a research study and agrees to take part in it.

inpatient: A person who is hospitalized for at least one night to receive treatment or participate in a study.

interface: Hardware or software that facilitates interaction between disparate components of a system.

interoperability: Refers to the ability of health information systems to work together within and across organizational boundaries in order to advance the effective delivery of healthcare for individuals and communities.

ionizing radiation: A type of electromagnetic radiation that can strip electrons from an atom or molecule—a process called ionization. Ionizing radiation has a relatively short wavelength on the electromagnetic spectrum.

laboratory results reporting (LRR): The transmission of laboratory results in an electronic format from a clinical laboratory to electronic health record system (EHRS) for association with a patient's electronic health record (EHR).

mammography: An X-ray imaging method used to image the breast for the early detection of cancer and other breast diseases. It is used as both a diagnostic and screening tool.

meaningful use (MU): Federal incentive program and regulations administered by CMS defining the minimum requirements that providers must meet through their use of certified EHR technology in order to qualify for the payments.

mesenchymal stem cells: A term used to define nonblood adult stem cells from a variety of tissues. However, it is not clear whether mesenchymal stem cells from different tissues are the same.

mHealth: An abbreviation for mobile health, which is the practice of medicine and public health supported with mobile devices such as mobile phones for health services and information.

microfluidics: A multidisciplinary field including engineering, physics, chemistry, and biotechnology involving the design of systems for the precise control and manipulation of fluids on a small, sub-millimeter scale.

microscopy: Using microscopes to view samples and objects that cannot be seen with the unaided eye.

minimal risk: It means that the probability and magnitude of harm or discomfort anticipated in the research are not greater in and of themselves than those ordinarily encountered in daily life or during the performance of routine physical or psychological examinations or tests.

minimally invasive surgery: A surgical procedure typically utilizing one or more small incisions through which laparoscopic surgical tools are inserted and manipulated by a surgeon. Minimally invasive surgery can reduce damage to surrounding healthy tissue, decrease the need for pain medication, and reduce patient recovery time.

nanoparticle: Ultrafine particles between 1 and 100 nanometers in size. The size is similar to that of most biological molecules and structures. Nanoparticles can be engineered for a wide variety of biomedical uses including diagnostic devices, contrast agents, physical therapy applications, and drug delivery vehicles.

nanotechnology: The manipulation of matter with at least one dimension sized from 1 to 100 nanometers. Research areas include surface science, molecular biology, semiconductor physics, and microfabrication. Applications are diverse and include device physics, molecular self-assembly, and precisely manipulating atoms and molecules.

near infrared spectroscopy (NIRS): A spectroscopic method that uses the near-infrared region of the electromagnetic spectrum for pharmaceutical and medical diagnostics, typically measurements of blood sugar, and blood oxygen levels.

neuroimaging: Includes the use of a number of techniques to image the structure and function of the brain, spinal cord, and associated structures.

nuclear medicine: A medical specialty that uses radioactive tracers (radiopharmaceuticals) to assess bodily functions and to diagnose and treat disease. Diagnostic nuclear medicine relies heavily on imaging techniques that measure cellular function and physiology.

optical coherence tomography (OCT): A technique for obtaining sub-surface images such as diseased tissue just below the skin.

optical imaging: A technique for noninvasively looking inside the body, as is done with X-rays. Unlike X-rays, which use ionizing radiation, optical imaging uses visible light and the special properties of photons to obtain detailed images of organs and tissues as well as smaller structures including cells and molecules.

personal health record (PHR): An electronic application through which individuals can maintain and manage their health information (and that of others for whom they are authorized) in a private, secure, and confidential environment.

photon: A particle of light or electromagnetic radiation. The energies of photons range from high-energy gamma rays and X-rays to low-energy radio waves.

placebo: An inactive pill. This is sometimes called a "sugar pill." In some studies, participants may be assigned to take a placebo rather than the study medication.

point-of-care: Testing and treating of patients at sites close to where they live. Rapid diagnostic tests are used to obtain immediate, on-site results. The success of the concept relies on portable, rapid diagnostic devices that provide results directly to the user, which allows healthcare workers in remote areas to test and treat patients at the time of the visit.

polymer: A large molecule composed of many repeating subunits. Polymers range from familiar synthetic plastics such as polystyrene to natural biopolymers such as DNA. Polymers have unique physical properties, including strength, flexibility, and elasticity.

positron emission tomography (PET): PET scans use radiopharmaceuticals to create three-dimensional images. The decay of the radiotracers used with PET scans produce small particles called positrons. When positrons react with electrons in the body they annihilate each other. This annihilation produces two photons that shoot off in opposite directions. The detectors in the PET scanner measure these photons and use this information to create images of internal organs.

progenitor cells: Progenitor cells are cells that are similar to stem cells but instead of the ability to become any type of cell, they are already predisposed to develop into a particular type of cell.

prosthetics: The design, fabrication, and fitting of artificial body parts.

radiation: The emission of energy as electromagnetic waves or as moving subatomic particles, especially high-energy particles that cause ionization.

radiopharmaceuticals/radioactive tracers: Radioactive tracers are made up of carrier molecules that are bonded tightly to a radioactive atom. The carrier molecule is designed to bind to the tissue being examined so that the radioactive atom can be scanned to produce an image from inside the body.

Raman spectroscopy: This technique relies on inelastic scattering of visible, near-infrared, or near-ultraviolet light that is delivered by a laser. The laser light interacts with molecular vibrations in the material being examined, and shifts in energy are measured that reveal information about the properties of the material.

regenerative medicine: A broad field that includes tissue engineering but also incorporates research on self-healing—where the body uses its own systems, sometimes with the help of foreign biological material to rebuild tissues and organs.

rehabilitation engineering: The use of engineering science and principles to develop technological solutions and devices to assist individuals with disabilities, and aid the recovery of physical and cognitive functions lost because of disease or injury.

scaffold: A structure of artificial or natural materials on which tissue is grown to mimic a biological process outside the body or to replace a disease or damaged tissue inside the body.

sensors: In medicine and biotechnology, sensors are tools that detect specific biological, chemical, or physical processes and then transmit or report this data.

single photon emission computed tomography (SPECT): A nuclear medicine imaging technique using gamma rays. SPECT imaging instruments provide three dimensional images of the distribution of radioactive tracer molecules that have been introduced into the patient's body.

spectroscopy: The branch of science concerned with the investigation and measurement of spectra produced when matter interacts with or emits electromagnetic radiation.

stem cell: An undifferentiated cell of a multicellular organism that is capable of giving rise to more of the same cell type indefinitely, and has the ability to differentiate into many other types of cells that form the structures of the body.

telehealth: The use of communications technologies to provide and support healthcare at a distance.

theranostics: The relatively experimental science of combining therapy and diagnosis into a single procedure or molecule. Toward this end, bioengineers are building multifunctional nanoparticles that can be introduced into a patient, find the site of disease, diagnose the condition, and deliver the appropriate, personalized therapy.

tissue engineering: An interdisciplinary and multidisciplinary field that aims at the development of biological substitutes that restore, maintain, or improve tissue function.

ultrasound: A form of acoustic energy, or sound, that has a frequency that is higher than the level of human hearing. As a medical diagnostic technique, high frequency sound waves are used to provide real-time medical imaging image inside the body without exposure to ionizing radiation. As a therapeutic technique, high-frequency sound waves interact with tissues to destroy diseased tissue such as tumors, or to modify tissues, or target drugs to specific locations in the body.

X-ray: A form of high-energy electromagnetic radiation that can pass through most objects, including the body. X-rays travel through the body and strike an X-ray detector (such as radiographic film, or a digital X-ray detector) on the other side of the patient, forming an image that represents the "shadows" of objects inside the body

Chapter 55

Directory of Agencies That Provide Information about Health Technology

Government Agencies That Provide Information about Health Technology

Agency for Healthcare Research and Quality (AHRQ)
Office of Communications and Knowledge Transfer
5600 Fishers Ln.
Rockville, MD 20857
Phone: 301-427-1364
Fax: 301-427-1873
Website: www.ahrq.gov

Centers for Disease Control and Prevention (CDC)
1600 Clifton Rd.
Atlanta, GA 30333
Phone: 404-639-3311
Toll-Free: 800-CDC-INFO
(800-232-4636)
Toll-Free TTY: 888-232-6348
Website: www.cdc.gov
E-mail: cdcinfo@cdc.gov

Resources in this chapter were compiled from several sources deemed reliable; all contact information was verified and updated in December 2017.

Eunice Kennedy Shriver
National Institute on
Child Health and Human
Development (NICHD)
P.O. Box 3006
Rockville, MD 20847
Phone: 301-496-5133
Toll-Free: 800-370-2943
Toll-Free TTY: 888-320-6942
Toll-Free Fax: 866-760-5947
Website: www.nichd.nih.gov
E-mail:
nichdinformationresourcecenter@
mail.nih.gov

Federal Trade Commission
(FTC)
600 Pennsylvania Ave. N.W.
Washington, DC 20580
Phone: 202-326-2222
Website: www.ftc.gov

Health Resources and Services
Administration (HRSA)
5600 Fishers Ln.
Rockville, MD 20857
Phone: 301-443-3376
Toll-Free: 800-221-9393
Toll-Free TTY: 877-897-9910
Website: www.hrsa.gov

Healthfinder®
National Health Information
Center (NHIC)
P.O. Box 1133
Washington, DC 20013-1133
Phone: 301-565-4167
Toll-Free: 800-336-4797
Fax: 301-984-4256
Website: www.healthfinder.gov
E-mail: healthfinder@nhic.org

National Cancer Institute
(NCI)
9609 Medical Center Dr.
Bethesda, MD 20892-9760
Phone: 240-276-6600
Toll-Free: 800-4-CANCER
(800-422-6237)
Toll-Free TTY: 800-332-8615
Website: www.cancer.gov
E-mail: cancergovstaff@mail.nih
.gov

National Human Genome
Research Institute (NHGRI)
National Institutes of Health
(NIH)
31 Center Dr. MSC 2152
Bldg. 31 Rm. 4B09
Bethesda, MD 20892-2152
Phone: 301-402-0911
Fax: 301-402-2218
Website: www.genome.gov

National Institute
of Arthritis and
Musculoskeletal and Skin
Diseases (NIAMS)
Information Clearinghouse
1 AMS Cir.
Bethesda, MD 20892-3675
Phone: 301-495-4484
Toll-Free: 877-226-4267
TTY: 301–565–2966
Fax: 301-718-6366
Website: www.niams.nih.gov
E-mail: niamsinfo@mail.nih.gov

National Institute of Biomedical Imaging and Bioengineering (NIBIB)
6707 Democracy Blvd.
Ste. 202
Bethesda, MD 20892-5469
Phone: 301-496-8859
Website: www.nibib.nih.gov
E-mail: info@nibib.nih.gov

National Institute of Diabetes, Digestive and Kidney Diseases (NIDDK)
Office of Communications & Public Liaison
31 Center Dr. MSC 2560
Bldg. 31 Rm. 9A06
Bethesda, MD 20892-2560
Phone: 301-496-3583
Toll-Free: 800–472–0424
Website: www.niddk.nih.gov
E-mail: niddkinquiries@nih.gov

National Institute of Standards and Technology (NIST)
100 Bureau Dr.
Gaithersburg, MD 20899
Phone: 301-975-2000
Website: www.nist.gov

National Institute on Deafness and Other Communication Disorders (NIDCD)
National Institutes of Health (NIH)
31 Center Dr. MSC 2320
Bethesda, MD 20892-2320
Website: www.nidcd.nih.gov
E-mail: nidcdinfo@nidcd.nih.gov

National Institute on Mental Health (NIMH)
6001 Executive Blvd. MSC 9663
Rm. 6200
Bethesda, MD 20892-9663
Phone: 301-443-4513
Toll-Free: 866-615-6464
Toll-Free TTY: 866-415-8051
TTY: 301-443-8431
Fax: 301-443-4279
Website: www.nimh.nih.gov
E-mail: nimhinfo@nih.gov

National Institutes of Health (NIH)
9000 Rockville Pike
Bethesda, MD 20892
Phone: 301-496-4000
TTY: 301-402-9612
Website: www.nih.gov
E-mail: nihinfo@od.nih.gov

National Science Foundation (NSF)
2415 Eisenhower Ave.
Alexandria, VA 22314
Phone: 703-292-5111
Toll-Free: 800-877-8339
TDD: 703-92-5090
Toll-Free TDD: 800-281-8749
Website: www.nsf.gov

Substance Abuse and Mental Health Services Administration (SAMHSA)
5600 Fishers Ln.
Rockville, MD 20857
Toll-Free: 877-726-4727
Toll-Free TTY: 800-487-4889
Fax: 240-221-4292
Website: www.samhsa.gov

U.S. Congressional Budget Office (CBO)
Ford House Office Bldg.
Fourth Fl. Second and D St. S.W.
Washington, DC 20515-6925
Phone: 202-226-2602
Website: www.cbo.gov
E-mail: communications@cbo.gov

U.S. Department of Energy (DOE)
1000 Independence Ave. S.W.
Washington DC 20585
Phone: 202-586-5000
Fax: 202-586-4403
Website: www.energy.gov

U.S. Department of Health and Human Services (HHS)
200 Independent Ave. S.W.
Washington, DC 20201
Toll-Free: 877-696-6775
Website: www.hhs.gov

U.S. Department of Justice (DOJ)
950 Pennsylvania Ave. N.W.
Washington, DC 20530-0001
Phone: 202-514-2000
Toll-Free TTY: 800-877-8339
Website: www.justice.gov

U.S. Department of Labor (DOL)
200 Constitution Ave. N.W.
Washington, DC 20210
Toll-Free: 866-4-USA-DOL
(866-4487-2365)
Toll-Free TTY: 877-889-5627
Website: www.dol.gov

U.S. Department of Veterans Affairs (VA)
810 Vermont Ave. N.W.
Washington DC 20420
Toll-Free: 877-222-VETS
(877-222-8387)
Website: www.va.gov

U.S. Food and Drug Administration (FDA)
10903 New Hampshire Ave.
Silver Spring, MD 20993
Toll-Free: 888-INFO-FDA
(888-463-6332)
Website: www.fda.gov

U.S. Library of Congress (LOC)
101 Independence Ave. S.E.
Washington, DC 20540
Phone: 202-707-5000
Website: www.loc.gov

U.S. National Library of Medicine (NLM)
8600 Rockville Pike
Bethesda, MD 20894
Phone: 301-594-5983
Toll-Free: 888-FIND-NLM
(888-346-3656)
Website: www.nlm.nih.gov
E-mail: custserv@nlm.nih.gov

Private Agencies That Provide Information about Health Technology

AdvaMed
701 Pennsylvania Ave. N.W.
Ste. 800
Washington, D.C. 20004-2654
Phone: 202-783-8700
Fax: 202-783-8750
Website: www.advamed.org
E-mail: info@advamed.org

American Academy of Family Physicians (AAFP)
11400 Tomahawk Creek Pkwy
Leawood, KS 66211-2680
Phone: 913-906-6000
Toll-Free: 800-274-2237
Fax: 913-906-6075
Website: www.aafp.org

American Academy of Pediatrics (AAP)
141 N.W. Pt. Blvd.
Elk Grove Village, IL
60007-1098
Toll-Free: 800-433-9016
Fax: 847-434-8000
Website: www.aap.org
E-mail: international@aap.org

American Association for the Advancement of Science (AAAS)
1200 New York Ave. N.W.
Washington, D.C. 20005
Phone: 202-326-6400
Website: www.aaas.org

American Federation for Medical Research (AFMR)
500 Cummings Center, Ste. 4400
Beverly, MA 01915
Phone: 978-927-8330
Fax: 978-524-0498
Website: afmr.org

American Heart Association (AHA)
National Center
7272 Greenville Ave.
Dallas, TX 75231
Toll-Free: 800-AHA-USA-1
(800-242-8721)
Website: www.heart.org

American Medical Association (AMA)
AMA Plaza 330 N. Wabash Ave.
Ste. 39300
Chicago, IL 60611-5885
Toll-Free: 800-621-8335
Website: www.ama-assn.org

American Optometric Association (AOA)
243 N. Lindbergh Blvd.
St. Louis, MO 63141
Toll-Free: 800-365-2219
Website: www.aoa.org

American Society of Health-System Pharmacists (ASHP)
4500 East-West Hwy
Ste. 900
Bethesda, MD 20814
Toll-Free: 866-279-0681
Website: www.ashp.org

American Society of Opthalmic Plastic and Reconstructive Surgery (ASOPRS)
1043 Grand Ave.
Ste. 132
St Paul, MN 55105
Phone: 612-601-3168
Website: www.asoprs.org/i4a/
pages/index.cfm?pageid=3504
E-mail: info@asoprs.org

Americans for Medical Progress (AMP)
444 N. Capitol St. N.W.
Ste. 417
Washington, DC 20001
Phone: 202-624-8810
Website: www.amprogress.org/
about/contact-us

Biotechnology Innovation Organization (BIO)
1201 Maryland Ave. S.W.
Ste. 900
Washington, DC 20024
Phone: 202-962-9200
Fax: 202-488-6301
Website: www.bio.org/contact-bio
E-mail: info@bio.org

Cincinnati Children's Hospital Medical Center
3333 Burnet Ave.
Cincinnati, OH 45229-3026
Phone: 513-636-4200
Toll-Free: 800-344-2462
TTY: 513-636-4900
Website: www.
cincinnatichildrens.org

Cleveland Clinic
9500 Euclid Ave.
Cleveland, OH 44195
Toll-Free: 800-223-2273
Website: www.
my.clevelandclinic.org

Drug, Chemical & Associated Technologies Association (DCAT)
One Union St.
Ste. 208
Robbinsville, NJ 08691
Phone: 609-208-1888
Toll-Free: 800-640-DCAT
(800-640-3228)
Fax: 609-208-0599
Website: www.dcat.org/Contact
E-mail: info@dcat.org

Health Volunteers Overseas (HVO)
1900 L St. N.W.
Ste. 310
Washington, DC 20036
Phone: 202-296-0928
Fax: 202-296-8018
Website: www.hvousa.org/
contact-us
E-mail: info@hvousa.org

The Healthcare Association of New York State (HANYS)
499 S. Capitol St. S.W.
Ste. 405
Washington, DC 20003
Phone: 202-488-1272
Website: www.hanys.org

Healthcare Information and Management Systems Society (HIMSS)
33 W. Monroe St.
Ste. 1700
Chicago, IL 60603-5616
Phone: 312-664-4467
Fax: 312-664-6143
Website: www.himss.org

Immunization Action Coalition (IAC)
2550 University Ave. W.
Ste. 415 N.
St. Paul, MN 55114
Phone: 651-647-9009
Fax: 651-647-9131
Website: www.immunize.org

Materials Research Society (MRS)
506 Keystone Dr.
Warrendale, PA 15086-7537
Phone: 724-779-3003
Fax: 724-779-8313
Website: www.mrs.org
E-mail: info@mrs.org

Mental Health America (MHA)
500 Montgomery St.
Ste. 820
Alexandria, VA 22314
Phone: 703-684-7722
Toll-Free: 800-969-6642
Fax: 703-684-5968
Website: www.
mentalhealthamerica.net

National Alliance on Mental Illness (NAMI)
3803 N. Fairfax Dr.
Ste. 100
Arlington, VA 22203
Phone: 703-524-7600
Toll-Free: 800-950-6264
Fax: 703-524-9094
Website: www.nami.org

National Safety Council (NSC)
1121 Spring Lake Dr.
Itasca, IL 60143-3201
Phone: 630-285-1121
Toll-Free: 800-621-7615
Fax: 630-285-1434
Website: www.nsc.org
E-mail: customerservice@nsc.org

National Scoliosis Foundation (NSF)
5 Cabot Pl.
Stoughton, MA 02072
Toll-Free: 800-NSF-MYBACK
(800-673-6922)
Fax: 781-341-8333
Website: www.scoliosis.org
E-mail: nsf@scoliosis.org

Palo Alto Medical Foundation (PAMF)
795 El Camino Real
Palo Alto, CA 94301
Phone: 650-321-4121
Toll-Free: 888-398-5677
Website: www.pamf.org

Pan American Health Organization (PAHO)
525 23rd St. N.W.
Washington, DC 20037
Phone: 202-974-3000
Fax: 202-974-3663
Website: www.paho.org/hq

Radiological Society of North America (RSNA)
820 Jorie Blvd.
Oak Brook, IL 60523-2251
Phone: 630-571-2670
Toll-Free: 800-381-6660
Fax: 630-571-7837
Website: www.rsna.org/
ContactUs.aspx

Index

Index

Page numbers followed by 'n' indicate a footnote. Page numbers in *italics* indicate a table or illustration. Page numbers in **bold** refer to information contained in boxes within the chapters or sections.

A

abnormal cell division, stem cell research 449
ACA *see* Affordable Care Act
access control tools, electronic health records 428
ACL reconstruction *see* anterior cruciate ligament (ACL) reconstruction
ADA *see* Americans with Disabilities Act
adipocytes, mesenchymal stem cells 456
adult stem cell differentiation, stem cell research 455
AdvaMed
  contact 493
  see also Advanced Medical Technology Association
advanced analytics, described 55
"Advanced Magnetic Imaging Methods" (NIST) 167n

Advanced Medical Technology Association (AdvaMed), telemedicine 16
advanced molecular detection (AMD), overview 116–8
"Advanced Molecular Detection (AMD)" (CDC) 116n
"Advances in Colorectal Cancer Research" (NIH) 122n
Affordable Care Act (ACA), health IT regulations 407
Agency for Healthcare Research and Quality (AHRQ), contact 489
alarm devices, assistive devices for communication 344
ALDs *see* assistive listening devices
ambulatory surgery centers, medical technology 4
AMD *see* advanced molecular detection
American Academy of Family Physicians (AAFP), contact 493
American Academy of Pediatrics (AAP), contact 493
American Association for the Advancement of Science (AAAS), contact 493
American Federation for Medical Research (AFMR), contact 493

American Heart Association (AHA), contact 493
American Medical Association (AMA), contact 493
American Optometric Association (AOA), contact 493
American Society of Health-System Pharmacists (ASHP), contact 493
American Society of Ophthalmic Plastic and Reconstructive Surgery (ASOPRS), contact 494
Americans for Medical Progress (AMP), contact 494
Americans with Disabilities Act (ADA)
  MeBot 315
  mobility devices 349
angiography, defined 479
animal studies
  induced pluripotent stem cells 459
  technologies in tumor surgery 224
anterior cruciate ligament (ACL)
  reconstruction, knee surgery 444, 465
antibiotic resistance
  advanced molecular detection 117
  infectious disease surveillance 112
arthritis
  assistive devices 340
  cartilage engineering 272
  rehabilitation medicine 289
  robotics in rehabilitation 312
  stem cell research 465
artificial brain, overview 437–9
"Artificial Brains Learn to Adapt" (NSF) 437n
artificial cloning 432
artificial intelligence (AI)
  advanced analytics 55
  described 56
artificial legs, rehabilitation engineering 284
artificial neural networks, described 437
artificial pancreas
  diabetes 209
  overview 205–9
"Artificial Pancreas Device System" (FDA) 205n

artificial retina, overview 299–302
asexual reproduction, cloning 431
assistive devices
  mobile assistive technologies 298
  overview 338–53
  rehabilitation engineering 284
  sensors in medical care 63
"Assistive Devices for People with Hearing, Voice, Speech, or Language Disorders" (NIDCD) 343n
assistive listening devices (ALDs) *see* hearing aids
assistive technology *see* assistive devices
astrocytes
  nanotechnology 253
  stem cell research 454
audit trail, electronic health records (EHRs) 428

B

BAN *see* body area network
"Basics of Health IT" (ONC) 362n
BASP *see* brush-arm star polymer
BCI *see* brain-computer interface
behavioral learning, artificial brains 438
"Benefits of Health IT" (ONC) 364n
"Benefits of Nanotechnology for Cancer" (NCI) 249n
Big Data
  advanced analytics 55
  infectious disease surveillance 111
  overview 107–10
biocompatibility
  defined 479
  nanotechnology 251
bioengineering
  defined 479
  electrical signals and stimulations 321
  rehabilitation medicine 288
biofeedback, robotics in rehabilitation 312
biofilms
  computational modeling 444
  surface plasmon resonance imaging 175

bioinformatics
  advanced molecular detection 116
  defined 479
biological neurons, artificial
  brains 438
biological sensors, sensors in medical
  care 63
biomaterial
  defined 479
  nonlinear optical imaging 172
  robotics in rehabilitation 308
  stem cell research 465
  tissue engineering 268
biomechanical modeling,
  rehabilitation medicine 288
biomedical imaging, defined 480
biomimetics, defined 480
biosensors, defined 480
Biotechnology Innovation
  Organization (BIO), contact 494
birth defects, stem cell research 448
blastocyst, stem cell research 448
Blue Button
  health IT 369
  overview 382–8
Bluetooth
  digital health 58
  remote patient monitoring 79
  wearables and safety 73
body area network (BAN)
  novel digital health 59
  overview 67–70
"Body Area Networks and Pervasive
  Health Monitoring" (NIST) 67n
bone marrow transplantation 47
bone marrow stroma, stem cell
  research 454
brain-computer interface (BCI)
  assistive devices 345
  defined 480
  electrical signals and
    stimulations 323
  functional near-infrared
    spectroscopy (fNIRS) 137
  rehabilitation medicine 290
  sensors in medical care 63
"Breast Cancer—Basic Information—
  What Is a Mammogram?"
  (CDC) 143n

brain surgery
  mini-heat pipes **225**
  surgical robots 212
brush-arm star polymer, metal-free
  magnetic resonance imaging (MRI) 163
"Bye-Bye Biopsies?" (NIH) 160n

C

C-reactive protein (CRP),
  cardiovascular diseases 126
"Can Light Therapy Help the Brain?"
  (VA) 277n
cancer screening
  health technology assessment 39
  overview 118–9
"Cancer Screening in a Briefcase"
  (NIH) 118n
cardiomyocytes, stem cell research 462
cardiovascular disease (CVD)
  artificial pancreas device system 205
  computational modeling 443
  defined 480
  diagnosis 126
carrier testing, genetic testing 124
CDS see Clinical Decision Support
cell culture
  artificial brains 439
  cancer therapy 238
  stem cell research 451
cell-based therapies, stem cell
  research 448
Center for Devices and Radiological
  Health (CDRH), defined 480
Centers for Disease Control and
  Prevention (CDC)
  contact 489
  publications
    advanced molecular
      detection 116n
    Big Data and genomics 107n
    mammogram 143n
    medical technology 3n
    wearable technology 73n
Centers for Medicare and Medicaid
  Services (CMS)
  electronic health records 391
  health IT regulations 408
  remote patient monitoring 76

cerebral palsy
  assistive devices 341
  medical treatment technology 197
  physical therapists 333
  rehabilitation for movement
    disorders 356
  rehabilitation medicine 289
CGM *see* continuous glucose
  monitoring
Cincinnati Children's Hospital
  Medical Center, contact 494
Cleveland Clinic, contact 494
Clinical Decision Support (CDS),
  defined 480
"Clinical Decision Support (CDS)"
  (ONC) 101n
"Clinical Video Telehealth (CVT)"
  (VA) 22n
Clonaid, cloning 433
cloning, overview 431–4
"Cloning" (NHGRI) 431n
clot-busting therapy, sensitive stroke
  detection 126
cloud, described 56
CMS *see* Centers for Medicare and
  Medicaid Services
cochlear implants
  assistive devices 346
  health technology assessment 38
  magnetic resonance imaging
    (MRI) 141
  overview 302–4
  rehabilitation engineering 284
"Cochlear Implants: A Different Kind
  of 'Hearing'" (FDA) 302n
cognitive rehabilitation, light therapy
  for brain 278
colorectal cancer
  diagnosis 122
  genomic medicine 195
computational modeling
  defined 480
  opioid alternatives **445**
  overview 441–5
computed tomography (CT) scan,
  defined 480
"Consumer Health IT Applications"
  (HHS) 366n

continuous glucose monitoring (CGM)
  artificial pancreas device system 205
  overview 81–4
  remote patient monitoring 78
contractile proteins, chronic
  wounds 444
contrast agents
  computed tomography 134
  defined 480
control group
  defined 480
  preventive medicine 79
  rehabilitation medicine 290
crowdsourced data, infectious disease
  surveillance 112
CRP *see* C-reactive protein
culture medium, stem cell
  research 451
CVD *see* cardiovascular disease
cybernetics, overview 306–10
"Cybernetics" (NNSA) 306n
cybersecurity, digital health 54

D

decellularization, stem cell
  research 464
deoxyribonucleic acid (DNA)
  advanced molecular detection 116
  cloning 431
  genetic testing 123
  genomics 107
  microchip technology 120
  radiation therapy 147
designated record set
  health information privacy law 404
  HIPAA privacy rule 412
  personal health records 423
diabetes
  computational modeling 443
  continuous glucose monitoring 81
  digital health records 395
  pancreas 205
  remote patient monitoring 10, 75
  telehealth 26
  telemedicine 17
diagnostic tests
  electronic health records 428
  medical technology 3

diagnostic ultrasound, overview 154–7
diffuse optical tomography (DOT),
  optical imaging 153
digital health, overview 53–9
digital imagery, telehealth 13
DNA *see* deoxyribonucleic acid
DNA microchip, overview 120–1
"DNA Microchip Technology"
  (NHGRI) 120n
DNP *see* dynamic nuclear polarization
DOT *see* diffuse optical tomography
Drug, Chemical & Associated
  Technologies Association (DCAT),
  contact 494
drug delivery systems
  defined 480
  nanotechnology 246
  overview 202–4
dynamic nuclear polarization (DNP),
  magnetic imaging methods 167

E

"E-Health and Telemedicine" (HHS) 9n
e-Health tools, health IT 363
"eHealth Tools You Can Use"
  (ONC) 377n
e-prescribing
  defined 363
  electronic health records 396
  medical technology 3
e-prescription
  digital health records 399
  healthcare quality 392
ECG *see* electrocardiogram
"Effects of Remote Patient Monitoring
  on Chronic Disease Management"
  (NIH) 75n
"Effects of Remote Patient Monitoring
  on Heart Failure Management"
  (NIH) 75n
EHRs *see* electronic health records
EHRS *see* electronic health record
  system
elastography, defined 481
electrocardiogram (ECG)
  body area network 67
  medical device data system 58
  overview 135–7

"Electrocardiogram" (NHLBI) 135n
electronic health records (EHRs)
  benefits 391
  Big Data 111
  defined 481
  health IT 362
  health technology assessment 38
  HITECH Act 407
  mobile apps 87
  mobile device communication 98
  personal health records 420
  telemedicine 19
electronic health record system
  (EHRS), defined 481
electronic medical records
  defined 481
  health IT 362
  medical technology 3
  teleconsultations 10
  trends 371
electronic personal health records,
  defined 367
electronic stethoscope, mobile
  apps 88
electronic storage, medical device data
  system 58
embryonic stem (ES) cells
  artificial cloning 432
  heart disease 462
  pluripotent stem cells 459
  research 448
embryos
  clones 431
  embryonic stem cell 451
  human cloning 433
  pluripotent stem cells 459
  stem cell research 448
emergency medical services (EMS),
  wireless patient monitoring 187
EMS *see* emergency medical services
endoscope, defined 481
endoscopy, described 152
endothelial progenitor cells, stem
  cells 462
engineered livers, 3D printing 464
"Engineering Cartilage" (NIH) 272n
enteroendocrine cells, stem cell
  differentiation 456

epilepsy
    artificial brain 439
    assistive devices 341
    medical spending 47
Eunice Kennedy Shriver National
    Institute on Child Health and
    Human Development (NICHD)
    contact 490
    publications
        rehabilitation medicine 287n
        rehabilitative and assistive
            technology 338n
evidence-based medicine
    health technology assessment 37
    described 109
exoskeleton, defined 481

F

"FDA Continues to Lead in Precision
    Medicine" (FDA) 198n
Federal Trade Commission (FTC)
    contact 490
    publication
        medical device privacy
            consortium 75n
feeder layer, embryonic stem
    cells 451
fibroblasts
    computational modeling 443
    tissue barriers 252
filtered light (polarized), cancer
    screening 119
fitness trackers, wearables 73
"Fixing Flawed Body Parts"
    (NIH) 447n
fluorescence, defined 481
fluoroscopy, defined 146
fMRI *see* functional magnetic
    resonance imaging
fNIRS *see* functional near-infrared
    spectroscopy
"Food Allergy Lab Fits on Your
    Keychain" (NIBIB) 183n
Food and Drug Administration Safety
    and Innovation Act (FDASIA),
    described 408
food irradiation, photonic
    dosimetry 476

"For Providers and Professionals—
    Benefits of Electronic Health
    Records (EHRs)" (ONC) 391n
"From Orbit to Operating Rooms,
    Space Station Technology
    Translates to Tumor Treatment"
    (NASA) 212n
functional magnetic resonance
    imaging (fMRI), defined 481
functional near-infrared spectroscopy
    (fNIRS), overview 137–9
"Functional Near-Infrared
    Spectroscopy (fNIRS) Cognitive
    Brain Monitor" (NASA) 137n
functional ultrasound, diagnostic
    ultrasound 154
functionality, defined 481

G

gamma ray, defined 482
gene cloning, artificial cloning 432
genetic testing
    health technology assessment 41
    overview 123–5
genetics, healthcare expenditure 46
genomic profiling, colorectal cancer 122
genomics
    Big Data 107
    medicine 194
growth factors
    cancer biomarker 182
    cartilage engineering 273
    computational modeling 444
    regenerative medicine 269
    stem cell research 465

H

"Health Communication and
    Health Information Technology"
    (HHS) 375n
health information exchange (HIE),
    defined 482
health information organization
    (HIO), HIPAA 415
health information technology (IT)
    benefits 364
    defined 482

health information technology (IT),
continued
digital health 53
electronic health records 391
integration 374
legislation 407
overview 362–3
telemedicine 15
"Health Information Technology"
(SAMHSA) 362n
Health Information Technology for
Economic and Clinical Health
(HITECH) Act
defined 482
electronic health records 391
regulations 407
Health Insurance Portability and
Accountability Act (HIPAA)
described 408
health IT 411
individual rights 423
personal health records 389, 419
privacy law 403
remote monitoring 81
security 428
trends 368
"Health IT Legislation and
Regulations" (ONC) 407n
health plans
electronic health records 396
health technology assessment 36
HIPAA 405
personal health records 389
security 428
Health Resources and Services
Administration (HRSA),
contact 490
health technology assessment (HTA),
overview 35–45
"Health, United States, 2009"
(CDC) 3n
Health Volunteers Overseas (HVO),
contact 494
The Healthcare Association of
New York State (HANYS),
contact 494
Healthcare Information and
Management Systems Society
(HIMSS), contact 495

"Healthcare Telehealth and Remote
Patient Monitoring Use in Medicare
and Selected Federal Programs"
(GAO) 75n
Healthfinder®, contact 490
hearing aids
cochlear implants 302
mobile apps 90
overview 346–8
"Hearing Aids—Other Products
and Devices to Improve Hearing"
(FDA) 346n
heart transplants, medicinal
technology 5
hematopoietic stem cells
adult stem cell differentiation 456
stem cells 450
HIE *see* health information exchange
HIO *see* health information
organization
HIPAA *see* Health Insurance
Portability and Accountability Act
"The HIPAA Privacy Rule's Right
of Access and Health Information
Technology" (HHS) 411n
HITECH Act, defined 482
"H.R.3498—Human Cloning
Prohibition Act of 2105"
(LOC) 431n
human cloning, law 433
Human Cloning Prohibition Act of
2105, described 433
human embryonic stem cells
defined 448
pluripotent stem cells 460
stem cells 452
human embryos
cloning 432
stem cells 448

I

identical twins, cloning 431
image-guided robotic interventions,
defined 482
imaging, MRI **142**
immune rejection
stem cell research 459
transplant 462

immune system
  bone marrow transplantation 47
  embryonic stem cell 453
  human stem cells 461
  intracellular delivery 203
  regenerative medicine 269
Immunization Action Coalition (IAC),
  contact 495
implantable defibrillators, medical
  technology 3
implantable devices, defined 482
implantable wireless sensors,
  described 68
in vitro
  adult stem cells 456
  defined 482
  kidney regeneration 272
  nanotechnology 256
  stem cells 448
  see also in vivo
in vivo, defined 482
Individual Access Principle,
  HIPAA 412
individual rights, described 423
"Individual Privacy and HIPAA"
  (HHS) 403n
induced pluripotent stem cells (iPSCs)
  defined 482
  described 459
informed consent, defined 482
inpatient, defined 483
insulin
  body area networking 67
  continuous glucose monitor 83
  human stem cells 461
  pancreas 205
  stem cell research 457
interface, defined 483
integrated sensor monitoring systems,
  epidemiological study **66**
interoperability, defined 482
intraoperative monitoring (IOM),
  described 10
"Introduction to Health Technology
  Assessment" (NLM) 35n
IOM *see* intraoperative monitoring
ionizing radiation, defined 482
ionizing radiation medical therapy,
  photonic dosimetry 476

iPSCs *see* induced pluripotent stem
  cells
"Is Genetic Testing Right for You?"
  (NIH) 123n

J

Jibo, robotics 261
joint replacements
  described 48
  medical technology 3
  rehabilitation engineering 284
Journal of Neurotrauma, traumatic
  brain injury 278

K

KI *see* knowledge integration
kinematics, rehabilitation
  engineering 284
knee injury
  computational modeling 443
  stem cell research 465
knowledge integration (KI),
  described 109

L

lab-on-a-chip, sensors 62
"Label-Free Imaging of Cells and
  Their Extracellular Matrix by SPR
  Imaging" (NIST) 174n
laboratory conditions, cloning 432
laboratory results reporting (LRR),
  defined 482
laparoscopy, robotic assisted
  surgery 214
live cell imaging, overview 170–2
"Live Cell Imaging of Induced
  Pluripotent Stem Cell Populations"
  (NIST) 170n
LRR *see* laboratory results reporting
lupus, rehabilitative medicine 289

M

magnetic particle imaging (MPI),
  described 168
magnetic resonance (MR) scanners,
  Internet-based computing 57

magnetic resonance electrography, overview 160
magnetic resonance imaging (MRI)
  autism 161
  cancer 222
  cerebral palsy 291
  ischemic stroke 125
  metal-free contrast agents 163
  overview 139–42
  pregnant women 133, 147
  surgical robots 212
  teleconsultations 10
  see also magnetic resonance electrography; virtual colonoscopy
malaria outbreaks, detection **114**
mammogram
  cancer 146
  defined 483
  overview 143–5
"Managing Diabetes—Continuous Glucose Monitoring" (NIDDK) 81n
Materials Research Society (MRS), contact 495
MBAN *see* medical body area network
MDDS *see* Medical Device Data System
meaningful use (MU), defined 483
"MeBot: Robotic Wheelchair Wows Judges in Scotland" (VA) 314n
"Medical Applications of 3D Printing" (FDA) 467n
medical apps policy, FDA regulation 87
medical body area network (MBAN), digital health 59
medical device communication, described 98
Medical Device Data System (MDDS)
  described 57
  mobile medical apps 90
  overview 91–5
"Medical Device Data Systems" (FDA) 91n
medical device interoperability, overview 97–9
"Medical Device Interoperability" (NIST) 97n

"Medical Device Privacy Consortium (MDPC)" (FTC) 75n
medical devices
  digital health 54
  medical technology 3
  mobile apps 58
  telemedicine 34
  see also wireless medical devices
"Medical Devices—Computer-Assisted Surgical Systems" (FDA) 220n
"Medical Devices—Digital Health" (FDA) 53n
"Medical Devices—Mobile Medical Applications" (FDA) 85n
"Medical Devices—Wireless Medical Devices" (FDA) 70n
medical encounter files 112
medical history
  Blue Button 383
  electronic health records 392, 428
  IT applications 366
  personal health records 368
Medical Industry Technology Alliance (MITA), telemedicine 16
medical management record systems, right of access 414
medical technology
  healthcare spending 47
  overview 3–7
"Medical Technology Spotlight" (DOC) 3n
medication errors, telemedicine 18, 28
Mental Health America (MHA), contact 495
mesenchymal stem cells
  cartilage engineering 273
  defined 483
  differentiation pathways 456
metal-free MRI contrast agent, overview 162–5
microbial resistance, 3D placenta **469**
microfluidics, defined 483
microscopy, defined 483
"Milwaukee VA Medical Center Zaps Germs with Robots" (VA) 261n
miniature human organ systems, diagnosis **121**
minimally invasive surgery, defined 484

minimal risk, defined 483
MITA *see* Medical Industry
  Technology Alliance
mobile health (mHealth),
  defined 483
mobile health data, wearable
  sensors 12
Mobile Medical App (MMA),
  described 58
molecular biology
  curative therapies 46
  drug delivery systems 202
molecular signatures, cancer
  screening 118
"More Sensitive Stroke Detection"
  (NIH) 125n
MPI *see* magnetic particle imaging
MR scanners *see* magnetic resonance
  scanners
MRI *see* magnetic resonance
  imaging
"MRI (Magnetic Resonance Imaging)"
  (FDA) 139n
MU *see* meaningful use
multiple sclerosis, rehabilitation
  technology 289, 341
multiscale modeling
  defined 441
  microbial biofilms 444
muscular dystrophy
  embryonic stem cells 453
  rehabilitation technology 289, 341

N

"Nanomedicine" (NHGRI) 200n
nanoparticles
  defined 484
  cancer treatment **204**
  nanomedicine 257
  passive tumor accumulation 250
nanotechnology, defined 484
"Nanotechnology at the National
  Institutes of Health" (NIH) 246n
"Nanotechnology for Treating
  Cancer: Pitfalls and Bridges on the
  Path to Nanomedicines"
  (NCI) 254n
NAS *see* network attached storage

National Aeronautics and Space
  Administration (NASA)
  publications
    functional near-infrared
      spectroscopy (fNIRS) 137n
    movement disorders
      rehabilitation 355n
    surgical robots 212n
National Alliance on Mental Illness
  (NAMI), contact 495
National Cancer Institute (NCI)
  contact 490
  publications
    benefits of
      nanotechnology 249n
    nanotechnology for cancer
      treatment 254n
    virtual colonoscopy 165n
National Eye Institute (NEI)
  publication
    blindness rehabilitation 296n
National Heart, Lung, and Blood
  Institute (NHLBI)
  publication
    electrocardiogram 135n
National Human Genome Research
  Institute (NHGRI)
  contact 490
  publications
    cloning 431n
    DNA microchip
      technology 120n
    genomic medicine 194n
    nanomedicine 200n
National Institute of Arthritis and
  Musculoskeletal and Skin Diseases
  (NIAMS), contact 490
National Institute of Biomedical
  Imaging and Bioengineering (NIBIB)
  contact 491
  publications
    cancer therapy 237n
    computational modeling 441n
    computed tomography
      (CT) 132n
    drug delivery systems 202n
    food allergy lab 183n
    image-guided robotic
      interventions 263n

National Institute of Biomedical
  Imaging and Bioengineering (NIBIB)
  publications, *continued*
    metal-free MRI contrast
      agent 162n
    microneedle patch 471n
    nuclear medicine 148n
    optical imaging 151n
    science education 283n
    sensors 62n
    telehealth 9n
    tissue engineering 268n
    ultrasound 154n
National Institute of Diabetes,
  Digestive and Kidney Diseases
  (NIDDK)
  contact 491
  publication
    continuous glucose
      monitoring 81n
National Institute of Standards and
  Technology (NIST)
  contact 491
  publications
    advanced magnetic imaging
      methods 167n
    body area networks 67n
    cardiovascular disease
      risk 126n
    live cell imaging 170n
    medical device
      interoperability 97n
    nonlinear optical
      imaging 172n
    photonic dosimetry 475n
    precision medicine 181n
    regenerative medicine 274n
    SPR imaging 174n
National Institute on Deafness and
  Other Communication Disorders
  (NIDCD)
  contact 491
  publication
    assistive devices 343n
National Institute on Mental Health
  (NIMH)
  contact 491
  publication
    mental health treatment 229n
National Institutes of Health (NIH)
  contact 491
  publications
    biopsies 160n
    build bones 275n
    cancer screening 118n
    colorectal cancer research 122n
    engineering cartilage 272n
    genetic testing 123n
    infectious disease
      surveillance 111n
    nanotechnology 246n
    neuroimaging technique 161n
    noninvasive spinal cord
      stimulation 326n
    nutrigenetics and
      nutrigenomics 241n
    point-of-care diagnostic
      testing 177n
    remote patient monitoring 75n
    robotic arm 322n, 333n
    robots for better health 260n
    sensitive stroke detection 125n
    stem cell 447n
    tumor surgery 222n
    voluntary movement 318n
    X-rays 145n
National Safety Council (NSC),
  contact 495
National Science Foundation (NSF)
  contact 491
  publication
    artificial brains 437n
National Scoliosis Foundation (NSF),
  contact 495
Nationwide Privacy and Security
  Framework for Electronic Exchange
  of Individually Identifiable Health
  Information 412
natural clones *see* identical twins
near infrared spectroscopy (NIRS),
  defined 484
neonatal intensive care
  genome sequencing 196
  healthcare spending 48
neuroimaging
  autism 161
  defined 484
  neuronal activity 137

"Neuroimaging Technique May Help Predict Autism among High-Risk Infants" (NIH) 161n

neuromodulation
    noninvasive stimulation 329
    spinal cord injury 285

"New Method Builds Bone" (NIH) 275n

"New NIST Tool Aims to Improve Accuracy of Test to Determine Cardiovascular Disease Risk" (NIST) 126n

"New Robotic Wheelchair in the Works at Pittsburgh Lab" (VA) 314n

"New Technology Isolates Tumor Cells from Blood to Optimize Cancer Therapy" (NIBIB) 237n

newborn screening
    defined 124
    whole genome sequencing 196

"NIH-Funded Researchers Develop Metal-Free MRI Contrast Agent" (NIBIB) 162n

"NIH-Led Effort Examines Use of Big Data for Infectious Disease Surveillance" (NIH) 111n

NIRS *see* near infrared spectroscopy

nonembryonic stem cells, cell proliferation 449

nonhematopoietic stem cells 454

"Noninvasive Spinal Cord Stimulation for Paralysis" (NIH) 326n

"Non-Linear Optical Imaging" (NIST) 172n

notice of privacy practices (NPP), described 424

NPP *see* notice of privacy practices

nuclear medicine
    defined 484
    Medicare 5
    overview 148–50

"Nutrigenetics and Nutrigenomics Approaches for Nutrition Research" (NIH) 241n

"Office of Research and Development" (VA) 322n

Office of the National Coordinator for Health Information Technology (ONC)
    publications
        benefits of health IT 364n
        Blue Button 382n
        ehealth tools 377n
        electronic health information 368n
        electronic health records 391n
        electronic prescribing 397n
        health information privacy law and policy 403n
        health IT 362n
        health IT legislation and regulations 407n

oligodendrocytes, non-neuronal cells 456

open-heart surgery, stem cells 463

optical coherence tomography (OCT)
    defined 484
    described 152

optical imaging, defined 484

optical imaging systems, oral cancer 118

optogenetics, defined 438

organ transplants
    medical technology 3
    transplantable tissue 272

OSCS *see* oversulfated chondroitin sulfate

osteoarthritis (OA)
    ACL reconstructive surgeries 444
    cartilage engineering 272
    microfracture surgery 271
    stem cells 461

osteoblasts
    defined 276
    differentiation pathways 456

oversulfated chondroitin sulfate (OSCS), sensor technology 64

"Overview of the Artificial Retina Project" (DOE) 299n

O

OA *see* osteoarthritis

OCT *see* optical coherence tomography

P

pacemakers
    computational modeling 445

pacemakers, *continued*
  Medicare 77
  MR environment 141
  patient monitoring 78
pain management, secondary disorder
  treatment 285
Palo Alto Medical Foundation
  (PAMF), contact 495
Pan American Health Organization
  (PAHO), contact 496
paneth cells, differentiation
  pathways 456
"Paralyzed Individuals Use Thought-
  Controlled Robotic Arm to Reach
  and Grasp" (NIH) 322n
paraplegia, electrical spinal
  stimulation 318, 326
Parkinson disease
  artificial prosthetics 439
  atomoxetine 4
  SPECT scans 149
  ultrasound 203
"Patient Consent for eHIE—Health
  Information Privacy Law and Policy"
  (ONC) 403n
patient-specific devices, defined 468
PDGF *see* platelet-derived growth
  factor
pericytes, defined 455
personal health records (PHRs)
  defined 484
  described 363
  HIPAA Privacy Rule 419
  mobile medical apps 87
  overview 389–90
  see also electronic personal health
    records
"Personal Health Records and the
  HIPAA Privacy Rule" (HHS) 389n
"Personal Health Records and the
  HIPAA Privacy Rule" (HHS) 419n
PET *see* positron emission
  tomography
PHI *see* protected health information
photoacoustic imaging, defined 152
photon, defined 485
"Photonic Dosimetry" (NIST) 475n
PHRs *see* personal health records
physical prosthetics, defined 284

"Pillars of a Smart Safe Operating
  Room" (HHS) 225n
placebo, defined 485
platelet-derived growth factor
  (PDGF), wound-healing
  approaches 444
point-of-care
  defined 485
  described 11
  improved healthcare quality 392
  overview 177–9
  sensor research 65
"Point-of-Care Diagnostic Testing"
  (NIH) 177n
polymer, defined 485
portable low-field NMR,
  described 168
positron emission tomography (PET)
  defined 485
  described 149
  medical technology 4
  multimodal imaging **142**
  see also nuclear medicine
"Precision Medicine for Cancer
  Diagnostics" (NIST) 181n
preimplantation-stage embryo *see* cell
  culture
prenatal testing, defined 124
"A Prescription for e-Prescribers:
  Getting the Most Out of Electronic
  Prescribing" (ONC) 397n
"Prevention and Chronic Care—
  Improving Primary Care Practice—
  Health Information Technology
  Integration" (HHS) 374n
privacy law, overview 403–5
privacy protections
  electronic health records 427
  health information 408
  personal health records 424
"Privacy, Security, and Electronic
  Health Records" (HHS) 427n
problem-oriented assessments,
  defined 38
progenitor cells, defined 485
project-oriented assessments,
  defined 38
"Prosthetic Engineering—Overview"
  (VA) 310n

511

prosthetic socket
  bubble pressure sensor 310
  described 306
  patient comfort 313
prosthetics
  assistive technology 290
  biological sensors 63
  cybernetics 306
  defined 485
  medical technology 3
  neural control 308
  see also physical prosthetics; sensory
    prosthetics
protected health information (PHI)
  HIPAA 404, 411
  personal health record 421
  use and disclosure 422
"Public Health Approach to Big Data
  in the Age of Genomics: How Can
  We Separate Signal from Noise?
  (CDC) 107n

Q

quality of life
  BrainGate 324
  medical care 63
  rehabilitation medicine 287
  remote patient monitoring 76
  vision loss 297

R

radiation, defined 485
radiation dose, medical X-rays 147
radiation emergency medical
  management (REMM), mobile
  medical apps 86
radiation therapy, medical X-rays 147
radio frequency identification (RFID),
  radio frequency (RF) wireless
  technologies 70
radioactive tracers, described 148
Radiological Society of North America
  (RSNA), contact 496
radiopharmaceuticals/radioactive
  tracers, defined 485
Raman spectroscopy
  defined 486
  described 153

real-time videoconferencing,
  telemedicine 28
reference workflow taxonomy,
  described 106
"Regenerative Medicine
  Biomanufacturing" (NIST) 274n
rehabilitation chair, biometric
  approach 335
rehabilitation engineering
  defined 486
  see also rehabilitation robotics
"Rehabilitation Medicine: Research
  Activities and Scientific Advances"
  (NICHD) 287n
rehabilitation robotics, rehabilitation
  engineering 284
"Rehabilitative and Assistive
  Technology: Condition Information"
  (NICHD) 338n
REMM see radiation emergency
  medical management
remote patient monitoring (RPM)
  overview 75–81
  telehealth technologies 10
reproductive cloning, artificial
  cloning 432
"Researchers Develop Microneedle
  Patch for Flu Vaccination"
  (NIBIB) 471n
retinal prosthesis, retinal
  implant 300
RF wireless technology, described 70
RFID see radio frequency
  identification
"Robotic Arms—Physical Therapists
  of the Future?" (NIH) 333n
"Robotic Surgery: Risks vs. Rewards"
  (HHS) 214n
"Robots for Better Health and Quality
  of Life" (NIH) 260n
RPM see remote patient monitoring

S

SaMD see Software as a Medical
  Device
SAN see storage area network
scaffold, defined 486
"Science Education" (NIBIB) 283n

"Science Education—Computational Modeling" (NIBIB) 441n

"Science Education—Computed Tomography (CT)" (NIBIB) 132n

"Science Education—Drug Delivery Systems: Getting Drugs to Their Targets in a Controlled Manner" (NIBIB) 202n

"Science Education—Image-Guided Robotic Interventions" (NIBIB) 263n

"Science Education—Nuclear Medicine" (NIBIB) 148n

"Science Education—Optical Imaging" (NIBIB) 151n

"Science Education—Sensors" (NIBIB) 62n

"Science Education—Telehealth" (NIBIB) 9n

screen-reading software, assistive technology 96

sensors, defined 486

sensory prosthetics, defined 284

SFT *see* store-and-forward

single photon emission computed tomography (SPECT)
  defined 486
  nuclear medicine 148

smartphone apps, wearable sensors 12

Software as a Medical Device (SaMD), described 55

software programs
  mobile apps 85
  speech-generating devices 343

"Space Technologies in the Rehabilitation of Movement Disorders" (NASA) 355n

SPECT *see* single photon emission computed tomography

spectroscopy, defined 486

spiking neural networks
  artificial brain 438
  artificial neural networks 437

spinal cord, electrical stimulation 318

spinal stimulation, overview 318–22

"Spinal Stimulation Helps Four Patients with Paraplegia Regain Voluntary Movement" (NIH) 318n

"Stem Cell Basics VII" (NIH) 447n

stem cell niche, adult stem cells 455

stem cell therapy, described 47

stem cells
  artificial cloning 432
  bones 475
  defined 486
  future treatment 462
  research 447

stents
  implanted devices 141
  medical technology 3

storage area network (SAN), medical device data system (MDDS) 94

store-and-forward (SFT)
  overview 26–7
  telehealth 13

stroke
  computed tomography scan 133
  magnetic resonance imaging (MRI) 125
  rehabilitation robotics 284
  stem cells 462

Substance Abuse and Mental Health Services Administration (SAMHSA)
  contact 491
  publication
    health IT 362n

super-resolution microscopy, optical imaging 153

surface plasmon resonance imaging, overview 174–5

T

tactile sensing, pressure measurement sensors 309

TBI *see* traumatic brain injury

"Technological Change and the Growth of Healthcare Spending" (CBO) 45n

"Technologies Enhance Tumor Surgery" (NIH) 222n

"Technology and the Future of Mental Health Treatment" (NIMH) 229n

technology-oriented assessments, health technology assessment (HTA) 38

telecommunications devices, augmentative and alternative communication devices, 343

teleconsultation, telehealth
  technologies 10
teleDermatology, described 26
telehealth
  defined 486
  overview 9–14
  remote patient monitoring 75
  telerehabilitation care 285
  Veteran Affairs 78
telehealth specialties, clinical video
  telehealth (CVT) 25
telehomecare (THC), telehealth
  technologies 10
telemedicine
  barriers 34
  benefits 4, 17
  challenges 19
  defined 16
  patient safety 27
  products and services 16
"Telemedicine: An Important Force in
  the Transformation of Healthcare"
  (DOC) 15n, 33n
"Telemedicine and Patient Safety"
  (HHS) 27n
teleMental health, clinical video
  telehealth (CVT) 24
teleRehabilitation, clinical video
  telehealth (CVT) 24
teleretinal imaging, described 27
telesurgery, clinical video telehealth
  (CVT) 24
terahertz tomography, optical
  imaging 153
teratoma, embryonic stem cells 453
THC *see* telehomecare
theranostics, defined 486
therapeutic cloning, artificial cloning 432
therapeutic ultrasound, medical
  ultrasound 156
tissue engineering
  cartilage replacement 272
  defined 487
  overview 268–72
  review 463
"Tissue Engineering and Regenerative
  Medicine" (NIBIB) 268n
TMS *see* transcranial magnetic
  stimulation

transcranial magnetic stimulation
  (TMS), stroke 340
transcription factors, laboratory
  tests 452
transdifferentiation, adult stem cell
  differentiation 456
traumatic brain injury (TBI)
  complex rehabilitative technology 341
  LED therapy 278
  rehabilitation medicine 287
  rehabilitation robots 333
"Trends in Consumer Access and Use
  of Electronic Health Information"
  (ONC) 368n

U

UDI *see* unique device identification
ultra-low field (ULF) MRI,
  described 167
"Ultrasound" (NIBIB) 154n,
  defined 487
ultra-wideband (UWB), body area
  network (BAN) 69
"Understanding the Heart's Electrical
  System and EKG Results"
  (NHLBI) 135n
undifferentiated cells, human
  embryonic stem cells research 452
unique device identification (UDI),
  medical device data system
  (MDDS) 94
unreviewable grounds for denial,
  Health Insurance Portability and
  Accountability Act (HIPAA) Privacy
  Rule 417
U.S. Congressional Budget Office
  (CBO)
  contact 492
  publication
    healthcare spending 45n
U.S. Department of Commerce (DOC)
  publications
    medical technology 3n
    telemedicine 15n, 33n
U.S. Department of Energy (DOE)
  contact 492
  publication
    artificial retina project 299n

U.S. Department of Health and
  Human Services (HHS)
  contact 492
  publications
    clinical decision support
      (CDS) 101n
    e-health and telemedicine 9n
    electronic health
      records 427n
    health communication 375n
    health information
      privacy 427n
    health IT applications 366n
    health IT integration 374n
    HIPAA privacy rule 419n
    individual privacy 403n
    personal health records 389n
    right of access and health
      IT 411n
    robotic surgery 214n
    safe operating room 225n
    telemedicine and patient
      safety 27n
U.S. Department of Homeland
  Security (DHS)
  publication
    wireless patient
      monitoring 187n
U.S. Department of Justice (DOJ)
  contact 492
  publication
    mobility devices 348n
U.S. Department of Labor (DOL),
  contact 492
U.S. Department of Veterans Affairs
  (VA)
  contact 492
  publications
    BrainGate 322n
    clinical video telehealth
      (CVT) 22n
    light therapy 277n
    polytrauma system of
      care 283n
    prosthetic engineering 310n
    robotic cleaners 261n
    robotic wheelchair 314n
    telehealth services 26n
    telehealth technology 22n

U.S. Food and Drug Administration
  (FDA)
  contact 492
  publications
    artificial pancreas device
      system 205n
    cochlear implants 302n
    computer-assisted surgical
      systems 220n
    digital health 53n
    hearing aids 346n
    magnetic resonance imaging
      (MRI) 139n
    medical device data
      systems 91n
    mobile medical
      applications 85n
    precision medicine 198n
    3D printing 467n
    wireless medical devices 70n
U.S. Government Accountability
  Office (GAO)
  publication
    remote patient
      monitoring 75n
U.S. Library of Congress (LOC)
  contact 492
  publication
    Human Cloning Prohibition
      Act of 2105 431n
U.S. National Library of Medicine
  (NLM)
  contact 492
  publication
    health technology
      assessment 35n
UWB *see* ultra-wideband

V

"VA Telehealth Services—Store-And-
  Forward Telehealth" (VA) 26n
vapor phase hydrogen peroxide
  (VPHP), sensors 64
vector, cloning techniques 432
"VHA Clinical Video Telehealth
  Technology" (VA) 22n
virtual colonoscopy, overview 165–6
"Virtual Colonoscopy" (NCI) 165n

virtual reality
  rehabilitative technologies 340
  virtual rehabilitation 284
viruses
  cartilage engineering 273
  cloning techniques 432
  induced pluripotent stem
    cells 459
"Vision Research Needs, Gaps, and
  Opportunities" (NEI) 296n
visual alert signalers, alerting
  devices 344
visual paired comparison (VPC),
  Alzheimer disease research 13
visually impaired
  assistive technology 296
  mobile assistive technologies 298
voice recognition, assistive
  technologies 339
VPC see visual paired comparison
VPHP see vapor phase hydrogen
  peroxide

W

walking assistance system, spinal
  cord injuries **342**
wearable computers, described 73
"Wearable Computers and Wearable
  Technology" (CDC) 73n
wearable sensors
  body area network 67
  telehealth 12
wearable technology, overview 73–4
wearables, monitoring **74**
"What Is Genomic Medicine?"
  (NHGRI) 194n
wheelchair
  assistive technology 338
  mobility aids 348
  rehabilitation medicine 288
  robotic wheelchair 314

"Wheelchairs, Mobility Aids, and
  Other Power-Driven Mobility
  Devices" (DOJ) 348n
Wi-Fi
  body area network 69
  mobile medical app 58
  remote patient monitoring 80
  wearable technology 73
wireless medical devices
  digital health 54
  overview 70–2
"Wireless Patient Monitoring" (DHS)
  187n
wireless technology
  medical devices 70
  radio frequency 72
  wireless patient monitoring 187

X

X-rays
  defined 487
  electronic health records 428
  mammogram 143
  mobile medical apps 90
  optical imaging 151
  photonic dosimetry 476
  sensitive stroke detection 126
  telehealth services 13
  virtual colonoscopy 165
"X-Rays" (NIH) 145n

Y

"Your Health Information Privacy
  Rights" (HHS) 427n
"Your Health Records—About Blue
  Button" (ONC) 382

Z

Zika, disease monitoring 112
Zykadia (ceritinib), target therapy 199